Praise for PCOS SOS

"Polycystic ovary syndrome (PCOS) is a complex condition that baffles many healthcare providers. This leads to missed diagnoses and a lack of options for those who are diagnosed. There is never a one-size-fits-all method to approaching and managing PCOS. Dr. Gersh's book provides a deep understanding of the condition and a variety of treatment options that will help both healthcare providers and patients think more holistically and strategically about PCOS care. PCOS SOS can help readers discover options and answers that they may not otherwise find. Dr. Gersh's work is a jewel!"

~ Sasha Ottey, M.H.A., M.T. (ASCP),
Founder and Executive Director of PCOS
Challenge, PCOS Advocate and Patient

"It's not an easy task for women to find the best physician to help them in their quest for better health. When it comes to PCOS, Dr. Felice Gersh is that specialist. Superbly trained in functional medicine and supremely gifted as an experienced communicator, she lays out the definitive plan for any woman with PCOS who wants to get started on a path to wellness."

~ Mark J. Tager, M.D.,
CEO of ChangeWell, Inc.

"Dr. Felice Gersh, an integrative gynecologist, is a gifted clinician who infuses her PCOS guide with passion, positivity, and information based on solid research. She is an ardent advocate for women with PCOS, and dispenses with the 'shame and blame' culture of conventional medicine. Dr. Gersh's book is a lifeline for anyone with PCOS."

~Katherine Sherif, M.D.,
Professor and Vice Chair of Academic Affairs at the Sidney
Kimmel Medical College at Thomas Jefferson University
and Director of Jefferson Women's Primary Care

"In this groundbreaking and highly readable book, Dr. Gersh gives us an explanation and solution to an all-too-common condition that is ignored or mistreated by mainstream medicine. Using the best of science along with her considerable clinical skills, Dr. Gersh describes how she helps women restore hormonal balance and thereby gain freedom from pain, infertility, obesity, and many of the challenging health issues that plague the modern-day woman. A must read!"

~Hyla Cass M.D.,
Author of 8 *Weeks to Vibrant Health*

"Dr. Gersh's deep understanding of PCOS shines through on every page."
~Lara Briden, Naturopathic Doctor,
Author of *Period Repair Manual*

"Dr. Felice Gersh is a rare combination of traditionally-trained OB/GYN and fellowship-trained integrative medicine physician. She provides insight and expertise into the latest medical PCOS research while also understanding the importance of natural healing modalities. As a woman who has successfully managed her own PCOS, as well as treated thousands of women in her practice, Dr. Gersh understands the pain and struggles of being diagnosed with PCOS, and her book provides an empathetic, science-based, root-cause healing approach to PCOS."

~Amy Medling,
Author of *Healing* PCOS and
founder of PCOS Diva

"PCOS SOS is an empowering new resource for women with PCOS who want to restore their health. Dr. Gersh's years of experience and masterful knowledge shine in this wonderful guide!"

~Dr. Fiona McCulloch,
Bestselling author of 8 *Steps to Reverse Your PCOS*

"Thank goodness Dr. Felice Gersh's book is finally here! Her depth of knowledge and passion for best-care practices make this an amazing book written by a powerhouse doctor. It is a dynamic read, resource, and tool for all living with, treating, and supporting patients with PCOS."

~Ashley Levinson,
PCOSgurl

"Dr. Felice Gersh's groundbreaking treatment shows women how they can treat all of their PCOS symptoms by treating the root cause."

~**Izabella Wentz, Pharm.D., FASCP,**
New York Times bestselling author of *Hashimoto's Protocol*

"Dr. Felice Gersh understands PCOS in a way that few doctors do. In this book she shares her incredible wisdom from years of clinical practice with a perspective that may surprise you, yet make you feel totally normal and NOT crazy. No matter what your symptoms, you'll appreciate how special you truly are and the steps you need to take to heal, once and for all. Enjoy the journey!"

~**Robin Nielsen, C.N.C.,**
Functional Hormone Expert

"Beautifully written and very informative! Dr. Gersh has written this book in a way that makes readers feel safe and secure because she understands how they are feeling. PCOS SOS is a great book for anyone who has PCOS and anyone who supports women with PCOS."

~**Megan M. Stewart,**
Founder of the PCOS Awareness Association

"A must read for any woman with PCOS wanting to reclaim her total health, not just fix her individual body parts. Dr. Gersh really is the leader in integrative medicine for PCOS!"

~**Angela Grassi, M.S., R.D.N., L.D.N.,**
Founder of the PCOS Nutrition Center and author of *The PCOS Workbook: Your Guide to Complete Physical and Emotional Health*

"My colleague, Dr. Felice Gersh, lectures extensively and I am always excited to learn critical new information about little-known issues relating to PCOS, such as the potential risks of metformin. Now, her wealth of knowledge is available in this outstanding book."

~**Walter Futterweit, M.D.,**
Clinical Professor of Endocrinology at the Mount Sinai School of Endocrinology, former president and active member of the Androgen Excess and PCOS Society

PCOS SOS

A Gynecologist's Lifeline

To Naturally Restore

Your Rhythms, Hormones,
and Happiness

Felice Gersh, M.D.
with Alexis Perella

Health Disclaimer

This book contains advice and information relating to health care. It should be used to supplement rather than replace the advice of your doctor or another trained health professional. If you know or suspect you have a health problem, it is recommended that you seek your physician's advice before embarking on any medical program or treatment. All efforts have been made to assure the accuracy of the information contained in this book as of the date of publication. The publisher and the author disclaim liability for any medical outcome that may occur as a result of applying the methods suggested in this book.

Printed in the United Kingdom
First Printing, 2019

ISBN 978-1-911443-11-7 (Paperback)
ISBN 978-1-911443-12-4 (eBook)

Right Angles
Suite 205, 15 Ingestre Place
Soho W1F 0DU
United Kingdom

www.right-angles.info

To my daughters and to all the strong women who
are finding their way with PCOS.

Contents

Foreword by
Felice Gersh, M.D.

Over the course of my life, I have watched from a front row seat as our understanding and treatment of PCOS have evolved.

When you have PCOS, it can feel like you are lost alone at sea. You collect symptoms that affect every aspect of your life, and there is no clear path to health. You send out an SOS call, but no one answers.

Most women see three or more doctors just to get a PCOS diagnosis. And it doesn't get better from there. Once diagnosed, most women are simply given drugs to treat their most pressing complaints. They don't receive information about the long-term risks associated with PCOS.[1] They are not taught how to actually heal. Not surprisingly, they quickly lose trust in their doctors.[2]

I have been there. I have PCOS, too, and I know what it's like to ask for help and be placated with ever more pills.

In high school, I developed terrible acne, worse than anyone else I knew. I was very self-conscious about it. I scrubbed my face with rubbing alcohol, hoping that if my face were cleaner, the acne would go away. But, scrubbing my skin didn't help. It just made it peel and crack — literally *crack*. And my face was still covered in so many pimples.

My periods were always irregular. I'd have a period for a few months, and then it would disappear for awhile.

Today, I know these symptoms indicate PCOS, but when I was a teenager, my doctor didn't have a diagnosis. He said, "Oh, you have acne and irregular periods. You'll grow out of it." I left with a skin cream that did nothing but sting and burn.

In college, I went to a gynecologist for the first time, hoping he could cure my crazy periods and ongoing acne, which made me feel self-conscious and unattractive.

He put me on the earliest form of birth control pills. This was the 1970's, so they were very radical, cutting edge, and strong. The pills lessened my acne and regulated my period, but they made me sick so I never stuck with them for long.

My doctor told me the birth control pills were hormones. I was too embarrassed to ask why I needed hormones in a pill and why my own hormones were messed up.

I went on to medical school. At that point, the pill made me nauseous all the time, and I stopped taking it. My period stopped for two whole years. I was living with Bob, my soon-to-be-husband, and even though we weren't ready to start a family yet, we did want to have children. I was terrified that I was infertile and would never be able to become pregnant.

Desperate for help, I went to one of the big shots in the OB-GYN department at my medical school. Surely, he would have some answers. But, no.

"What's your problem? Just go back on birth control pills," he said. "There's another drug you can take to get pregnant later on."

Out of options, I reluctantly went back on the pill. Even though it made me nauseous, the pill restored my period and I powered through medical school.

At the end of medical school, I decided to become an OB-GYN. I was personally and professionally interested in female reproduction, and I was passionate about caring for women as they navigated the emotional and medical ups and downs of building their families.

I easily connected with women as I helped them through fertility challenges, pregnancy, sometimes pregnancy loss, and post-pregnancy care. I loved delivering their babies. I was a skilled surgeon. I could act quickly in an emergency. I saved lives.

While I did my residency, I diagnosed myself with PCOS. I hadn't known about PCOS before and no one diagnosed me because I didn't meet the strict Stein-Leventhal criteria. You had to be really obese and I was tiny. I didn't have thick facial hair; I had maybe a few faint wisps. Mostly I had acne and irregular cycles. And I probably had cystic ovaries, but nobody did ultrasounds in those days. I theorized that PCOS was a spectrum disorder and that I had a mild version. I wondered if someday I could help develop a cure.

I was still an intern when Bob and I decide to start our family. Everyone told me to wait, but I was so scared I wouldn't be able to have children. I was 26 years old and had been married for nearly three years.

The standard fertility treatment for all women with missing or irregular cycles, including PCOS women, was to induce ovulation with the drug Clomid, so that's what I did.

At first, it didn't work, and I panicked. I took ever higher doses, until finally, I got pregnant and gave birth to my daughter, Alexis (who is now writing this book with me!)

I completed my OB-GYN residency and launched my own medical practice, Women's Medical Group of Irvine. It was a revolutionary practice at the time, one run by women, for women. My practice included

OB-GYNs, internists, and family doctors. Even back then, I believed that the best healthcare experience was a combination of traditional and alternative healing practices, so I also had nutritionists, psychologists, aestheticians, Chinese Medicine practitioners, and massage therapists.

For the next 25 years, I was a full time OB-GYN and the director of my unique practice.

Sometimes, when I look back, I don't know how I built a thriving, successful medical practice while raising a family. I went on to have three more children. It was all-consuming. Several times each week, I'd put my four kids to bed and race to the hospital to deliver babies. I'd reappear at home in the early morning, sleep a bit, get the kids ready for school, and head off again to start my work day. Bob was the behind-the-scenes hero who kept things running, picked up the slack, and filled in all the gaps.

I'd disappear at night and on holidays. I'd sneak out of recitals and soccer games, and sneak back in as soon as I could. I felt like I had an amazing, exhausting, secret life.

And this went on for 25 years!

Then in 2006, I retired from obstetrics, and an incredible thing happened. I got some sleep. It was as if my brain woke up, and I began reexamining how I was caring for my GYN patients — the ones who were not having babies.

I felt like the only tools I had were pharmaceuticals and surgery. And, while these were wonderfully powerful treatments for some conditions, they failed miserably with others. Women would come in with things like endometriosis, fibroids, and, of course, PCOS. We really didn't have much to offer except birth control pills, other drugs, or surgery. So, until they got really sick, it would be, "Okay, we'll just watch you."

I began to wonder what the point of all of my training and experience was. All I could do was jot down prescriptions and perform surgeries, and most of the time, that was for late-stage disease. What could I do for people before they reached a crisis?

Around this same time, several of my own family members were struggling with PCOS symptoms and trying to start their families. They had been diagnosed much earlier than I had because we now know that PCOS is genetic and passed down through families. I felt powerless to help them. Why were we stuck with the same treatments doctors gave me in the 70s? Was there nothing new?

I felt lost and started looking for answers in all the usual places.

First, I turned to the pharmaceutical companies. I had trusted them in the past, so it seemed logical to dig a little deeper into their research. Maybe I just wasn't aware of newer insights and better treatments. I asked all of the pharmaceutical reps who came to my office (and there was a parade of them) to show me their latest studies on female health. I'd never asked the drug companies to "prove" anything. I just believed whatever the sales reps told me without asking them to show me the data.

The data was eye-opening and not in a good way. I was not impressed. Often, the numbers appeared to be manipulated to show that the drug being tested made a difference — no matter how small — from the placebo. Or it would look like a drug was starting to show a lot of side effects, but then the study would end.

So, that's when I started losing my faith and confidence in big pharma completely. Basically, I had a midlife doctor crisis.

Now, as I mentioned earlier, I always felt that there was much more to healthcare than just giving a pill or doing surgery. From the inception of my practice, I had what I called ancillary services in my office. I had a Chinese medicine practitioner with me. She just retired, but she was with me for over 20-something years. I've had nutritionists and psychological counselors. I've had biofeedback. I've had the same massage therapist now for probably 15 years.

But I myself had no specific training in anything but the conventional. So I went on a journey. I started randomly taking courses. I had no mentor and no guidance. But in 2008, I ended up at a conference in Portland, Oregon with a bunch of naturopathic doctors. I had never even heard of a naturopathic doctor at the time. But they introduced me to a healthcare approach that I found very compelling.

I attended a lecture by Dr. Low Dog, the fellowship director from the Center of Integrative Medicine at the University of Arizona. I discovered that integrative medicine is a science-based approach to medicine founded on principles similar to those of the naturopaths: With proper tools, the body can heal itself; lifestyle and diet can create a path to health; the doctor and the patient are a team of equals.

The integrative approach emphasizes open-mindedness, evidence-based interventions, and a whole-body approach to wellness. Integrative doctors search for the root causes of illnesses instead of simply treating visible symptoms.

Starry-eyed, I introduced myself to the lecturer, and said, "Dr. Low Dog, I am here because I found this course online. I didn't know what to expect, but now I know that this is how I want to practice medicine. I want to learn how to help my patients before they get really sick. I want to use therapies that heal without hurting. I want to figure out how to treat chronic diseases that, up until now, I've just been covering up."

She replied, "In two weeks, the Fellowship of Integrative Medicine will begin another class at the University of Arizona School of Medicine. Why don't you join us? Just apply."

So I got home, I applied, and two weeks later I was in Tucson. Two years later, I graduated. Now I'm a fellowship-trained, double board-certified Integrative OB-GYN. There are very few of us in the world.

And since then, I haven't looked back. I've taken dozens of courses that I wish were offered in medical school but are not. I've learned cutting-edge cell biology, biochemistry, and physiology. I've studied environmental medicine and the impact of endocrine disruptors and environmental toxins.

With this up-to-date scientific knowledge, I developed models for the cellular, genetic, and environmental pathways of chronic diseases.

Then I created treatment protocols that go beyond pharmaceuticals and surgery to include lifestyle, nutrition, targeted supplements, acupuncture, massage, IV therapies, mind-body medicine, and exercise, all of which are based on research studies and successful real-world use.

I renamed my practice: Integrative Medical Group of Irvine. Even though most of my patients, doctors, and staff are still women, I dropped "women" from the name because so many of my patients began bringing in their husbands, and I wanted them to feel comfortable, too.

When I decided to become an OB-GYN all those years ago, one of my dreams was to find a cure for PCOS. And that has become the primary focus of my research.

Every night, I scour all the latest medical articles. I read the environmental literature and the gynecology, endocrinology, and cardiovascular journals. I look across all areas of medicine to really put everything together and understand what's going on in PCOS.

Because I have no funding, I'm not beholden to anyone. My only agenda is to understand the truth so I can help women with PCOS. Women like me, my family, and my patients.

And that's what this book is — years of research into the latest, cutting-edge understanding of PCOS. I've studied PCOS on a cellular, hormonal, and physiological level. I've explored how it relates to our environment, our changed diet, our altered lifestyles, and everything that has come together to create what's really now a worldwide epidemic of PCOS.

Based on my research, I've put together a treatment plan that gives your body everything it needs to heal itself.

In this book, I lay out the protocol that I teach to women and doctors around the world and use with my own patients today — one that is not founded on pharmaceuticals and surgery, but on healthy living and natural supplements that support the body's normal rhythms and processes.

I live my life by the strategies in this book, and I look and feel the best I ever have. I have shared this knowledge with my patients and all of my female relatives to help them control their weight and acne, to restore their rhythms and fertility, and to heal their PCOS.

If you feel adrift in a sea of PCOS symptoms, this book is an answer to your SOS call.

As I learned from Dr. Low Dog at the beginning of my integrative journey; The body knows what to do. Give the body what it needs and let it heal itself. Doctors are teachers. We are helpers. We can't heal anybody. Everyone has to heal themselves.

So, really, that's what this book is — your lifeline — so that you can rescue yourself and begin your own journey towards health.

Foreword by Alexis Perella

When I was a teenager, PCOS was a small backstory to my life. My mom is a doctor with PCOS, so even though she wasn't my OB-GYN (boundaries!) she made sure I saw an OB-GYN and got diagnosed early. I went on the birth control pill because that's what everyone with PCOS did. This was before my mom knew anything about integrative medicine and more effective treatments for PCOS.

I loved birth control. It totally cured my acne, and my periods were completely predictable.

I ignored my blood tests showing high cholesterol. I didn't worry that I was tired all of the time or that I had hypoglycemic episodes where my hands would shake and I couldn't think straight. I never told my mom. I just ate a lot of candy. That was my normal.

I stayed on birth control for years and years and never gave my PCOS a second thought.

Then I got married. A few years later, my husband and I wanted to start our family. And everything changed.

The enormity of PCOS hit me. Most obviously, as soon as I went off of the pill, my acne came back with a vengeance. I was 30 years old and had the skin of a 15-year-old.

But more than that, I didn't have a single period.

I wasn't ovulating. At. All. Not once.

So, I couldn't get pregnant. And I couldn't get help because my doctor wouldn't officially diagnose me as infertile until my husband and I had tried to get pregnant for one year.

That was a long, sad, lonely year.

When my doctor finally started discussing infertility, she looked at my test results and flat out told me I would never get pregnant without Clomid.

That's when I finally asked my mom for help.

I was afraid of Clomid and its risks of ovarian hyperstimulation and a multiples pregnancy. So I texted her.

Between the tulip and hug emojis, she suggested that I try taking a supplement called myo-inositol. Being the rebellious daughter, I had always rolled my eyes at her supplements. But this time, I gave it a try. And holy cow, my mom was right!

Three weeks later, I ovulated.

And then I got pregnant.

I was over the moon. I held my tiny miracle in my womb. I cried. All of the time.

At my six week appointment, I gushed to my doctor that I owed it all to an incredible supplement. Even though it was supposed to be impossible, I had started ovulating soon after taking it. But my doctor wasn't impressed. She didn't believe in supplements.

I was deflated. I had hoped that once she knew about this treatment, she'd enthusiastically share it with her other PCOS patients.

Thirty-six weeks into my pregnancy, I gave birth to a premature but healthy baby girl.

Three years later, I was following more of my mom's lifestyle and diet advice. I was still taking myo-inositol plus a bunch of other amazing supplements, and I felt great. I gave birth to my son — a full-term healthy boy.

My mom, with her neverending research, her dedication to kinder and better treatments, and her passionate exploration of supplements, circadian rhythm, and the gut microbiome, gave me my fertility. She also cured my acne and brought my cholesterol levels way down into the healthy range. I haven't had a low blood sugar spell in years.

Today, more than ever, I love my body. I feel strong and healthy. Yeah, I tweeze a couple of hairs here and there. I get the odd pimple. Sometimes my period is off by a week. But every human body has its unique challenges. My body has carried me through 40 years of life and two pregnancies, and for that I am eternally grateful.

When my mom asked if I'd help her write this book, I was honored. Her advice gave me my health and my babies, and I feel privileged to help her share this wisdom with every woman who needs it.

Dr. Gersh may not be your mom, but now you have all of her advice right here in one place.

And to my mom, I'd like to say, "Thank you from the bottom of my heart!"

Prologue

S ince life first formed on earth, our planet has been spinning on its axis and orbiting the sun. A day has been 24 hours and a year has been 365 days.

All of life has evolved in sync with these natural rhythms. Animals, plants, and trees change their behaviors with the seasons. Birds migrate; bears hibernate; trees lose their leaves in the winter, and new growth emerges in the spring.

As the Earth spins, every creature has its own 24-hour cycle. We call this "circadian rhythm." Some animals are active during the day, some at night, and some, like the mosquito, are most active at dawn and dusk. Even plants and single-celled microorganisms have their own 24-hour cycles.

Humans evolved within this natural dance of day and night.

However, unlike every other creature on earth, we humans have the ability to change our experience of the Earth's 24-hour rotation. During the day, we can shield ourselves from the sun, hiding inside our houses and office buildings. We can extend the light of day far into the night with light bulbs, computers, and televisions. We can eat whenever we want and as often as we want. We can hit the gym after work as the sun goes down.

What happens when we live this way? What happens when we pretend that we somehow exist outside of the natural rhythms of the world?

Consider this: Starting a few thousand years ago, we humans began collecting wild animals and putting them in zoos. And what did our ancestors discover when they locked animals in cages? They found that they would not reproduce. They became antisocial. They got fat and lazy and had a lot of anxiety. And they died.

So what did humans do? As soon as drugs became available, we began slipping animals antidepressants and sleeping pills. Humans actually did this. We had zoos full of sick, sedated animals. And then someone clever said, you know what? Maybe we could create living environments for the animals that resemble their natural habitats. And that's what the new, more modern zoos do, right? They take the animals out of barred cages and put them into enclosures that mimic their original homes. The animals are much healthier. They even have babies.

That's what we need to do for ourselves. We need to emerge from the self-imposed cage of modern life that keeps us from living in sync with our bodies' natural rhythms. When we are out of sync, is it any wonder we are anxious, can't sleep, and have fertility problems? We've allowed ourselves to become like the caged animals in the zoo, and now we have the same problems.

So, we medicate. We take drugs. Lots and lots of drugs. We take drugs to help us sleep, treat our depression, heal our digestion, and enable us to get pregnant. We take drugs for *everything*.

If you have PCOS, this story is familiar. We PCOS women have lots of problems and we get prescribed lots and lots of drugs.

But these drugs don't work, not really. None of these drugs address the real problem — that we are living out of touch with our natural cycles —

and all of them cause a whole slew of side effects and new problems. For which we take more drugs.

We have to stop this cycle. We have to return to our natural habitat and live in sync with the 24-hour day. Only then will we thrive.

This is true for all people, and it is especially true for women with PCOS.

PCOS, at its core, is a rhythm problem. Our hormones don't rise and fall properly with the 24-hour day, and they don't cycle with the months of the year. The female body depends on these rhythms, and when we don't have them, we get sick.

But, when we live in accordance with the the natural cycles of the Earth, when we use the spinning of this planet to reset the rhythms in our bodies, we can get well.

This is not a hand-wavy, mystical book. This is a book based on science and hundreds of pages of research. It only sounds "woo-woo" because we are so used to thinking of ourselves as being outside of the natural order of the universe.

Once we accept that we need to live in harmony with our environment, we can open the door to healing PCOS in a natural way that doesn't rely on pharmaceuticals to simply cover our symptoms. We can heal from the inside out and be fully healthy.

Introduction

$\mathcal{I}$ am so excited you are here. You may feel excited, nervous, curious, skeptical, or guardedly optimistic.

One thing you are not: alone. I have helped thousands of women take the journey you are about to begin.

No two women are the same. No two cases of PCOS are the same. And no two PCOS treatment plans are the same. But they all have deep similarities. And they can all end with health.

Let's start yours.

Is this book for you?

PCOS (PEE-see-oh-ehs) is the acronym for polycystic ovary syndrome.

> I'm including all of the medical terms for the conditions described in this book along with pronunciations because health literacy empowers patients to better advocate for themselves and their families. It's easier to Google when you know the proper name for something, and it's easier to discuss a symptom with your doctor when you know you are saying its name correctly.

If you have PCOS, you probably have a bunch of symptoms, and you may be wondering if this book will address your version of PCOS.

The short answer is, yes!

This is an integrative approach to healing that gets at the root causes of PCOS. So, no matter what your PCOS symptoms are and which ones are the most severe, they will get better when you treat the underlying causes of PCOS.

You are probably familiar with the typical medical approach. You decide what symptom is currently bothering you the most. Then you pick out the doctor who usually deals with that part of the body. If you have irregular menstrual cycles or fertility problems, you go to your gynecologist because she knows about uteruses. If you have acne, you go to your dermatologist, who knows about skin. If you have sleep problems, anxiety, or depression, which are very common, you go to a psychiatrist or therapist. If you have gut problems, such as irritable bowel syndrome (IBS) or acid reflux, you go to the gastroenterologist.

Each doctor prescribes a treatment plan and likely gives you medication. None of them talk to each other. No one sees the whole picture.

In modern medicine, we treat the body like a series of parts. That's not what I do.

I am an integrative gynecologist, a rare breed of doctor who has trained to diagnose and treat your body as the whole, integrated, complex system that it is.

When I began practicing medicine this way, I was amazed that I could help my patients resolve a wide array of seemingly unrelated symptoms throughout their whole bodies by addressing deep, underlying health issues.

That's what this book does.

First, I will explain the underlying causes of PCOS and how they lead to all of the symptoms you are experiencing. Then, I will help you address those causes, and no matter what your PCOS symptoms are, they will get better.

It took me years to understand the body this way, so if you are feeling skeptical, I totally understand. I'll show you the research and data, and you can come to your own conclusions.

One of the tenets of integrative medicine is that a patient and her doctor are a team. I can't tell you what to do and I can't heal you. I can only work with you to create a path that we both believe will lead to health and wellness.

Everything in this book is based on scientific studies, often studies that were done in the last two to three years. Unless your doctor is obsessed with reading scientific journals every night the way I am, she probably hasn't heard much of this information yet. All of my resources are listed in the back of the book so you can check them out, analyze the findings, and share them with your doctors.

See what you think and then make the best decisions for you.

Structure of this book

The organization of this book will guide you, step-by-step, on your journey.

Part 1 provides everything you need to know about PCOS: what it is, how you got it, and how it works. I'll show you how this condition is caused by a simple hormonal irregularity that cascades into an incredibly complex condition. And I'll explain how restoring circadian rhythm, gut microbiome health, and clean living can be your keys to restoring your hormones, fertility, and health.

Part 2 offers all of my concrete advice for how to heal your PCOS, organized into seven practical steps. Steps one, two, and three focus on circadian rhythm. Steps four and five heal your gut microbiome. Step six gets endocrine disruptors out of your life. And step seven helps you fine-tune your wellness plan to meet your specific needs.

As my patients and kids can confirm, I give out a lot of advice. Most of it focuses on lifestyle and diet. Some of it includes supplements. I also cover a wide range of traditional treatment options, including the pharmaceuticals that I do and don't recommend.

I have laid out this treatment plan in a sequence that works well with my patients. It's logical and it focuses on some of the easier changes first so you can get started on your path to health right away.

But the recommendations are not hierarchical. The last ones are as critical to healing as the first ones. Depending on your particular PCOS, one section may prove more relevant than another, but at the end of the day, you will get the best results when you read all of the sections and adopt all (well, let's be realistic — *almost all*) of the tips together.

What is integrative medicine?

As a gynecologist, before I discovered integrative medicine, I was an expert in vaginas, uteruses, and the reproductive stages of a woman's life. I wasn't responsible for my patients' diabetes, heart disease, or autoimmune disorders. Other doctors took care of that. Just tell me what's wrong with your uterus, and I bet I have a pill or a surgery to make it better!

Integrative medicine takes a completely opposite approach. When I became an integrative gynecologist, I began looking at my patients' entire medical history because I learned how every system of the body affects every other system. Diabetes affects fertility. Acne is a sign of hormonal imbalance. Hypothyroidism can signal PCOS.

I also consider a much broader range of treatment options. There are definitely times when surgery, pharmaceuticals, and other medical interventions are the best course of action. I am a classically trained medical doctor, and I use these tools when they are appropriate.

But my toolbox is now much bigger. I also prescribe diet, lifestyle changes, acupuncture, supplements, exercise, laser treatments, and massage. When done properly in ways backed by rigorous scientific studies, these are powerful interventions that can change the course of a disease and a person's life.

A foundational theory of integrative medicine is that, because everything in the body is interrelated, we cannot just tinker with one part of the body. We cannot stop ovulation with birth control pills or stop stomach acid production with proton pump inhibitors without changing anything else. When you change one bodily system, you are inevitably affecting a bunch of other systems and organs. No treatment does just one thing. This is why pharmaceuticals have so many side effects.

On the positive side, when you fix one thing, you'll often find that you unintentionally fix a lot of other problems. You lose weight and your acne clears up. You get daylight in the morning so you sleep better at night, and your eating disorder goes away. You eat less sugar so your blood sugar levels go down, and you start ovulating more regularly.

Your body is amazingly complex and we are only beginning to understand how it works. What we do know is that healing cascades into healing. This is what an integrative doctor specializes in. This is why I became an integrative gynecologist. And this is what I bring to you.

Let's talk about fertility

This is not a how-to-get-pregnant book, per se. But if you are hoping to get pregnant as soon as possible, or even a little further down the road, this book will help because the plan laid out here will help you reclaim your total health. Female fertility is inextricably linked to female health.

I want to say that again, because it's one of the most important takeaways from this book: Your natural menstrual cycle is a vital sign of health.

Messed up periods and infertility are signs of other health problems. Stress (mental and physical) triggers the body, as one of its most basic survival mechanisms, to shut down reproductive functions. People who are starving or under extreme stress, for example, are less fertile. So are people who have hormonal and metabolic dysfunctions, which are some of the underlying conditions of PCOS.

The solution to an irregular menstrual cycle is not to treat the symptoms by prescribing birth control pills or powerful fertility drugs. The solution is to address the root causes and restore total health so that natural reproductive functions start back up again.

Let's talk about weight loss

This is also not a weight-loss book, but if you are overweight (and at least 70% of women with PCOS are overweight or obese[1]), then you will probably lose weight on this protocol. It wasn't my intention to create a weight-loss program. I don't care about your dress size. All women are beautiful and powerful. You are amazing as you are, and you are allowed to take up as much space in this world as you need.

But every single symptom of PCOS is worse for heavier women. Losing weight is one of the most powerful ways to restore your health. Losing weight indicates that the protocol is working and that you are regaining metabolic health. And losing weight will simultaneously magnify the positive benefits you are experiencing.

I talk a lot about metabolism (meh-TAB-oh-lizm), which is how your body makes, uses, and stores energy. We usually think of metabolism in term of weight-gain (storing energy as fat) and weight-loss (burning fat as energy). But it's more complicated than that. Metabolism relies on hormonal messengers. It includes every organ in the body, especially the liver, pancreas, and hypothalamus. It occurs primarily on a cellular level, with individual cells absorbing or repelling sugars and fats circulating in the blood to use for fuel. And it incorporates the health and lifespan of those cells. If you have metabolic health, all of these organs and processes work smoothly together.

Study after study shows that for women with PCOS, losing 5% to 10% of body weight improves fertility, improves metabolic health, and substantially reduces the risks of heart disease, diabetes, and cancer[2].

I hope you will get to a healthy weight because I want you to be healthy, but I will not ask you to diet, at least not in the typical sense of the word. I will never ask you to count calories.

Traditional dieting does not work, and besides, dieting is crappy. Yes, if you cut calories, you can lose weight. But your body is designed not to lose weight.

Throughout human history, starvation has been a greater threat than obesity, so human bodies are optimized to guard their extra weight as an insurance policy against the next famine. This has been a great survival strategy for the past 100,000 years or so, but it's less helpful now that humans have invented grocery stores, fast food restaurants, donuts, and chocolate bars (my favorite!). So even when women lose weight while dieting, they typically gain it all back.

The only sustainable way to lose weight is to reset your metabolic functions so your body naturally gravitates to a lower weight. Healthy eating (Is that a diet if you can still eat as much as you'd like?) will help. But it's not the whole plan. It's not even the main part of the plan.

The strategies for long-term weight loss are the same strategies for reining in your PCOS, and they are the same strategies for establishing long-term, whole-body health.

They are:

1. Reduce inflammation
2. Normalize your hormones and their rhythms
3. Increase insulin sensitivity

What is inflammation?

Inflammation is your immune system's way to fight infections and heal wounds. When a part of your body is injured, immune cells rush to the site, and the resulting increase in blood causes redness and swelling. This works great to heal acute injuries. Unfortunately, the body treats chronic conditions like PCOS as chronic injuries, and you get chronic inflammation. Instead of healing, chronic inflammation makes you sick. It causes diabetes, heart disease, cancer, and weight gain.

What are hormonal rhythms and balance?

Hormones are chemical messengers that tell your body what to do and when to do it. PCOS is an endocrine disorder because so many of our hormones are out of balance. We don't have the right levels of each hormone and our hormones don't behave the way they are supposed to. Testosterone, cortisol, and insulin are too high. Estrogen and serotonin are too low. And on top of that, these hormones don't cycle up and down properly with the 24-hour day, which causes anxiety, sleep disorders, infertility, and, yes, weight gain.

What is insulin sensitivity?

Insulin sensitivity is your body's ability to see and respond to insulin, a hormone that regulates blood sugar. Insulin plays such a critical role in PCOS symptoms that, even though it is part of hormonal balance, I want to call out insulin sensitivity as a unique piece of the PCOS puzzle.

PCOS makes you insulin resistant, which means your body can't react to insulin and your blood sugar goes up and down more than it should. This is the same condition that leads to type 2 diabetes. Additionally, insulin resistance causes inflammation and heart disease. It raises your testosterone levels, which exacerbates acne. And it keeps your body in fat storage mode, so you perpetually gain weight and never burn it.

How do I lose weight?

Losing weight is not about optimizing a calories-in-calories-out equation. It is about resetting the systems in your body so you use fat and sugar as fuel for your cells the way you are supposed to. It is about reducing inflammation and improving insulin sensitivity. It is about restoring hormonal rhythms and balance throughout your body. In short, you lose weight by healing PCOS.

Let's talk about health

I have PCOS. I have Hashimoto's thyroiditis. I am insulin resistant. I have androgenic alopecia and mild hirsutism. I am postmenopausal. I think of myself as adorably chubby, but really, I should lose another 10 pounds.

I am healthy.

Health is a feeling. It is the flexibility and resilience to recover from the challenges we experience while living life.

It is not a number, a dress size, a distance of miles run. Thank goodness!

It is not even the absence of disease. Today, anything that isn't "normal" or "ideal" is either a disease, a condition, or a syndrome. Everyone has something.

Health is a relationship to our bodies, our lives, our fellow creatures on this planet, and our environments. Health is an ability to move through the world with flexibility, strength, happiness, and confidence. It is physical, emotional, and social. And it is a dynamic process, not a finish line.

We don't get health. We live with health.

Consequently, it is totally possible to have PCOS and be healthy. Truly, gloriously, wonderfully healthy.

I hope you will come with me on this journey. You deserve to feel good in your body.

PART ONE

What you need to know

CHAPTER 1

———

Get started right now

$\mathcal{T}$he first thing you need to know is that this protocol works. The best way to prove this is for you to start right away and see for yourself that it works.

Here are a few things to do now to jumpstart your journey to health.

This quickstart won't solve everything. That's what the rest of this book does! But if you follow it, you should see some improvements in the following weeks and months. Your menstrual cycle may become more regular. Your acne may ease up. You may find fewer new hairs on your chin and a little more hair on your head. You may start losing weight.

Establish your baseline

To monitor your progress as you move through this book and your health journey, you need to establish your baseline.

Your menstrual cycle

First of all, make sure you are tracking your menstrual cycle. I recommend that you do this on your phone. Seriously, there's an app for that.

My favorite menstrual cycle tracker for PCOS women is Life. It's the best one I've seen for monitoring irregular periods. It has a period analysis graph that compares the length of each cycle so it's really easy to see changes. And it's not an in-your-face fertility tracker. It does track ovulation and peak fertility days, but it's not as emphasized in Life as in some other apps, so you can still use it for all those times when you're not trying to make a baby.

For premium pricing, Life lets you track other fitness stats, but the core functionality is free.

Obviously, this is more meaningful for women not on hormonal birth control, but even if you are taking the pill, you should track your period as a good habit.

Your basic stats

Take a moment to gather these measurements. You can write them right here in the book, but again, I think you should keep them in your phone. I have an iPhone and the built in Apple Health app is fine for tracking simple health data. You can also use a Fitbit or other fitness tracker of your choice.

Stat	How to measure	Your measurements
Weight	All you need is a simple bathroom scale. For best results, weigh yourself in the morning, naked, after you have used the toilet.	
BMI	Find an online calculator. You'll need your weight and height.	* Optimal is 18.5-24.9.
Waist circumference	This is the number of inches around your middle, measured just above your belly button line.	
Hip circumference	This is the number of inches around your hips, measured at your largest spot.	
Waist to hip ratio	Divide your waist measurement by your hip measurement.	* Optimal is below 0.8.
Blood pressure	You can find free blood pressure machines at most drug stores and pharmacies, or you can buy your own cuff. For best results, take your blood pressure at 8 PM.	* Optimal is less than 120/80

You should measure your weight every morning and track it digitally (or on a piece of graph paper, if that works better for you). Women who weigh themselves daily are more successful at losing weight and then maintaining a healthy weight.[1]

Use your weight to calculate your body mass index (BMI). It's imperfect because it doesn't take into account muscle mass, fitness level, and bone density, but it's still a helpful metric to track for most people. Find a BMI calculator online.

- Less than 18.5 is underweight.
- Between 18.5 and 24.9 is ideal.
- Between 25 and 29.9 is overweight.
- Over 30 is obese.

Once a week, check your waist to hip ratio. This measurement specifically looks at whether you are carrying extra weight in your belly (dangerous) or in your hips (better). A higher ratio corresponds to a higher risk of a cardiovascular event like a heart attack or stroke. Divide your waist by your hips. For example, if your waist is 30 inches and your hips are 36 inches around, your ratio is 30/36=0.83.

- Below 0.8 is low risk.
- 0.8 to 0.89 is moderate risk.
- 0.9 or above is high risk.

Many people think they can shrink their waistline by doing sit ups. Sadly, it doesn't work this way. There are two ways to lose belly inches. One is to lose weight throughout your entire body. The other is to reprogram your metabolism to store excess weight in your hips instead of your midsection. Both are helpful and the protocol in this book will do both.

Once a week after dinner, measure your blood pressure. I recommend that everyone purchase their own blood pressure cuff. The digital wrist cuffs are easy to use and you can buy them online or in your local drug store. These days, most pharmacies and drug stores also have a free blood pressure machine.

Your blood pressure is comprised of two numbers: The top number is your systolic blood pressure and the bottom number is your diastolic blood pressure. For both numbers, lower is better. The cut-offs for hypertension (high blood pressure) were recently revised, so even if you think your blood pressure is okay, you should double check.[2]

Systolic (top number)		Diastolic (bottom number)	
Less than 120	with	Less than 80	is ideal.
120-129	with	Less than 80	is elevated.
130-139	or	80-89	is high, stage 1.
140 and above	or	90 and above	is high, stage 2.
Above 180	or	Above 120	is hypertensive crisis. **Call your doctor right away!**

High blood pressure means that your arteries are stiff and indicates cardiovascular disease. You should try to bring these numbers into the ideal range, preferably without medication. If you are already taking blood pressure medications, then be diligent about tracking your blood pressure while you follow the protocol in this book. Your blood pressure should improve, and you will likely need to adjust your medication. Hopefully, you can get off of blood pressure pharmaceuticals entirely!

Medical tests

Blood tests and other medical tests, combined with clinical observation and basic PCOS statistics, will allow you and your doctor to create a highly personalized medical plan. Tests provide a window into how your body is operating, so you and your doctor can prioritize treatments that target your greatest current health needs and proactively minimize your risks for future disease.

I highly recommend you set up an appointment with your doctor and have her order these tests. Get them done sooner rather than later so you know where you are today, your starting point. Then repeat them every 6 to 12 months to track your progress.

The tests listed here are the most basic and affordable tests I recommend, and they should be available virtually everywhere. They provide critical information about your overall metabolic and hormonal health and will provide insight into your long-term health risks. These tests also create a picture of your specific version of PCOS so you and your doctor can make informed decisions about your healthcare.

Test	What it shows	Your results
Antinuclear Antibody Panel (ANA)	If it is high, it indicates a potential autoimmune disease or an elevated risk for a future autoimmune disease.	
Basic Hormones: · Estradiol · Total Testosterone · DHEA-S · FSH · LH	Can help diagnose PCOS, identify your specific type of PCOS, and provide information on your PCOS severity.	
Basic Nutrients: · Ferritin (as a marker for iron levels) · Vitamin D (as a 25 OH Vitamin D test)	Nutrient deficiencies lead to poor health. Iron and vitamin D deficiencies are common, especially among PCOS women.	* Vitamin D: Optimal is 40-60 ng/mL.
Complete Blood Count (CBC)	Can identify blood disorders, anemia, and immune system disorders.	
Comprehensive Metabolic Panel (CMP), preferred to do fasting	Assessment of overall body health. Can identify underlying metabolic disorders such as kidney disease, fatty liver disease, and diabetes.	
Lipid Panel: · Total cholesterol · LDL (low-density lipoprotein) · HDL (high-density lipoprotein) · ApoA1 · ApoB · Triglycerides	This test assesses the health of your cardiovascular system. High triglycerides can also indicate liver dysfunction or fatty liver disease.	

| Thyroid Panel:
• TSH
• Free T4
• Free T3
• Anti TPO
• Thyroglobulin antibodies | Thyroid disorders are common among PCOS women so all PCOS women should be periodically tested. | |

There are dozens of additional tests that can provide highly detailed and valuable information about your health. I highly recommend that you check out the lab tests section in Appendix A (page 313) and discuss with your doctor what additional tests might be helpful.

Take these core supplements

Supplements fill in the gaps and imperfections in our lifestyle and diet. They provide essential nutrients and extra support to fragile systems like our immune system, digestive system, and reproductive system. And they can minimize or reverse harmful feedback loops, particularly those based on inflammation.

If you walked in the door of my practice today with PCOS, I would put you on the following supplements right away. Feel free to consume them at whatever time of day is most convenient to you. Most people incorporate their vitamins and supplements into their morning or evening routine. Taking these now will get your body going in the right direction and make all of the other recommendations in this book more effective.

Supplement	Dosage	What I give my patients
Myo-inositol	4 g of powder daily, mixed in water or juice	Pure Encapsulations Inositol (powder) 2 scoops daily
Quercetin	1000 mg daily	Pure Encapsulations Quercetin 4 capsules daily
N-acetyl cysteine (NAC)	1800 mg daily	Pure Encapsulations NAC 600 mg 3 capsules daily

Supplement	Dosage	What I give my patients
Curcumin	750-1500 mg daily	Pure Encapsulations CurcumaSorb 3-6 capsules daily or Thorne Meriva 500-SF Curcumin Phytosome 2-3 capsules daily
Vitamin D3	2000 IU daily	Pure Encapsulations Vitamin D3 1000 IU 1-2 capsules daily, depending on what's in your multivitamin or Thorne D-1000 1-2 capsules daily, depending on what's in your multivitamin
Multivitamin	Daily	Pure Encapsulations O.N.E. Multivitamin 1 capsule daily or Thorne Basic Nutrients 2 capsules daily
Probiotic	Daily	Ortho Molecular Products Ortho-Biotic 1 capsule daily or Pure Encapsulations Probiotic-5 1 capsule daily
Omega-3s	EPA 600 mg, DHA 400 mg daily	Pure Encapsulations O.N.E. Omega 1 soft gel daily or Metagenics EPA-DHA 720 2 softgels daily

Here's a bit more about each of the supplements. If any of this sounds like gibberish, don't worry. I go into depth on all of these topics elsewhere in the book.

Myo-inositol (my-oh-in-AW-si-tall)

If you only take one supplement, it should be myo-inositol, a sugar alcohol that plays a critical role in glucose metabolism.

Specifically, myo-inositol reduces insulin resistance, which is a central characteristic of PCOS and one of the root causes of nearly every symptom you are experiencing.

Myo-inositol is so effective that among women who take this supplement daily, 70% will begin having regular menstrual cycles. Myo-inositol reduces your lifelong risk of developing diabetes and cardiovascular disease. If you choose to have a baby, myo-inositol improves your egg quality and reduces your risk of developing gestational diabetes.[3,4,5]

A powder that you can mix into water or juice, it's slightly sweet but otherwise tasteless. This is a powerhouse supplement that can change your life.

Quercetin (KWAIR-si-tin)

Quercetin is a flavonoid found in a variety of plants, including green apples and red wine. Like myo-inositol, quercetin improves insulin resistance, and additionally, it improves adiponectin (ad-i-pah-NEK-tin) receptors. Adiponectin is good; it's a hormone critical for burning fat and maintaining metabolic health. So, quercetin makes adiponectin work better and helps with weight loss and maintenance. It also decreases testosterone and improves ovarian health and function.[6,7,8]

Quercetin has the added benefit of stabilizing mast cells. These are specialized immune cells that initiate a cascade of inflammatory reactions. Stabilizing mast cells reduces inflammation.

N-acetyl cysteine (NAC)

NAC is an antioxidant. In women with PCOS, NAC improves egg quality, normalizes ovulation, and increases the chances of both getting pregnant and having a live birth. NAC supports healthy glucose metabolism and is the precursor to the production of glutathione (gloo-tuh-THEYE-own), known as the master antioxidant and detoxifier of the body. It also protects the liver from fatty liver disease, which is a leading cause of liver failure. Women with PCOS have high rates of fatty liver disease, so we want this protection.[9,10,11]

Curcumin (ker-KYOO-men)

This polyphenol is the active component in turmeric. Another anti-inflammatory, it protects against many of the long-term health conditions that PCOS can lead to. It reduces insulin resistance and the risk of diabetes. It protects the liver from fatty liver disease by decreasing liver inflammation. It lowers hypertension and protects against heart attacks. It reduces the risk of cancer. It's also great for brain health.[12]

Vitamin D₃

The sunshine vitamin, vitamin D has risen in popularity because of its critical role in proper immune health. But it does much more than prevent colds. Vitamin D is essential for blood sugar regulation, ovarian function, cancer prevention, and sleep, all things that women with PCOS struggle with.

As many as 85% of women with PCOS are vitamin D deficient, and treating this deficiency improves a wide array of PCOS symptoms. On top of that, it really does prevent colds.[13,14,15,16]

Multivitamin

If you go into any pharmacy, you'll find dozens upon dozen of multivitamins. Look for a pharmaceutical grade multivitamin to be sure that the vitamins and minerals in the supplement are bioavailable, in a form that your body can absorb.

Your multivitamin should have, at a minimum, the recommended dietary allowance (RDA) for the included vitamins and minerals.

The B vitamins should be methylated (METH-ill-ate-ed). For example, instead of folic acid, also known at vitamin B9, your multivitamin should include a folate such as methylfolate. For vitamin B12, it should have methylcobalamin, not cyanocobalamin. Many people have a genetic mutation that makes it difficult to methylate B vitamins. Methylation is a critical part of the vitamin metabolism process, and when you take premethylated B vitamins, your body can better utilize them.

Be very careful when you take a multivitamin that you don't unknowingly double up on some vitamins. For example, in this section, I recommend 2000 IU of vitamin D. If your multivitamin already has 1000 IU, then you only need to add 1000 IU. If you take 2000 IU on top of what's in your multivitamin, you'll be taking 3000 IU total. Some women need higher doses of Vitamin D, but it's best to use the higher doses after confirming you truly need them. In many cases, vitamins can become problematic or even toxic at high levels. Be especially careful not to overdose on vitamin A, vitamin E, iron, and zinc.

Vitamin overdoses are rare, but they are possible, so just be sure you know how all of your vitamins add up.

Probiotics (pro-by-AW-ticks)

Probiotics are live bacteria that benefit your gut microbiome.

They are great for improving digestive and intestinal function. Many women with PCOS suffer from irritable bowel syndrome (IBS) and probiotics can treat a wide range of IBS symptoms.

Additionally, probiotics help with a whole host of other hormonal and metabolic functions. In women with PCOS, daily probiotics improve weight loss, triglycerides, cholesterol, and insulin resistance. They reduce testosterone levels and improve hirsutism (the irritating dark hairs you may have on your chin, chest, and back). They also enhance mood, and in pregnancy, they reduce the risk of preeclampsia and preterm birth.[17,18,19,20]

Omega-3 fatty acids

Primarily found in fatty fish, omega-3s reduce inflammation and improve immune system functioning. There are two main types, Eicosapentaenoic Acid (EPA) and Docosahexaenoic Acid (DHA). There is another type, Alpha-Linolenic Acid (ALA) that comes from plants, but to use ALA, we humans first need to convert it to EPA and DHA, and we aren't very good at it.

Omega-3's are particularly useful for preventing heart disease and autoimmune diseases, which PCOS otherwise increases your risk for. They also support brain health, improving mood and cognitive functions.[21,22,23]

The best way to get your omega-3s is to eat fatty fish like wild salmon or sardines twice per week. Unfortunately, many fish are contaminated with mercury and other toxic compounds, so I recommend eating fish only once or twice per month and taking fish oil supplements.

Better together

It may seem like many of these supplements do the same thing, but they work through different pathways. I highly recommend that you take all of them.

I've indicated the specific brands I give to my patients because I know they are high quality and work well. Good supplements deliver exactly what's on the label in the advertised dosages, and they are free from impurities and toxins.

I really like Pure Encapsulations (full disclosure: I have a professional relationship with them, but I work with them because I like their products). I also like Thorne Research, Douglas Laboratories, Designs for Health, Metagenics, and Ortho Molecular Products. There are other great products out there, but these are the companies I know and trust.

Healthy habits to get you started

At the end of most chapters, I have a short section with little habits that can help you make the healthy changes I recommend throughout the book.

Change is hard. These little habits make it easier. Check them off as you adopt them. They don't cover everything you'll need to do to get healthy, but they definitely get you moving in the right direction.

Here are a few that you can start today.

- ☐ Put the Life app on your phone and enter the dates from your last six menstrual cycles.

- ☐ Buy a scale and put it on the floor of your bathroom.

- ☐ Weigh yourself every morning and track your weight and BMI.

- ☐ Buy a tape measure (the soft kind for sewing, not the stiff kind for home improvements) and store it with your scale.

- ☐ Take your waist and hip measurements and find your waist-to-hip ratio.

- ☐ Buy a blood pressure cuff.

- ☐ Begin tracking your blood pressure.

- ☐ Make an appointment with your doctor to order your blood tests.

☐ Buy your supplements online or at your local naturopathic pharmacy, if you have one. You can also buy them at my website: www.felicelgershmd.com.

☐ Use a pill organizer to lay out all of your vitamins for the week in one go. Keep it with your toothbrush. Set a calendar alert on your phone to remember to do this every Sunday.

CHAPTER 2

_____

What is PCOS?

*P*COS is a syndrome, not a disease, because it's diagnosed by identifying a specific collection of symptoms and ruling out other potential causes. There is no single PCOS blood test, just a long list of symptoms and test results that create a specific profile labeled PCOS.

A fair amount of controversy surrounds the exact collection of symptoms needed to make a PCOS diagnosis. So, if you hear that anywhere from 5% to 20% of all women may have PCOS, that's because different definitions lead to different estimates.

However, everyone agrees that PCOS is the most common female endocrine disorder seen in women today. It is the leading cause of female infertility. And, it is more than an infertility disorder. It is more than a gynecological disorder. It is a systemic, whole-body disorder that affects metabolism, the immune system, the cardiovascular system, the gut, the skin, the mind ... really, truly the whole body.

Your endocrine (EN-duh-krin) system is the collection of glands that make hormones, chemical messengers that travel throughout the body. An endocrine disorder is any ailment that involves the over- or under-production of hormones or any part of the transport, reception, and elimination or hormones.

How does it do that? Well, to understand and treat PCOS, first we need to agree on what it is.

The definition that I find most useful is the one developed by the Androgen Excess and PCOS Society. This definition was recently reaffirmed at an international symposium hosted by the Centre for Research Excellence in Polycystic Ovary Syndrome in 2018. According to the AE-PCOS Society and the CRE PCOS, a woman has PCOS if she has:

#1) hyperandrogenism (hy-per-AN-dro-jen-izm), an above average level of androgens, which are male sex hormones such as testosterone. This is a required symptom.

Hyperandrogenism can be documented through a blood test or by observing symptoms of elevated androgen levels, such as acne, unwanted hair in places where normally only men get it (face, chest, back), and thinning hair on the scalp.

We call hormones "male" and "female" but that's not really accurate. Everyone has the same hormones, just in different amounts. It's more like male-dominant and female-dominant.

Androgens are commonly thought of as male sex hormones because men have about ten times the amount that women do.

Testosterone is the most common and well-known androgen. Dehydroepiandrosterone-sulfate (DHEA-S) is another androgen that is elevated in a small subset of PCOS women. For simplicity and readability, I often refer to androgens as testosterone, even though in some cases, there could be a DHEA-S component.

Additionally, for a PCOS diagnosis, a woman must have one or both of the following symptoms:

#2) an irregular or absent menstrual cycle (in women of reproductive age). An irregular cycle is anything less frequent than once every 35 days, anything more frequent than every 21 days, a cycle that varies in length by more than a few days, or a cycle where bleeding lasts longer than 7 days.

#3) polycystic ovaries, as seen on an ultrasound. This isn't as scary as it sounds. What this means is, due to hormonal imbalances, the ovaries contain many small follicles.

All women's ovaries are full of follicles, tiny fluid-filled sacs that each have a single, immature egg. When ovulation occurs properly, one follicle grows and develops each month until the egg bursts from the follicle (ovulation!) and travels down the fallopian tube into the uterus. If it is not fertilized by sperm, then it disintegrates or leaves the body along with the lining of the uterus (menstruation!).

At the start of a normal menstrual cycle, many follicles begin to develop, but only one is recruited to fully develop and release its egg. When that follicle is chosen, the other follicles regress, or shrivel up. In a healthy ovary, you may see several tiny follicles or one larger, more mature follicle.

In women with PCOS, no specific follicle gets recruited to be the one to ovulate, and so a large number of developing follicles continue to exist.

These follicles are sometimes described as a "string of pearls" because they form along the outer rim of the ovary.

These cysts are not dangerous. But when no single egg fully matures and bursts from its sack, ovulation does not occur. And then a woman doesn't get her period regularly. Lack of regular ovulation is a major cause of the infertility suffered by so many women with PCOS.

Polycystic ovaries are diagnosed through a transvaginal ultrasound and are evidence of the broken ovulation process. They don't cause PCOS. They are a symptom of PCOS.

And that's it.
If you have hyperandrogenism, plus irregular periods and/or polycystic ovaries, then you are in the same boat as me and approximately 10% of all women around the globe.[1] Welcome to the club!

Please don't diagnose yourself with PCOS. Remember, PCOS is a diagnosis of exclusion. There are other conditions, really serious conditions, that can look like PCOS. Only a doctor can rule out endocrine tumors, Cushing's Syndrome, congenital and acquired adrenal hyperplasia, and other endocrine disorders.

But, if your doctor can't find anything else causing these symptoms, and you meet the definition, then it's pretty safe to assume you have PCOS.

PCOS (in)famous symptoms

So, what are all of the symptoms that we PCOS ladies share, to some degree or another? Well, here are the most common ones that are likely to send you to a doctor, or at least to Dr. Google.

I know this section can get a little depressing. But don't worry. My protocol will show you how to combat all of these symptoms. I am right-now-as-we-speak successfully treating the causes of this syndrome with my own patients. I refuse to play symptom whack-a-mole, and you should, too.

But first, let's get on the same page regarding what PCOS looks like. Every woman has her own version of PCOS so you may not have all of these symptoms, but here's what you might be experiencing.

Acne

These are pimples, including the red ones, the white-capped ones, and the deep, hard nodules called cystic (SIS-tic) acne. We often think of acne as a skin problem, but it's really a hormone and inflammation condition. High testosterone levels plus inflamed skin lead to excess oil and an altered skin microbiome, the collection of bacteria that reside on our skin and protect it. The result is oily, inflamed skin covered in unfriendly bacteria, a sure-fire recipe for frequent breakouts.

Alopecia (ah-loe-PEE-shah)

Caused by high levels of testosterone, androgenic (an-droe-JEN-ic) alopecia is thinning scalp hair or scalp hair loss somewhat similar to male-pattern baldness.

Here's a personal "fun" story. I suffered hair loss many years ago and I tried to reverse it with what was then a revolutionary new drug, Rogaine. It did make hair grow on my head, but also all over my hands and face! My kids quickly noticed, and called me a werewolf. Let me tell you, treating PCOS with lifestyle, diet, and supplements is so much better! Luckily, when I discontinued the Rogaine, the hair on my hands and face fell out ... along with the new growth on my head.

Hirsutism (HER-soo-tizm)

Elevated testosterone levels trigger the hair follicles on your face, abdomen, legs, chest, and back to sprout dark hair, just as they would if you were a man.

Infertility

PCOS is a leading cause of female infertility. The primary challenge is irregular or absent ovulation. But it's more complicated than that. Women with PCOS have a variety of hormonal and inflammation dysfunctions. So, even with fertility treatments, women with PCOS are less likely to get pregnant than non-PCOS women.[2,3]

Menstrual dysfunction

A woman with regular periods will menstruate cyclically and predictably, about once every 28 days, give or take a week, and her period will last four to five days. Many women with PCOS have a menstrual cycle that is irregular in at least one of the following ways.

A cycle shorter than 21 days is called polymenorrhea (pol-ee-men-uh-REE-uh).

A cycle longer than 35 days is called oligomenorrhea (ol-ee-goh-men-uh-REE-uh).

If your cycle length frequently varies by more than 8 days, you have an irregular cycle length. There's not a fancy term for this.

If you go 90 days or more without a period, that's called amenorrhea (eh-men-uh-REE-uh). See a doctor as soon as you can because this increases your risk for endometrial cancer.

If your period is exceptionally heavy, that's called menorrhagia (men-uh-RAY-jee-uh). Signs of menorrhagia are: using more than one sanitary product every two hours, simultaneously using multiple sanitary products, passing clots larger than an inch, or frequently staining clothes.

Miscarriage

A miscarriage is a spontaneous, unplanned pregnancy loss. Some people will call a pregnancy loss after 20 weeks a stillbirth.

30% to 50% of PCOS pregnancies end in miscarriage. PCOS causes imbalances in many hormones, including testosterone, estrogen, insulin, progesterone, and luteinizing hormone. Additionally, there are challenges involving the health of the placenta, the vascular system, the liver, and more — all of which increase the risk of pregnancy loss.[4]

Before you get pregnant, I strongly advocate treating the root causes of PCOS and getting systemically healthy. You are more likely to get pregnant (maybe naturally!) and stay pregnant for a full 40 weeks.

Obesity

Obesity is defined as a body mass index (BMI) of 30 or higher. 70% of PCOS women are overweight or obese. And no matter what you weigh, compared to a non-PCOS woman who weighs the same as you, you are more likely to carry visceral fat. That's the belly fat that gives you the infamous "apple shape" associated with higher rates of heart disease, fatty liver, and diabetes.[5,6]

Lesser known (not-too-scary) symptoms

Here are a few more annoying symptoms that you may be experiencing that you (and maybe your doctor!) didn't know were connected to PCOS.

Acanthosis nigricans (ah-can-THO-sis NEE-gree-cans)

These patches of velvety, darkened skin are often caused by insulin resistance. The good news is that they usually fade once your insulin levels are back under control.

Gingivitis (jin-juh-VAHY-tis) and periodontal (per-ee-uh-DON-tl) disease

Gingivitis is a mild form of periodontal disease, which is red swelling of the gums in your mouth right around the base of your teeth. Women with PCOS have an altered oral microbiome (the bacteria that live in our mouths), and this causes us to have much higher rates of gum disease than women without PCOS.[7,8,9]

Irritable Bowel Syndrome (IBS) and Gastroesophageal Reflux (GERD)

IBS consists of any combination of frequent abdominal pain, bloating, gas, diarrhea, and constipation. GERD involves stomach acid coming up into the esophagus from the stomach and creating a burning sensation. Basically, PCOS dysregulates your entire gastrointestinal tract, from the mouth all the way down and through the large intestine, and that makes it hard to keep things moving smoothly, regularly, and in the right direction.

Skin tags

These little nubs of excess skin look like little balloon moles, usually attached to your skin by a tiny stalk. They are annoying but totally benign, which means they virtually never turn into cancer. They are related to insulin resistance, so once you get that under control, fewer new ones should grow. But for the ones you already have, if they bother you, the best option is to have a doctor remove them.[10]

Sleep disorders

Women with PCOS have higher rates of sleep disorders than women without PCOS. Insomnia (in-SOM-nee-ah), which is difficulty falling or staying asleep, is extremely common. PCOS women metabolize melatonin and cortisol, two hormones critical to the sleep-wake cycle, at abnormal levels and off-rhythm with the 24-hour day. Insomnia is exacerbated by depression and anxiety, which are also linked to PCOS.[11,12,13]

Additionally, regardless of weight, women with PCOS are more likely suffer from sleep apnea (AP-nee-ah), which is when a person momentarily stops breathing in her sleep.[14]

Sleep disorders affect your sleep quality and can lead to chronic fatigue. They also contribute to a wide array of chronic health conditions, including high blood pressure, diabetes, obesity, and mood disorders.[15]

Silent, long-term (scary!) risks

This is the scary stuff. This is why I don't think symptom whack-a-mole is an acceptable treatment plan for women with PCOS.

Most women with PCOS have underlying, chronic inflammation, insulin resistance, gut dysbiosis, and hormonal imbalances that most treatment protocols don't address. Over time, these conditions progress to long-term health conditions.

One reason that PCOS research is underfunded is that most of the symptoms I've already listed won't put you in the hospital. They might impact your self-esteem and your quality of life. They might make you feel crummy. They might break your heart. But they won't kill you.

Well, as hard as it is for me to say this, there are some conditions associated with PCOS that can make you extremely sick and might actually kill you.

If you have any of the conditions below, or if you think you might but have never been diagnosed, make an appointment with your doctor right away. They are serious and potentially life-threatening.

Autoimmune disease

In an autoimmune disease, your body's immune system has trouble distinguishing your own body's cells from foreign molecules like bacteria and toxins. Your body makes antigens to destroy the foreign molecules, but these antigens also attack your healthy cells. The specific antigen and the tissue it attacks determine what autoimmune disease you get diagnosed with.

Women with PCOS have higher rates of virtually all autoimmune diseases, especially Hashimoto's thyroiditis (haw-she-MOE-toes THY-royd-aye-tis), where the body's immune system attacks and destroys a person's thyroid gland.[16,17,18]

Cancer

Women with PCOS have 2.7 times the risk of developing endometrial (en-doe-MEE-tree-all) cancer, a cancer of the uterine lining. Risk factors are estrogen and progesterone imbalances and stretches of amenorrhea, when you miss your period so the endometrial lining of your uterus hangs around longer than it should. Many women with PCOS experience both of these.

For some women, fertility drugs also increase their risk of ovarian cancer.[19,20,21]

Cardiovascular disease

Cardiovascular disease is a catch-all term for several conditions affecting your circulatory system. It includes hypertension (high blood pressure), heart disease, heart attack, and stroke.

Women with PCOS have chronic inflammation that extends throughout the circulatory system. Additionally, we have low nitric oxide, a signalling molecule that relaxes blood vessels and improves oxygen and blood flow. Low nitric oxide plus inflammation causes arteries to harden and accumulate plaque. This is called atherosclerosis (ath-uh-roh-skluh-ROH-sis), which leads to hypertension and coronary artery disease and raises your risk for a heart attack or stroke.

Diabetes (dy-ah-BEE-teez)

Type 2 diabetes is a metabolic disease that occurs when the body loses its ability to regulate blood sugar. Under normal circumstances, when blood sugar increases, the pancreas releases insulin, a hormone that binds to cells throughout the body and signals that they should absorb sugar to use as energy. If a person becomes insulin resistant, their cells have a hard time binding with insulin. The cells don't "eat" the sugar, so blood sugar levels climb higher. The pancreas releases even more insulin until eventually the cells "see" the insulin, eat the sugar, and blood sugar goes back down. Over time, the pancreas wears out and can no longer produce enough insulin to overcome the insulin resistance. Blood sugar gets out of control and damages nerves, blood vessels, and organs. At this point, you officially have diabetes.

Type 2 diabetes always starts with insulin resistance, and women with PCOS are all insulin resistant to varying degrees. Consequently, PCOS women are four times more likely to develop full-blown diabetes than non-PCOS women, and on average, they develop it four years earlier.[22]

Unlike type 2 diabetes, type 1 diabetes is an autoimmune condition that a person is born with. In type 1 diabetes, a person's immune system produces antigens that destroy the pancreas and make it unable to produce insulin. This also leads to uncontrolled high blood sugar.

PCOS and insulin are so intertwined that type 1 diabetes actually causes PCOS in many women.[23]

Fatty liver

Did you know that your liver can get fat? We used to think of fatty liver as a disease that only alcoholics got, but women with PCOS often get it, too, even without drinking alcohol.[24,25]

Your liver is a metabolic workhorse that controls digestion, detoxification, blood clotting and hundreds of other critical jobs in your body. When it's full of fat cells, it does all of these jobs poorly, and eventually, you get sick.

The medical term for this condition is non-alcoholic fatty liver disease (NAFLD). In its early stages, fatty liver is silent and asymptomatic, but if left untreated, it can progress to non-alcoholic steatohepatitis (NASH). When you have NASH, your liver becomes inflamed, which damages the liver cells and leads to scarring, called fibrosis (fy-BRO-sis). NASH can then progress to full-blown cirrhosis (sir-OH-sis), where the liver is so scarred that it begins to fail.

Obesity is a major risk for non-alcoholic fatty liver disease, but women with PCOS seem to develop fatty liver at higher rates and at lower body weights than non-PCOS women. Even normal weight PCOS women are at risk of developing NAFLD.[26]

Mood disorders

A mood disorder is a condition where your mood frequently doesn't match your environment. You are too happy or too sad for what's going on around you.

A large percentage of women with PCOS struggle with at least one mental health condition. We have five times the rate of anxiety and ten times the rate of depression as non-PCOS women. Alarmingly, women with PCOS are seven times more likely to commit suicide than non-PCOS women.[27,28]

Mood disorders are tightly linked to eating disorders. PCOS is specifically associated with binge eating disorder and bulimia (bull-EE-me-ah) nervosa. A woman with binge eating disorder will repeatedly eat large quantities of food to the point that she is physically uncomfortable. In bulimia, a woman will follow a binge eating episode with purging, which is vomiting, exercising, or using laxatives to rid her body of the calories she just consumed. Both disorders are characterized by an out-of-control feeling and may include feelings of shame and guilt.[29]

If you have a mood disorder or an eating disorder, it is not "in your head." These problems are caused, at least in part, by hormonal imbalances throughout your body. If you are in crisis, seek help immediately.

My protocol will help with the hormonal imbalances, but mood disorders are complex and dangerous. If you are struggling, you need to be under the care of a trained physician.

If you might harm or hurt yourself, call the National Suicide Prevention Lifeline:

1-800-273-8255. Counselors are available 24/7.

If you have an eating disorder and you need help getting treatment, call the National Eating Disorders Association: 1-800-931-2237. They are open Monday through Friday during normal business hours, ET.

Pregnancy complications

Women with PCOS have higher rates of many pregnancy complications. We have three times the risk of preeclampsia, three times the risk of gestational diabetes, and two times the risk of delivering prematurely.[30]

Preeclampsia (pree-i-KLAMP-see-uh) is a dangerous condition where a woman's blood pressure rises rapidly in the second half of pregnancy.

Gestational (jeh-STAY-shun-all) diabetes is a type of diabetes that develops during pregnancy and usually resolves soon after the baby is born.

A premature delivery is any birth occurring before 37 weeks. Babies born prematurely are much more likely to need treatment in the neonatal intensive care unit (NICU).

During delivery, women with PCOS are more likely to have a cesarean section (c-section), which is a surgical delivery.

Babies are often large for their gestational age, a condition called macrosomia (mack-reh-SO-mee-ah), which can complicate deliveries. And the babies of PCOS women are more likely to have health complications themselves.[31]

Pregnant women with PCOS need to pay special attention to their health and monitor their vital signs carefully.

Macrosomia describes any baby born weighing more than 8 pounds 13 ounces. For PCOS women, this large birth weight is caused by insulin resistance. I wish I'd known how to control my blood sugar when I was having my babies. I'm 5'1" and my four babies ranged in weight from eight and a half pounds to nine and a half pounds! They were all delivered vaginally. It was not fun.

The common links

This is a long list of symptoms, and if you treat your PCOS symptom-by-symptom, you could end up taking a lot of drugs: birth control pills for your menstrual cycle, statins for high cholesterol, metformin for diabetes, spironolactone for high testosterone, antidepressants, sleeping pills, and on and on. These pharmaceuticals all have side effects, some of which exacerbate other PCOS symptoms.

Birth control pills increase hypertension and depression. Antidepressants can cause insomnia and weight gain. Statins and metformin can cause irritable bowel symptoms. So, sometimes, you think you are treating PCOS but you are actually treating a side effect of another drug you are taking.

There is a better treatment strategy. It's my protocol (surprise!).

All of these PCOS symptoms, every single one, can be tied to just a few underlying conditions.

1. Inflammation
2. Hormonal dysregulation
3. Insulin resistance

When we recognize this, we find hope. Because we don't need to treat every single symptom, one at a time. Instead of treating over a dozen symptoms, we only need to treat a few underlying conditions.

And the great news is that there are three things — your circadian rhythm, your gut microbiome, and the health of your environment — that powerfully regulate all of these conditions.

In the next chapter, I'll explain the underlying mechanics of PCOS, according to the most recent and cutting-edge research. Then I'll show you how to use circadian rhythm, your gut microbiome, and a clean environment to fix all of your PCOS symptoms.

CHAPTER 3

_____

What causes PCOS?

*P*COS is an ancient syndrome. Really ancient. Hippocrates likely penned one of the earliest descriptions of PCOS way back around 400 BC. But even at that point, PCOS wasn't new.

Rates of PCOS are consistent among all racial groups, which implies that it predates the development of racial diversity. That puts it at more than 50,000 years old.

Which is awe-inspiring on one hand and completely implausible on the other. How could a condition that impedes fertility persist in about 10% of the female population? How were all of these infertile women passing down their genes for infertility?!

Well, the fact is, ancient PCOS rarely looked like modern PCOS. In general, it was a relatively mild, inherited condition that bestowed many advantages on your ancestors who had it. Due to slightly higher-than-normal testosterone levels, your female ancestors had more muscle mass and denser bones that made them stronger than average women.

PCOS gave your ancestors a greater ability to store fat, so even though they were only slightly heavier than average women, their "thrifty genes" helped them survive famines. PCOS gave them mild inflammation, which helped them combat disease. And it created mild infertility, which in an age of high maternal mortality, meant that your female ancestors would have had fewer pregnancies that were better spaced, increasing the likelihood that they survived their pregnancies to nurture the babies they did bear.

Your female ancestors, and mine, were fabulously adapted to early hunter-gatherer nomadic lives. And when they settled down on farms, they continued to pass on their PCOS genes because these women were still hardier and better able to survive famines than their slightly more fertile sisters.

But you and I are not hunter-gatherers. And we are not in the midst of a famine. And so our PCOS looks very different from the PCOS of our foremothers.

Aromatization ... What?

On a molecular level, the very root cause of PCOS is a problem with a process called aromatization (uh-ROH-mah-tize-ay-shun).

All women (and men) create estrogen from androgens such as testosterone. The conversion of an androgen to estrogen is called aromatization. Here's how it works.

Your ovaries make testosterone. Who knew, right? Your ovaries also make an enzyme called aromatase. When the testosterone meets the aromatase, it gets transformed into estrogen. That's where your estrogen comes from.

Poor aromatization is caused by abnormalities in the granulosa cells of the ovary. These are the specific cells in the ovaries where aromatization takes place. In women with PCOS, granulosa cells produce less aromatase, and they respond improperly to a hormone called FSH. Additionally, there are structural and behavioral differences in the granulosa cells in women with and without PCOS.[1,2,3]

We know that poor aromatization is linked to granulosa cell abnormalities, but the exact mechanism is poorly understood. Consequently, there is no PCOS granulosa cell therapy, at least at this time.

Most of your estrogen is aromatized in your ovaries, but your brain, gut, uterus, lungs, and fat cells also make aromatase and convert androgens into estrogen because estrogen is that important.

In summary: androgen → aromatization → estrogen

That's how it's supposed to happen, but for a woman with PCOS, that process doesn't work as efficiently as it should. It works, just not that well.

So, poor aromatization is the very first piece of the PCOS puzzle.

The result of inefficient aromatization is that women with PCOS generally have lower than normal levels of estrogen. The brain senses this estrogen deficiency and it cues the body to make more testosterone to be converted into estrogen. So, the body makes more testosterone. But because aromatization is sluggish, estrogen levels never quite catch up.

What are "normal" estrogen levels?

If your estrogen levels are measured with a blood test, they will likely fall into the "normal" reference range. The reference range for estradiol (es-truh-DIE-all), the predominant estrogen type made by ovaries, is huge because the levels of estradiol in a normally menstruating woman vary greatly over a 28-day menstrual cycle. Having estradiol levels in the reference range does not indicate normal cyclic estradiol production.

The levels of estradiol in women with PCOS tend to be at the lower end of the reference range and do not peak appropriately to signal ovulation. When I say women with PCOS have low estrogen, what I mean is their estrogen level is at the lower end of normal all the time, and this isn't enough estrogen to trigger ovulation or for the body to function optimally.

Chronically low estrogen causes the brain to continually request more testosterone.

Hello, high testosterone.

Oh, and hello, mustache! Hello, acne! Hello, male-pattern baldness! These are the trifecta symptoms of hyperandrogenism, one of the hallmark indicators of PCOS.

High testosterone harms estrogen receptors

High testosterone is the next piece of the PCOS puzzle. Excess testosterone damages your estrogen receptors.[4,5]

Estrogen is a hormone, a chemical messenger, and it communicates with cells and organs throughout your body by binding with estrogen receptors.

> Hormones communicate with cells by locking into specially designated receptors on the surface of those cells. You can think of each hormone as a key. Any cell that responds to that hormone will have a receptor for that hormone, which is like a lock that fits the hormone key. When a hormone connects with a receptor, it unlocks a behavior in that cell.
>
> In this way, hormones control hunger, sleep, mood, digestion, metabolism, reproduction — pretty much everything that our bodies do.

In a woman, there are estrogen receptors on almost every single cell in every organ and system throughout her body. Yes, there are estrogen receptors in your vagina, uterus, and breasts.

But estrogen is not simply a reproductive hormone. You have estrogen receptors in your brain, in the lining of your colon, in your liver, on your fat cells, and on your immune cells. The list goes on and on.

When high testosterone levels damage estrogen receptors, your cells can't respond to estrogen. You already have low estrogen because of poor aromatization. When your cells can't "see" the estrogen you have, they tell your brain you need more. So you produce more testosterone to try and meet your body's need for estrogen.

This exacerbates hyperandrogenism.

In the meantime, while your cells are starving for estrogen, none of your organs can operate optimally. One organ in particular, your brain, desperately needs estrogen. You have estrogen receptors on part of the brain that syncs all of your organs together.

When your brain is low in estrogen, your organs and systems don't work properly, and equally importantly, they don't work properly together.

Low estrogen and damaged estrogen receptors are the next pieces of the PCOS puzzle. This estrogen shortage leads to a cascade of systemic problems throughout your body.

Estrogen is awesome, when you have it

Estrogen is the first and oldest hormone on Earth. It evolved in early invertebrates approximately 500 million years ago. For reference, Tyrannosaurus rex was stomping around about 65 million years ago. T-rex definitely had estrogen. 500 million years ago, Earth was in the Cambrian period. The only multicellular lifeforms were bizarre, ancient sea creatures, and they were the first animals that evolved to have estrogen.

Ancient estrogen likely existed in similar amounts in males and females. It regulated metabolic functions and cued sexual maturation for both male and female creatures. It was only about 50 million years ago that androgens evolved, and estrogen became a female-dominant hormone while androgens became male-dominant hormones. But in all vertebrates, estrogen has remained critical to metabolic health.

In the female human body today, estrogen is the master hormone, overseeing all metabolic, immunological, cognitive, gastrointestinal, cardiovascular, pulmonary, dermal, and urological functions. Reproduction is just one small piece. There's a receptor for estrogen in virtually every cell of the body.

Here are just a few of the amazing things that estrogen does.

Not surprisingly, the ovaries have estrogen receptors and estrogen plays a critical role in egg maturation and ovulation.[6]

The cells in the pancreas that produce insulin also have estrogen receptors. Without estrogen, these cells cannot respond properly to blood sugar levels and produce the correct amount of insulin.[7]

The liver has estrogen receptors and they are part of the pathway that communicates whether the liver should store or release fats and sugars into the bloodstream. This process is a critical step in the fat-storing to fat-burning transition.[8]

Your intestines have estrogen receptors. Estrogen is critical to maintaining the health and integrity of the intestinal lining, and it protects against inflammatory bowel disease and colon cancer.[9]

Estrogen modulates inflammation. Every immune cell in the body has an estrogen receptor, and estrogen regulates the production of inflammatory cytokines (sy-teh-KINES).[10] These molecules cause inflammation that protects the body from bacteria, viruses, and injuries. Estrogen also keeps this inflammation from getting out of control. So, without estrogen, you get get chronic, systemic inflammation.

There are estrogen receptors in your heart, lungs, and skin.[11,12]

And, as I mentioned, there are estrogen receptors in your brain that keep all of the systems in your body coordinated with each other by keeping your body's circadian rhythm in sync with the 24-hour day.

Your circadian rhythm is an umbrella term for all of the rhythms in your body that follow a 24-hour cycle. Obviously, this includes your sleep-wake cycle and your hungry-full cycle. But there are also daily rhythms to your immune system, your metabolism, your reproductive system, and your mood.

Circadian rhythm

The primary timekeeper in your body is a part of the hypothalamus (hy-poe-THAL-uh-muhs) in your brain called the suprachiasmatic nucleus, nicknamed the master clock. It has estrogen receptors, and without proper estrogen, the master clock drifts.

Your organs and other cells have clock genes known as peripheral clocks. Estrogen helps set them every day by syncing them to the master clock. Without proper estrogen, they also drift, becoming out-of-sync with the master clock, each other, and the 24-hour day.

Consequently, low estrogen causes circadian rhythm dysfunction. This is the next enormous piece of the PCOS puzzle.

You have circadian rhythm dysfunction and your ancestors did not.

Ancient women's lives were so connected to the rhythms of their environment — the cycling of days, nights, months, seasons, and years — that even with low estrogen and damaged estrogen receptors, their bodies stayed on the beat. Today, that connection is much weaker and it is easy to get out of sync.

When's the last time you stayed up past midnight, had late night munchies, or felt tired when you woke up in the morning? These are all common signs of circadian rhythm dysfunction.

Circadian rhythm dysfunction is terrible for women with PCOS. It exacerbates insulin resistance and contributes to diabetes, heart disease, cancer and mood disorders. It encourages weight gain, which in turn, further amplifies all of the conditions it's already caused. It increases androgens, which disrupts other hormonal systems, increases insulin resistance, and promotes even more acne, hirsutism, hair loss, and fertility problems. It triggers chronic inflammation and gut dysfunction.

All of these problems feed into each other in a downward spiral, until you end up with:

1. Inflammation
2. Hormonal dysregulation
3. Insulin resistance

And these lead to all of the serious symptoms of modern-day PCOS.

Circadian rhythm dysfunction is the special sauce that takes the normal, mild PCOS of our grandmothers and turns it into the monster condition it is today.

Gut dysbiosis and endocrine disruptors

The final pieces of the PCOS puzzle are gut dysbiosis (dis-by-OH-sis) and exposure to endocrine disruptors.

Gut dysbiosis

Your gut really is a second brain and the community of tiny microbes living in your intestines, your gut microbiome, do all of the thinking. You need the right bacteria in the right amounts to have a healthy gut microbiome.

Comprised of trillions of bacteria, your gut microbiome does more than digest your food and make your poop. It produces hormones, influences circadian rhythm, and modulates inflammation.

When you have the wrong bacteria in your gut, what we call gut dysbiosis, they mess up your whole metabolism. They maximize your body's ability to extract calories from food and store those calories as fat. They release toxins into your blood that trigger even more inflammation. And they disrupt your hormonal rhythms and balance.

Diet is yet another difference between modern PCOS women and our PCOS ancestors.

Appropriately nicknamed SAD, the modern Standard American Diet leads to the modern standard American gut microbiome, which lacks diversity and certain critically beneficial bacteria and instead contains an overabundance of dangerous, pathogenic bacteria.

Gut dysbiosis is a modern condition that powerfully reinforces the underlying conditions of PCOS.

Endocrine disruptors

Endocrine disruptors are a specific type of toxic chemical found throughout our modern environment that disrupt normal hormonal functions. These chemicals look very similar to your actual hormones so they can lock into hormone receptors on your cells. But they are different enough that they don't unlock the cells' correct behaviors.

The most damaging ones for women with PCOS are estrogen mimickers. They are everywhere in our environment and you've probably heard of many of them — bisphenol A (BPA), phthalates, and dioxins are just a few. These endocrine disruptors are similar in structure to estrogen, so they fit into your estrogen receptors. But they don't trigger the same actions as real, human-made estrogen. Instead, they interrupt natural estrogen pathways and block proper estrogen responses.

In a woman with PCOS, this is devastating. You already have low levels of estrogen and damaged estrogen receptors. The last thing you need is fake estrogen messing things up even more.

Endocrine disruptors are found in processed food, personal care products, plastics, and cleaning products and they are another new factor in the development of modern PCOS. They further amplify the hormonal dysregulation that PCOS already causes.

Long story short

PCOS starts with an impaired ability to aromatize testosterone into estrogen. This leads to chronically low estrogen and elevated testosterone.

A high testosterone level damages estrogen receptors throughout your body, which causes your cells to send a message to your brain that they need more estrogen. The brain relays this message back to the ovaries, which pump out more testosterone. High testosterone, which we call hyperandrogenism, causes acne, hirsutism, and alopecia.

At the same time, every organ system in your body is a little short on estrogen so they aren't functioning optimally.

In particular, the master clock in your brain can't keep your circadian beat in sync throughout your body. So your whole body drifts out of sync with the 24-hour day.

You are set up for circadian rhythm dysfunction by your low estrogen, but what really pushes you over the edge is a modern, first-world lifestyle that isolates you from the rhythms of the natural world.

A disrupted gut microbiome and exposure to endocrine disruptors exacerbate hormonal imbalances, contribute to insulin resistance and inflammation, and generally increase the severity of PCOS.

Your body gets out of balance and off the beat, and this converts your PCOS from a mild condition into a really terrible condition.

This is how we as a society have taken what was once a natural female variant, full of evolutionary advantages, and turned it into a life-changing medical condition that negatively impacts your appearance, fertility, and long-term health.

The good news is that once we understand this, we can undo it.

CHAPTER 4

How do I heal?

*N*ow that we understand the PCOS puzzle, the trick is figuring out how to take it apart.

The first piece of the puzzle is aromatization. Today, we cannot fix aromatization. I wish we could convert the testosterone in your body into estrogen, but we can't.

Next, we have the damaged estrogen receptors. Today, we cannot physically fix estrogen receptors.

The next puzzle pieces are high testosterone and low estrogen.

We actually can lower testosterone with pharmaceuticals such as birth control pills and spironolactone, but these drugs come with side effects and neither can be used during pregnancy. Additionally, lowering testosterone doesn't raise estrogen, and most of the worst symptoms of PCOS stem from low estrogen. Lowering testosterone is an incomplete and imperfect solution at best.

Can I just take estrogen?

Examining this research, I always think, "Wait a minute. If all of this dysregulation is caused by low estrogen, why can't I just take estrogen?"

I deeply, truly believe that in the future, rhythmic, bioidentical estrogen therapy will be the key to reversing all of the symptoms of PCOS. But we desperately need studies to prove that it works and to evaluate dosing levels.

To have studies, we have to have funding. And right now, the funding isn't there. But I am working to change that!

I've got a whole section in the appendix (page 319) about research and studies that I'm excited about and other studies that I want to help fund.

But today, I can't prescribe estrogen for PCOS.

What about birth control?

Most people think that birth control pills are estrogen. They are not. They are estrogen- and progesterone-mimicking endocrine disruptors.

The primary estrogen in your body is estradiol. Birth control pills contain ethinylestradiol. Ethinylestradiol is very similar to estradiol, but it is different in a few key ways. Consequently, birth control pills and other "hormonal" contraception increase your risk of depression, suicide, high blood pressure, cardiovascular disease, and blood clotting — conditions that PCOS already raises your risk of. I don't like birth control pills for PCOS women because I don't believe it is safe to further magnify these risks.[1,2,3,4]

This book is not an anti-birth control pill manifesto, but I think that women with PCOS should think very carefully about using synthetic, hormone-mimicking chemicals.

Circadian rhythm is the key

Consequently, the best strategy I have found to heal PCOS is to reestablish a strong circadian rhythm. This is the first piece of the PCOS puzzle that we can effectively, safely treat with zero unwanted side effects.

A healthy circadian rhythm is amazingly effective at re-establishing whole-body health because when all of the cells and organs in your body work together, your entire body experiences a reduction in physiological stress. This sets off a cascade of healing.

When your circadian rhythm gets back on the beat, your insulin levels and your insulin resistance drop. Your inflammation levels drop. And this, in turn, reduces your risk of heart disease, diabetes, and cancer.

Improved circadian rhythm lowers cortisol levels and restores the cortisol rhythm. This improves depression and anxiety and counteracts sleep disorders. It allows your body to transition from fat-storing to fat-burning mode.

Improved insulin sensitivity, lower inflammation, and properly cycling cortisol also lead to weight-loss (sometimes a lot!) and a drop in testosterone, which improves your hyperandrogenic symptoms like acne, hirsutism, and hair loss.

And all of this combined improves your fertility.

When we get our bodies back on the beat, every symptom of PCOS improves.

A case study in circadian rhythm dysfunction

One of the best ways to understand the profound impact of circadian rhythm dysfunction is to study shift workers. These are people like doctors, nurses, and security guards who work at night and sleep during the day.

They almost universally develop what's now called shift work disorder, especially if they only work the night shift on a rotating basis. Workers who are only partially shifted and work late into the night or start early in the morning are also highly susceptible to shift work disorder.

Nurses have been particularly well-studied. Compared to their day shift-only peers, night and rotating shift nurses suffer from more:

- Sleep disorders, including insomnia, daytime fatigue, and mental fog
- Mood disorders, particularly depression and anxiety
- Weight gain and obesity
- Cancer
- High blood pressure and heart disease
- Autoimmune disease, particularly Hashimoto's hypothyroidism
- Diabetes
- Early death from all causes[5,6]

Recent studies from Harvard University have also linked shift work to a range of fertility issues, including irregular menstruation, reduced egg quality, and higher rates of miscarriage.[7]

If you look at this list, you'll see that it's basically identical to the list of health conditions that women with PCOS suffer from, minus the hyperandrogenism.

This is because low estrogen initiates a feedback loop that directly causes circadian rhythm dysfunction. PCOS circadian rhythm dysfunction looks, from a health risk point of view, exactly like the circadian rhythm dysfunction of a shift worker.

Circadian rhythm is *that* powerful.

Can you feel the rhythm?

The evolution of circadian rhythm is an amazing, romantic story. All life forms on Earth have evolved for survival. And, not surprisingly, survival on Earth means working in harmony with the planet's 24-hour rotation on its axis. Every living creature is wedded to the Earth, and we are all dancing together to this beat that we call the circadian rhythm.

Certain lifeforms evolved to be active during the daytime and some are active at night. When they are not active, all lifeforms are resting, rejuvenating, and repairing. Humans are no different. Think of humans as two different creatures, a day creature and a night creature.

During the day, we can see, we can move, we can hunt and farm and build. We are hungry for food and our immune systems are primed for action in case we get a cut or an infection. Our bodies are optimized for energy — for consumption of energy and production of energy. That's your daytime metabolism.

At night, our bodies repair themselves. Our whole metabolism changes; it slows way down. Our temperature drops. Our heart rate and breathing slow. Our digestion slows. All of this happens so that damaged cells can break down and reform themselves. While we sleep, we build neural pathways. Our liver detoxifies our blood. Our immune system replenishes. Our body heals, on a cellular level, from the work of the day.

Everything about us is different. And so we are supposed to behave differently. Our bodies expect us to stop moving, to stop eating. Our bodies need us to retreat into darkness and sleep.

When we talk about circadian rhythm, we are talking about this day-night, wake-sleep beat. And we are also talking about all of the cycles and rhythms that occur within our bodies to support this 24-hour cycle. Every organ in your body, from your brain to your stomach to your liver, has a 24-hour rhythm. These rhythms change from day to night. But not just that; they change by the hour, bit by bit, throughout the day and night. Your hormones are all timed. They rise and fall in an intricate, 24-hour dance. Your metabolic processes and your immune system ramp up and down throughout the day. Nothing in your body is stable.

These rhythms are immutable. They are programmed in your genes, and these genes regulate how proteins are produced and how your cells actually work.

Human circadian rhythms evolved over many, many millenium. But today, we do not live in sync with the 24-hour day. We don't wake up to the sunrise and turn in at sunset; we don't hunt and gather food during the day and rest at night. And because we are not in sync with our environment, our organs and our metabolic processes are not in sync with each other. Our world has changed but our genes have not.

As a result, we get sick. For all people, circadian rhythm is the foundation for good health. Circadian rhythm dysfunction, living off the beat of the natural 24-hour day, causes many surprisingly serious medical problems. Obviously, it causes sleep disturbances. But it also causes weight gain. And depression and anxiety. It causes irritable bowel syndrome (because your digestive tract needs to be in sync). It causes heart disease and diabetes. And it causes a significant increase in your risk of autoimmune disease and cancer.[8,9,10]

For us PCOS women, the consequences are magnified because low estrogen makes our circadian rhythms more fragile.

It's almost unbelievable that the way you time and shape your day can have such a profound impact on your overall health.

But it is believable once you realize that circadian dysfunction causes hormonal dysregulation. Your hormones, the messengers in your body, get out of sync with each other. This, in turn, causes your organs to get out of sync with each other, and this causes systemic stress because each organ needs to work a little harder to do its job. Stress causes inflammation, and inflammation causes insulin resistance. Over time, chronic dysregulation throughout your body causes chronic diseases like diabetes, heart disease, and cancer.

I know it can sound far-fetched. Does your pancreas really need to know what time it is?! And if it's so important (which it is), why can't your pancreas just get its act together? Why is something that should be natural now broken?

Let's be serious, our ancestors didn't need to worry about whether or not their organs were keeping good time. That's because our ancestors were so totally controlled by their environments in a way that we no longer are. They couldn't get out of sync because they couldn't create limitless light and warmth. They didn't have pantries full of instantly available food. They didn't have entertainment available around the clock. So they went to bed when it got dark. They woke up when it got light. They worked during the day, often getting lots of exercise, and then they slept at night. They ate meals made from whole foods because that's all there was. They couldn't just unwrap a granola bar at the first pang of hunger.

And this rhythm, this timing for everything, kept their bodies in sync.

There were lots of things that our ancient ancestors died from. But, for the most part, they didn't die of heart attacks. Type 2 diabetes was rare. Cancers were rare. These are modern diseases created by our modern lifestyles. And circadian disruption is the key.

Our health depends on the 24-hour circadian rhythm. It's time we learned that we, like our ancestors, and like every other creature on Earth, have to live with our beat, with our inherent rhythms.

A path forward

So, what do we do?

No one can cure your PCOS because it isn't a disease. It is a natural female genetic variant. Under natural conditions, it is actually an advantage. But in our unnatural, modern society, your PCOS makes you highly vulnerable to a whole slew of terrible side effects that are triggered by circadian rhythm dysfunction coupled with a poor diet and exposure to endocrine disruptors.

The goal is to wind back the clock and to return your PCOS to its more natural, mild form — the form that made your grandmothers strong and powerful.

We do this by getting back in touch with the rhythms of the natural world. By reconnecting with the turn of the earth and the rise and set of the sun. By eating clean, natural food and by using clean, natural products.

We do this by living a smart, vibrant, human life.

The seven steps of my protocol will help you.

Steps one through three show you how to restore your circadian rhythm.

Steps four and five help you nurture a healthy gut microbiome.

Step six helps you find and eliminate endocrine disruptors.

Step seven provides resources so you can customize your personal wellness plan to meet your needs and better treat your most frustrating and hard-to-heal symptoms.

Healthy PCOS living

We cannot cure PCOS, but we can bring it under control and return it to its ancient, mild form.

We can strengthen your circadian rhythm and get you back on your natural, 24-hour beat.

We can heal your gut.

We can balance your hormones.

We can minimize your acne and the masculinizing symptoms of hyperandrogenism.

We can assuage your depression and anxiety.

We can improve your metabolism and achieve a healthier weight.

We can restore your digestive health.

We can reduce your risk of cancer and chronic disease.

And, whether this is critically important to you or not, we can increase your fertility.

We probably cannot perfectly treat every PCOS symptom because even mild, ancient PCOS had some symptoms. But health isn't about being perfect in every way. Neither is life.

What we can do is heal. We can nurture a body that is healthy, strong, vibrant, and fertile.

And it begins with light. Just as each new day begins with the light of the rising sun, so does your journey to optimal health.

PART TWO

What you need to do

CHAPTER 5

STEP 1:
Step into the light

Our ancestors stayed in sync with the 24-hour day by watching the rise and set of the sun. On Earth, the sun is the primary timekeeper that distinguishes day and night. So it's not surprising that it is the primary timekeeper for our bodies as well.

One of the most influential inventions of modern times is the electric light. Access to artificial light creates a paradoxical environment where people habitually get less light intensity exposure throughout the day because they experience less bright sunlight than our ancestors did. And, they simultaneously get increased quantity of light exposure because they have access to electric lights long after sunset.[1]

Light-emitting devices like televisions, computers, cell phones and tablets exacerbate this problem. Off-rhythm light exposure results in both a weaker circadian rhythm and a delayed circadian rhythm that encourages late bedtimes and makes getting up in the morning tough.

Does this sound like you? It definitely describes me. I'm a total night owl (maybe that's why I always loved delivering babies in the middle of the night but my kids were always late to school in the morning).

You might be a night owl, too, since most women with PCOS have a delayed circadian rhythm.[2]

Fortunately, there are easy and enjoyable things we can do to realign our circadian rhythms with the sun and the moon. All of the tips in this chapter will make you feel good, both while you are doing them and as they improve your overall health.

Hello, master clock

You are healthiest when you awaken with the growing brightness of the rising sun and fall asleep shortly after the sun goes down. The bright light of day and the darkness of night are environmental triggers that directly set your circadian rhythm.

They do this by setting your master clock.

Your master clock is a part of your brain located in the hypothalamus. It sits directly on top of the optic nerve, which is the nerve that travels from your eye to your brain.

The master clock has one job. It senses light and dark and transmits that information throughout the body. There are special receptors in the retina of your eyes that detect light and send out a signal that goes just to the master clock. The master clock establishes the body's primary circadian rhythm and uses hormones, along with neural and systemic signals, to broadcast that rhythm to every cell, organ, and system in the body. They, in turn, set each of their own peripheral clocks to this master signal.

Now, weirdly enough, the natural circadian rhythm of a human being is approximately, but not exactly, 24 hours. When scientists study people who are isolated from external time cues like daylight, people naturally fall into a daily rhythm that spans somewhere between 23.5 hours and 24.5 hours. Because of this, without external cues like the sun, your master clock will drift and slowly become out of sync with the Earth's day.[3]

So, every single day, your master clock must be entrained (that's the medical term, entrained) to the 24-hour day. You do this by seeing the bright sun in the morning.

Morning sun is a powerful timekeeping cue. It literally wakes up your body, entrains your master clock to the Earth's clock, and syncs up your body's rapid transition from nighttime metabolic processes to daytime metabolic processes.

Throughout the day, your master clock monitors the changing light levels. In the afternoon, as the sun tracks lower in the sky, the level of light dramatically decreases and the color of the light warms from blues to yellows. This triggers a new set of cues to your master clock that night is coming, and your body begins to synchronously prepare for another cycle of sleep.

So, one obvious way we can disrupt our circadian rhythms is by changing the times, intensities, and colors of our light exposure. When we spend our mornings indoors and don't get our dose of bright, blue-hued, morning sunshine, our master clock doesn't get a strong entrainment signal. When we stay up late in our well-lit homes watching TV or working on our computers, our master clock misses the afternoon dim light cue, and our bodies don't properly wind down from the day and prepare for sleep.

If you have PCOS, your estrogen levels are low and your estrogen receptors don't work properly, so your master clock is harder to entrain and more likely to drift. That's why we PCOS women usually stay up late, wake up tired, and aren't hungry for breakfast but get famished later in the day. Our master clocks are chronically behind the beat of the 24-hour day.

Hello, peripheral clocks

Approximately one-third of all the genes in the human body are clock genes and there are hundreds, maybe thousands, of documented circadian rhythms. Pretty much every cell in your body has its own clock.

This is why living off-beat affects more than just big daily rhythm things like hunger and sleep. It affects the metabolism of every cell in your body.

We call these cellular genes peripheral clocks and most of them set their time primarily off of the signals coming from the master clock. When everything works properly, these cells are beautifully coordinated, all moving to the same beat.

Take your digestive system, for example. In the morning, your stomach is ready for a big meal so the nerves become less sensitive, allowing your stomach to comfortably expand, encouraging you to eat more. In late afternoon, your stomach's nerves sensitize to stretching, which triggers your "I'm full" feeling with less food so you don't eat as much at night. In the morning, your cortisol levels are high to make you feel awake and hungry, and your insulin sensitivity is high so you can efficiently metabolize fats and sugars. This is all coordinated with your hunger hormones, ghrelin and leptin. Ghrelin triggers hunger and rises before anticipated meals. Leptin suppresses appetite and rises after meals to keep you full until the next mealtime. Your liver is a workhorse for digestion and detoxification. During the day, your liver actually increases in size as it produces proteins, digestive enzymes, and bile, and then it shrinks again at night.

At night, everything is quiet. Your stomach, liver, and pancreas are asleep and you should be, too. Then, when you wake up again in the morning, your intestines spring into action, digesting nutrients, moving waste along for your morning poop, and getting ready for the new day.

When this coordinated process becomes even a little unsynced, your health suffers. If you produce stomach acid on an empty stomach, you get heartburn. If your intestines move too fast, you get diarrhea, and if they move too slowly, you get constipation. If your liver is poorly timed, you get fatty liver disease, high blood sugar, and insulin resistance. And if your hunger and satiety hormones aren't coordinated, you overeat and gain weight.[4]

All of this dysfunction happens when you disrupt your circadian rhythm. And similar dysfunctions happen in every single organ and system in your body.

This is why a silly thing like staying up too late can make you sick. And conversely, it's why simple changes like eating breakfast by a sunny window can make you healthy.

A path forward

The solution is to go on a light diet where you control the brightness, color, and timing of the light you see. The goal is to experience a strong daily light rhythm that mimics as much as possible what is going on with the light outside, and ideally what the light does on a nice, bright day.

You can entrain your master clock and get your body on the Earth's clock.

Low estrogen means your master clock doesn't entrain as easily as it should, so you need an extra strong signal. Bright needs to be bright. Dark needs to be dark. And you need to get this signal every day, at the same time every day, or as close to that as you can.

"Watch" the sunrise

One of the most powerful ways to start your day is with the sunrise. When researchers expose people to the growing lights and colors of the sunrise, they see a 50% drop in mood disorders, an increase in morning alertness, and a phase advance of circadian rhythm. This means that people have fewer depression and anxiety symptoms. In the evening, they are able to fall asleep earlier, and they generally sleep better and longer. They feel good when they wake up in the morning.[5,6,7,8,9]

Now, if you're not a morning person (and most women with PCOS are not), here is some incredible news. You don't actually need to "watch" the sunrise.

When researchers perform these studies, they expose subjects to a dawn simulator, a light that mimics sunrise, during the 30 minutes before they wake up. Subjects experience the dawn simulator while they are still asleep. This is because our bodies are supposed to experience the sunrise through still-closed, still-sleeping eyelids.

As an added bonus, waking up gradually this way protects against morning cardiovascular events. Most heart attacks happen in the morning, and morning heart attacks are generally the most severe. So experiencing dawn could both set your circadian rhythm and save your life.[10,11]

Here are a few products to help you experience dawn.

Dawn simulator

Since real dawn doesn't always happen at a convenient time, I prefer a dawn simulator. This is an alarm clock-type device that will simulate sunrise for 30 minutes, starting at whatever time you choose.

Purchase one that produces a nice, diffuse, bright light as it simulates dawn. I love my Philips Wake-up Light and keep it on my night table.

Smart light bulbs

Install smart bulbs in your bedroom and program them to simulate dawn in the morning. As a bonus, you can dim them in the evening, which is a recommendation I'll cover in a little bit.

Philips Hue bulbs are the industry leaders in programmable, full spectrum light bulbs. They sell a smart bulb starter kit so you can try them out before you replace every bulb in your house.

Automatic window blinds

Install automatic window blinds in your bedroom and program them to open in the morning so you can experience the actual dawn and close them in the evening so your room is super dark at night.

Get morning light

Once you are up, you need 20 to 30 minutes of sunshine at the start of your day. You need to get a strong dose of bright morning light, the sooner the better.

So, open the shutters as soon as you wake up. Eat breakfast in a bright, sunny spot.

Going outside is best because even on a cloudy day, it's usually brighter outside than inside. So walk your dog, walk your kids to school, or just take a walk. Do a little morning gardening. But however you do it, get some sunshine. And, this is important, do not wear sunglasses.

Remember that your master clock needs to see the light for it to work, so you need that sunshine to go into your eyes. Don't look at the sun. That's dangerous. But for 20 to 30 minutes every morning, be in sunshine.

Bright morning light creates a strong circadian rhythm synchronization, so we see hormonal levels across the board start doing what they are supposed to do when they are supposed to do it.

One of the first things we see when people get bright light in the morning is that their morning melatonin (sleepy hormone) levels go down and their cortisol (wakeful hormone) levels go up. This makes it easier to wake up and start your day. And, this is exactly how your body is supposed to start your day, hormonally speaking.[12]

Morning light increases insulin sensitivity. Remember, insulin resistance is a major cause of weight gain and metabolic dysfunction, so improved insulin sensitivity is great. It allows people who get bright morning light to lose weight.[13]

Researchers at Northwestern University recently tracked 54 adults' exposure to morning light. They found that people who got bright light earlier in the morning had lower body mass indexes. This trend was strong even after they accounted for how many calories people consumed and how much they exercised, and it held for people of all ages and genders. Bright morning light, as close to your wake up time as possible, equals a healthier metabolism and a healthier weight, even if you make zero changes to your diet and exercise routine.[14]

Most or all mood disorders have a circadian rhythm component because our mood is strongly influenced by hormonal cycles. In head-to-head studies, people getting morning light therapy report more improvements in depression and anxiety symptoms than people taking antidepressants. For people who need medication, studies show that antidepressants work far better in conjunction with light therapy than they do on their own.[15]

This is profound because 60% of women with PCOS have at least one mood disorder, and we are four times as likely as non-PCOS women to suffer from anxiety or depression.[16,17]

One more benefit of morning light: sleep. Bright morning light corresponds to a forward shift in circadian rhythm by as much as an hour or more, and people who get bright morning sunshine report fewer sleep disturbances. At the end of the day, you will fall asleep faster and sleep better.[18,19]

Remember when I said circadian rhythm was powerful?

Getting morning sun is one of the healthiest daily habits you can adopt. Make it a priority to set your circadian rhythm every single day. For the price of 30 minutes of morning sun, you will feel better all day long and you will enjoy better health, pretty much across the board.

Get some midday sun, too

Sometime around lunch, you need another dose of light. Get out in the sun — no sunglasses, no sunscreen, with as much skin showing as the weather and propriety allow.

Now, exposure to sunshine is a balancing act. We all know that too much sunshine causes sunburns, wrinkles, and skin cancer. But the right amount of sunshine is excellent for your health.

One reason is that daytime light exposure leads to stronger circadian rhythms, more nighttime melatonin production, and better immune system function.[20]

Daytime sunshine helps your body produce vitamin D, the so-called "sunshine vitamin." Most cells and tissues in your body have vitamin D receptors, so it isn't all that surprising that vitamin D deficiency is an independent risk factor for death from all causes, including cancer, heart disease, depression, autoimmune disease, and even falls and fractures.[21]

We PCOS women need our vitamin D because 85% of us are vitamin D deficient. Getting some sunshine exposure on our skin everyday is critical.[22]

You should be taking 2000 mg of vitamin D every day. And even with that, you should still get sunshine on the days you can because it's more than just vitamin D.

Sunshine causes skin to release nitric oxide, a hugely beneficial signaling molecule that decreases blood pressure and improves the flexibility of your blood vessels. Women with PCOS have lower levels of nitric oxide, so this extra dose from the sun helps protect you against heart disease and stroke, which PCOS increases your risk of.[23,24,25]

On top of all that, sunshine reduces systemic inflammation, protecting you from autoimmune diseases and diabetes, which you are also at risk of.

The right amount of sunshine at the right time of day is fabulous for your health.

So, how much is the right amount? Well, it depends on your skin tone, where you live, the time of year, and even your age. That's a lot of factors!

Here's a rule of thumb: Get as much as you can without getting even a little bit pink.

In the summer, I recommend that people go outside for 10 to 20 minutes around 11AM or 3PM to avoid the brightest part of the day. But in the winter, aim for the sunniest time and go for as long as you can, up to two hours. If your skin is darker, you'll need more sun and if your skin is extremely fair, you'll need less. Additionally, you lose 30% of your ability to make vitamin D from sunshine as you age, so older people need more time in the sun to get the same results as younger people.[26,27]

Go catch some rays, but not too many!

Use a light therapy lamp

If you don't have access to year-round sunshine, you may want to get a light therapy lamp, also called a light box. They were originally developed to treat Seasonal Affective Disorder (SAD), which is winter-time depression, and they are highly effective. That's because, as its name implies, seasonal affective disorder is a circadian rhythm disorder caused by lack of exposure to sunshine during the darker, colder months of winter. Well, we now know that all forms of depression are at least in part a circadian rhythm dysfunction, and they all respond to a light therapy lamp.

If you can't get your daily dose of bright morning light from the sun every day, then you should get it from a light therapy lamp.

The standard dosage is 10,000 lux for 30 minutes.

Buy a lamp that can actually emit 10,000 lux. A lot of lamps produce less light, so you'd need to use them for longer every day. And who has time for that?

Sit by your 10,000 lux lamp for 30 minutes every morning as near to when you wake up as possible. When you use your lamp, position it about two feet from where you are sitting. You want it to be slightly above your head and off to the side a bit, aimed down towards your eyes. Make sure you use it every day because consistency is important.

Watch the sunset

Just as the colors of dawn get you going in the morning, the colors of the sunset wind you down in the evening. So, watch the sunset. Isn't that amazing? The warm colors of the sunset — the oranges, the reds, and the yellows — program our brain to prepare for evening and sleep.

Receptors in our eyes are highly sensitive to the color of light. When they are exposed to daytime light, which we see as blue light, these receptors convey that information to the master clock, which blocks the production of melatonin. But in the evening, when the intensity of the blues decreases and the color of the light warms, the receptors in our eyes cue our body to start producing melatonin again.

This initiates dim light melatonin onset, a critical part of the evening when your body begins producing melatonin and transitioning from daytime metabolism to nighttime metabolism.

If you miss your dim light melatonin onset, your entire sleep cycle gets delayed. Sunset is the best way to trigger this key phase of your circadian rhythm.

So, take a little time out of your day to enjoy one of Mother Nature's daily miracles, the beauty of the sunset.

Limit evening light

As evening advances and the light outside dims, the light inside needs to do the same. Now, this is really, really hard. Our homes are like perpetual daytime bubbles. They never get dark. And they need to.

Remember, light stops your body from producing melatonin. This is a great tool in the morning to get you up. But it is terrible in the evening when our bodies need to produce melatonin so we can fall asleep.

Under natural lighting conditions, your body begins producing melatonin around sunset. The amount of melatonin in your bloodstream slowly increases, reaching its peak at 2AM. Then, melatonin levels slowly fall as your body transitions to morning.

To get the recommended eight hours of sleep each night, we should all go to bed between 10PM and 11PM and wake up between 6AM and 7AM. If you wake up earlier, then go to bed earlier. But this is the rough schedule that most people find comfortable.

According to this sleep and wake schedule, you should start transitioning to dim light mode between 6PM and 8PM.

How can we possibly do that?

Table lamps

As the sun goes down, turn off bright, overhead lights and use only dimmer, warm-toned area lamps. Outfit these lamps with light bulbs that emit fewer than 1000 lumens, and then make sure they go under a lampshade, which further decreases their lumenocity.

Check your bulbs' Kelvin rating, which indicates the color temperature of your lights. Higher numbers, for example 5000 Kelvins, are daylight blue. For evening lamps, choose bulbs with lower Kelvin ratings, around 2700 or less. Sometimes called "soft white" or "warm white," these bulbs emit light on the warmer end of the color spectrum.

Dimmable lights

For areas where table lamps don't work, use dimmable lights. These can be controlled with a dimmer switch. If your lights aren't wired to a dimmable switch, you can install a wireless dimmer. Or swap your regular light bulbs for smart bulbs like Philips Hue that you can program to dim at a set time.

Night shift for screens

Light-emitting electronic devices like computers, tablets, and cellphones emit blue light, which suppresses melatonin and keeps you feeling awake long into the evening. However, many have a built-in night shift function. Turn it on. In the evening, your devices will automatically dim their screens and color shift to warmer tones.[28]

Screens off

And then, two hours before bedtime, turn your screens off. I know, I know! I love to watch CSI at night, too! It's painful. But your screens are ruining your sleep, even if you don't know it. And it's not just because they emit blue light and inhibit melatonin. They are also highly stimulating and wake your brain up. Screens are so stimulating that they draw our attention, even when they are off. So, if you sleep with screens in your bedroom, whether it's a TV on the wall or a cellphone on your night table, it will disrupt your sleep even if you don't use it. So, turn them off, and don't take them to bed.[29,30]

Amber glasses

If you just have to use your screens at night, get amber-tinted glasses to filter out the blue light. They are by far the cheapest and simplest solution for protecting yourself from blue light in the evening.

In a recent study, night owls who wore amber glasses in the evening were able to fall asleep more than two hours earlier than their habitual bedtimes.[31,32]

You can wear amber glasses anywhere, even when you are out and about. And, you can actually find a few that are reasonably stylish, although, sadly, most were not made with fashion in mind.

Sleep in the dark

When you go to bed, you need to sleep in a very dark room. Most people's rooms are not dark enough. Even a little bit of light coming through your eyelids while you sleep suppresses melatonin and disrupts your sleep quality. And that impacts your metabolism. It sounds crazy, but night time light exposure during sleep dramatically increases insulin resistance. So we all need to figure out how to make our sleeping environments as dark as possible.[33,34]

Blackout curtains

Install blackout curtains or blinds to block light from outside. These come in a lot of different styles and price points. Even the cheap paper blackout blinds work well. The key is preventing light from seeping in around the edges of your window treatments.

Sneaky light sources

Find all of the sources of light in your bedroom and turn them off. That includes the light on the power strip, the light on the charger, and the little blinky light by the dresser. If you can't turn them off, cover them with electrical tape.

Red light

If you need an alarm clock with glowing numbers (are you sure you need it?), get one with red numbers. Red light doesn't inhibit melatonin the way that blue, green, and white lights do. So if you need light at night, go for red.[35]

This holds true for night lights, too. If your kids need a night light or if you do (15% of adults are afraid of the dark, so you're in good company if that's you), then choose the dimmest red night light you can find.[36]

Sleep mask

I love sleeping with a sleep mask. Sleep masks are cheap, extremely effective at blocking light, and they travel. They come in a lot of different styles, so I'm sure you can find one that will work for you.

I tried and tried, but I simply could not get my bedroom dark enough. Also, I travel a lot and I can't always get hotel rooms dark enough either. A sleep mask works great for me.

The only downside of a sleep mask is that it blocks out the light of a dawn simulator so you have to pick one or the other. For me, since I live in a very sunny place, it's easier to get bright light during the day and harder to get darkness at night. So, I usually choose the sleep mask.

Go camping!

If your circadian rhythm is really messed up, you should go camping. In a tent. Out in nature where it gets really dark at night and you can do something fun outside during the day. Camping in an RV with electrical lights next to a 24-hour diner doesn't count.

Researchers at the University of Colorado Boulder have found that camping in a tent with a campfire as the only source of evening light will reset your circadian rhythm in just one weekend. The more of a night owl you are, the more effective it is.

When people go camping and they spend their days out hiking or playing in nature and their nights sleeping in a tent, they are exposed to at least four times more daylight during the day than they normally are, especially during those critical morning hours when the master clock is entrained. Also, not surprisingly, campers are exposed to exponentially less light after sunset.

Most people who go camping advance their circadian rhythms by about two hours. They go to bed earlier, shortly after sunset, and wake up earlier, shortly after sunrise. Additionally, their melatonin levels sync with what we call solar night, the time when the sun is down. Melatonin levels begin to rise at sunset and peak in the middle of solar night. But the most interesting thing is what happens to melatonin in the morning.

Melatonin offset is the time in the morning when your body stops making melatonin. For most of us living in the modern world, melatonin offset happens after we wake up. This is why we feel groggy in the morning and need to hit snooze on our alarm clocks. Our bodies are still in sleep mode even though the clock says, "Time to get up!"

Well, when you go camping, melatonin offset shifts forward and occurs almost one hour before you wake up. This pairs with a morning increase in cortisol, your wake-up-and-eat-breakfast hormone. So, even though you've been sleeping in a tent, you wake up feeling awake. It's incredible. Imagine actually wanting to get up in the morning.[37,38]

If camping is something you already do, keep it up. But if you are like me and you are more of a sleeps-in-beds type of person, then check out "glamping." Glamorous + camping = glamping, and it's wonderful. You can get most of the comforts of a hotel and most of the benefits of camping, so long as you find a location that limits your exposure to light. And the internet is full of places to go glamping.

The real trick is to use camping (or glamping) to reset your circadian rhythm and then keep it that way after you get home. You'll need a great light diet of daytime sun, evening dim light, and nighttime darkness to keep your healthy, new circadian rhythm on the beat.

And you might just need to go camping every so often. Or glamping.

Troubleshooting

If you go on a light diet and you don't get the improvements you are hoping for, there may be a few things working against you. Here are some challenges you might encounter and what to do about them.

I wake up earlier than I want to.

Most women with PCOS have Delayed Sleep Phase Syndrome (DSPS). This is when your circadian rhythm is shifted later and you are a night owl. But a minority of women have Advanced Sleep Phase Syndrome (ASPS). These reluctant early birds wake up early, before 6AM, and simply can't fall back asleep, even though they are still tired.

If you think you have ASPS, you should do everything mentioned above and you need to add one more thing: In the evening, you need another dose of bright light to push back your melatonin onset time.

Now, here's the thing about evening light treatments. Unlike morning light, which is pretty impossible to overdose on, evening light therapy is very dose and time dependent. I recommend that you work with a trusted sleep medicine specialist and use a light therapy lamp so you can control your dose.

You should start your evening light therapy around 7PM. Start with five to ten minutes at 10,000 lux, or longer if you have a weaker lamp. Go to bed at the same time as usual and see what time you wake up. Do this every day for a few days and then assess.

If you want to sleep longer, add another five minutes of light. Keep adding light in five minute increments until you are waking up at a time that works for you. Depending on when you are currently going to bed and when you'd like to go to bed, you may be able to push back your bedtime. But if you get to a point where you are having trouble falling asleep, back off on the amount of evening light you are getting.

My job requires shift work.

If you work off-hours or you take rotating nights, my best advice is to do this for as few years as possible. It just isn't good for you. But while you are doing it, you need to do everything within your power to keep your clocks synced with each other, even though they are not synced to the sun.

In terms of light, this means artificially creating your day and night light conditions. Be as consistent as you can. If you work nights during the week, don't shift back to a day schedule on the weekend. If you take a night shift here or there, treat it like travel. In the next chapter, I talk about how to use melatonin to adapt to new timezones (page 112). You can use the same strategy for your shifted schedule days.

And then make sure you rigidly adhere to timed schedules for sleeping and eating, and you carefully nurture your gut microbiome. You'll learn all about sleeping in step two of my protocol. Timed eating is step three. And I'll show you how to care for your gut microbiome in steps four and five. These chapters are important for all PCOS women, but they are critically important for PCOS women who work a shifted schedule.

We can't totally offset the health risks of shift work, but for many people shift work is their reality. If this is you, please take all of the advice in this book to heart. This won't make things perfect for you, but these strategies will keep you healthier than you otherwise would be.

I take birth control pills.

There is evidence oral contraceptives change the way a woman responds to light. A study published in 2017 found that women on birth control pills don't benefit from light therapy the way that women who are not taking hormonal contraceptives do.[39]

By the way, I say "hormonal contraceptives" because that is what they are commonly called. But please remember that these pharmaceuticals do not contain any hormones. They contain endocrine disruptors that work by disrupting normal hormonal pathways.

We know that chemical contraceptives disrupt normal estrogen production and function and that estrogen is essential for proper circadian rhythm function. More studies need to be done to understand how contraceptives influence a woman's ability to properly respond to environmental light cues.

In the meantime, if you are taking oral contraceptives or are using another form of "hormonal" birth control and you are not responding to light therapy, your birth control might be the culprit.

A quick summary

In the modern world, we spend significant parts of our days surrounded by artificial light and isolated from the natural light of the outside world. Our master clock in our brain cannot stay entrained to the Earth's 24-hour day and all of the circadian rhythms in our body drift.

PCOS and low estrogen make us highly susceptible to drifting.

To get back on the beat, we need to experience natural lighting rhythms by getting strong, bright light during the day and retreating to darkness at night.

- Watch the sunrise.
- Get morning light.
- Get another good dose of light around midday.
- Watch the sunset.
- In the evening, dim your lights and cut out blue light, in particular.
- Sleep in a dark, dark room.
- Reset your circadian rhythm quickly by going camping.

Healthy habits to get you started

- [ ] Open all of the shades in your bedroom as soon as you wake up.

- [ ] Buy a dawn simulator.

- [ ] Find a sunny spot for breakfast.

- [ ] Buy a light therapy lamp.

- [ ] For every chair you sit in during the day, move it as close to a window or bright lamp as possible.

- [ ] Take phone calls outside.

- [ ] Go for a walk outside at lunch.

- [ ] Every evening, take five minutes to share the sunset with your family and friends.

- [ ] Outfit your main living spaces with dim light options.

- [ ] Set up the night shift function on all of your electronic screens.

- [ ] Buy amber glasses for late night work.

- [ ] In the evening, replace TV, computer, and cellphone entertainment with reading physical books and magazines.

☐ Hang blackout shades in your bedroom.

☐ Darken all light sources in your bedroom.

☐ Buy a sleep mask.

☐ Replace all of your normal night lights with red bulbs.

☐ Put a red night light in your bathroom so you don't need to turn on the main light for middle-of-the-night trips.

☐ Plan a camping (or glamping!) trip.

CHAPTER 6

STEP 2:
Get some sleep

*W*e spend one-third of our lives asleep.

We may think of sleep as down-time, hours of nothing but lying in bed. When all goes well, other than the odd dream, we don't remember sleeping, and it can feel like lost time.

But, during those hours when your consciousness winks off, your body and mind undergo essential physical changes. Your immune system regenerates. Your cells make critical repairs. Your wounds heal and your organs clear out waste products produced by the metabolic processes of the preceding day. While you sleep, your brain organizes and stores new information, strengthening neural connections to memories worth recalling and dissolving connections to information you don't need.

Sleep is one-third of our circadian rhythm and its primary purpose is rejuvenation. Good sleep facilitates thinking and learning, restores your body's resiliency, and is foundational to good health.

When you experience good sleep, you fall asleep within about 30 minutes of going to bed. If you wake up, it's only once per night and you are able to fall back asleep within twenty minutes. You snuggle up in a dark, cool room, and while you sleep, your temperature drops. Your breathing and heart rate slow. You naturally transition back and forth between dreaming REM (Rapid Eye Movement) sleep and deep, slow brainwave non-REM sleep. You breathe easily. Your body relaxes. In the morning, you wake up gently, feeling refreshed and ready to start your day.[1]

If this is how you normally sleep, congratulations. You get great sleep.

If this is not you, then you are like me and most women with PCOS. Sleep is hard.

PCOS, the great sleep thief

Women with PCOS are twice as likely as non-PCOS women to struggle with sleep disturbances, and 80% of us have accompanying daytime fatigue.[2,3]

Most women with PCOS have delayed sleep phase syndrome. Because of our low levels of estrogen, our whole sleep-wake cycle shifts later and we are night owls. We go to bed late, and we're not actually done sleeping when it's time to get up in the morning. We frequently feel groggy, to say the least.

But our sleep problems go beyond estrogen and our master clock.

Women with PCOS have abnormalities in a wide range of hormonal levels and rhythms. Two hormones, melatonin and cortisol, orchestrate our sleep-wake cycle. Not only are they delayed, they both act in surprising, unusual ways in PCOS women.

Melatonin regulates sleep. It rises at night to induce sleep and then drops in the morning when we wake up. It stays low throughout the day, and then begins to rise again around sunset to prepare for the next sleep cycle.

In our bodies, nothing does just one thing and melatonin is no exception. This "sleep hormone" is also a powerful antioxidant. At night when levels are high, melatonin aggressively scavenges your body for free radicals that would otherwise damage your cells' DNA. It protects your body from oxidative stress, a destructive process implicated in cancer, cardiovascular disease, neurological disease, and autoimmune disease.[4]

Women with PCOS are twice as likely as non-PCOS women to suffer from sleep disturbances, and we have abnormally high levels of oxidative stress. It would be natural to conclude that we have low levels of melatonin. But, here is the unbelievable thing. Around the clock, at all stages of the melatonin cycle, our levels of melatonin are higher than non-PCOS women. Somehow, our high melatonin levels are not giving us good sleep and are not protecting our cells from oxidative stress. At this point, no one knows for sure why, although one theory is that our melatonin receptors, like our estrogen receptors, are damaged and functioning suboptimally.[5,6,7,8]

Cortisol is the hormone that controls the wake portion of your sleep-wake cycle. Cortisol is supposed to be low at night so you can fall asleep and stay asleep. It slowly rises in the early morning to peak around the time you wake up. In addition to waking you up, this high morning cortisol stimulates your appetite for a big breakfast. After you eat and start going about your day, your cortisol level slowly drops until it hits its lowest point in the evening, and cortisol remains low as you move through your next sleep cycle.

That's what cortisol is supposed to do, but for us PCOS women, it doesn't work quite that smoothly. Throughout this cycle, our cortisol levels are abnormally elevated.[9]

Cortisol does double duty as a stress hormone, so high cortisol during the day makes you feel anxious and easily overwhelmed. It's an appetite stimulant, so high cortisol makes you abnormally hungry around the clock, which contributes to weight gain. And, not surprisingly, high cortisol at bedtime makes it hard to wind down and fall asleep.[10,11]

Melatonin and cortisol irregularities cause insomnia, which is loosely defined as trouble falling or staying asleep. In the general population, around 30% of people experience symptoms of insomnia at least once per month. Rates of insomnia for women with PCOS are anywhere from 4 to 10 times as high![12,13,14]

On top of that, women with PCOS are 30 times more likely to suffer from sleep apnea than women without PCOS. Sleep apnea, which is often but not always accompanied by snoring, occurs when a person temporarily stops breathing while asleep. When you stop breathing, you don't get enough oxygen and you wake up frequently. Everyone needs to breathe all night long, and waking up multiple times per night increases inflammation and contributes to heart disease.[15,16]

By the way, most people with sleep apnea don't know that they do this, especially if they don't snore.

Excess weight increases your risk, but even lean PCOS women have high rates of sleep apnea. This may relate to abnormal estrogen receptors within the sleep centers of the brain. Many women going through menopause, another low estrogen state, develop sleep apnea, and hormone replacement therapy dramatically lowers the risk.[17]

PCOS causes melatonin and cortisol irregularities that delay your sleep cycle and increase rates of insomnia and sleep apnea. Long story short: PCOS makes it hard for a girl to get a good night's sleep.

You really need sleep

What happens when you don't get enough sleep? Obviously, you feel crappy. You're tired and irritable. You don't think as well. Your reaction time goes down, which can make driving dangerous. And you get lovely, baggy, bloodshot eyes.

But it's more than that. Lack of high-quality sleep, especially when it's chronic over months and years, will make you sick. Eventually, really sick.

Sleep is critical and lack of sleep triggers a cascade of health events. This is what happens to your body when you don't get enough sleep.

Weight gain

The first thing lack of sleep does is make you gain weight. Why? Well, there are several weight gain pathways that all get triggered when you miss out on sleep.

First off, sleep deprivation causes you to release more insulin, leading to insulin resistance. Insulin resistance causes high blood sugar and the sugar in your blood gets stored in your fat cells, particularly as visceral fat in your belly. More fat in your fat cells equals weight gain. At the same time, your cortisol levels go up even higher. Cortisol causes you to store more fat, and it makes you hungry so you eat more. Simultaneously, your ghrelin levels go up. Ghrelin also triggers hunger, so now you're even hungrier. And your body becomes more leptin resistant. Leptin is your I-feel-full hormone. When you are leptin resistant, your body can't hear the I-feel-full signal, so you keep eating.[18]

Lack of sleep makes you eat more and store your calories as fat.

Diabetes

The same insulin resistance that causes weight gain increases your risk of developing type 2 diabetes. Every hour below seven hours of sleep per night increases your risk of diabetes, and people who sleep less than five hours per night double their risk of diabetes. Even periodic late nights are bad for you. In a recent study, just one night of sleep deprivation triggered the same degree of insulin resistance as six months on a high fat diet.[19,20]

Cardiovascular disease

Lack of sleep hurts your cardiovascular health. People who sleep less than six hours a night have higher blood pressure. They have stiffer arteries. They have higher cholesterol and triglyceride levels. And sadly, they are much more likely to have a heart attack or stroke.[21]

Mood disorders

Depression and anxiety lead to sleep disturbances. And lack of sleep causes depression and anxiety. The two virtually always go together in one way or another. As many as 80% of people who are depressed have insomnia. And people who have insomnia often develop depression.[22]

Cancer

A good night's sleep is critical to proper immune system functioning. It only take one night of reduced sleep to cause a 70% drop in our killer T cells, the immune cells that seek out and kill cancer cells. Sleep deprivation also causes systemic inflammation. And it is often accompanied by an overall drop in melatonin levels. Melatonin is such a powerful antioxidant that having too little is likely a cancer risk factor all on its own.

Consequently, people who sleep less have higher rates of all types of cancer and in many cases, their cancer is more aggressive. The link is so strong the the World Health Organization recently classified night shift work as a probable carcinogen.[23]

Autoimmune disease

Another frequent result of an impaired immune system plus chronic inflammation is autoimmune disease. People who are chronically sleep deprived are at much higher risk of developing virtually all types of autoimmune diseases, and they develop these diseases younger than the general population.[24]

Aging

Lack of sleep ages your body prematurely.

While you sleep, your skin repairs and regenerates, and sleep-induced high levels of melatonin combat oxidative stress. When you don't get enough sleep, your melatonin levels get suppressed and your skin can't rejuvenate. The result? Wrinkles.[25]

Chronic lack of sleep is also linked to premature hair loss, dry skin, and poor skin tone. Conversely, people who sleep well actually rate themselves as more attractive than people who sleep poorly.[26]

Beauty sleep is a real thing.

And what happens to your skin also happens to all of the organs inside your body, even your brain. Poor sleep in your middle-aged years prematurely ages your brain, dramatically increasing your risk of dementia later on.[27]

Death from all causes

So maybe it's not surprising that poor sleep increases your risk of dying, period. A recent study showed that self-identified night owls (like me!) are more likely to be generally sicker, and we have a 10% increased risk of dying overall compared to people with normally-timed circadian rhythms. This is true for men and women of all ages.[28]

A path forward

So, on that cheerful note, what do we do? We know that PCOS causes circadian rhythm dysfunction. PCOS and circadian rhythm dysfunction cause melatonin and cortisol dysfunction, and that causes sleep disruption. Sleep disruption cycles back to create more melatonin, cortisol, and circadian rhythm dysfunctions.

PCOS and chronic sleep deprivation share a similar chronic health risk profile — weight gain, mood disorders, metabolic syndrome, cancer, and autoimmune disease.

And there's your good news!

Yet again, we have linked all of the most serious symptoms of PCOS back to circadian rhythm.

Poor sleep is a critical component of circadian rhythm dysfunction, so if you can get the right amount of quality sleep, you can undo the cascade that triggers these terrible diseases.

You can lose weight (even without dieting!). You can lower your risk of heart disease, diabetes, cancer, and autoimmune disease. You can treat your depression and anxiety.

And science definitely says that you'll feel more beautiful.

All you need to do is get a good night's sleep!

Which, because you have PCOS, is much easier said than done.

Well, here's how you do it.

Go on a light diet

Did you read the last chapter? If you haven't gone on a light diet yet, you really should. It feels good, and it sets your circadian rhythm for the day and the night. Go do that, especially the bright morning light and dim evening light parts.

Schedule your sleep

Next, make it a priority to go to bed at the same time every night. In the grand scheme of the universe, there are very few times that the can't-wait, gotta-do-it-now thing we do late at night is actually more important than our health and happiness.

So go to bed, every single night, between 10PM and 11PM.

Set an alarm. Set your TV on a timer. Do what you need to do to make it happen.

My iPhone has a bedtime function that I've set to play a little melody at 10PM so I can (almost) always get to bed before 11PM.

And then wake up between 6AM and 7AM. This will help you hit the sweet spot of seven to eight hours of sleep per night. This is the amount of sleep that is associated with the best health. Any less (or any more) and you will see your risk of chronic disease rapidly rise.[29]

Avoid weekend social jet lag

Don't change your routine on the weekend.

We call this social jet lag. Everybody knows that if you fly across many time zones, you will get jet lag, which is just another name for circadian rhythm disruption. But we don't think about self-imposed jet lag. This where you stay up really late on the weekend and then sleep late to make up for it.

What you are really doing is trying to change your clock. It doesn't work that way. You can't reprogram your clock genes just for the weekend. They are embedded into us.

Weekend social jet lag doubles your risk of diabetes and metabolic syndrome, and it's particularly damaging for people younger than 60. So try to keep the same rhythm, even on the weekend.[30]

Practice good sleep hygiene

Millions of people have written about sleep hygiene, so I'm just going to touch on it briefly. You need to create the conditions that promote restorative sleep.

Start relaxing a good two hours before bed. Dim the lights. Stop doing things that make you anxious or get you riled up. Avoid screens two hours before bed. Definitely avoid the news.

Stop eating. We'll talk about this more in the next chapter, but your stomach and pancreas need their sleep, too. You can drink some calming herbal tea, just nothing with caffeine or calories.

And then, when you go to bed, go to sleep. Your bed should only be for sleeping and sex. If you want to read or watch TV (not before bed!), go do it somewhere else.

Sleep in a cool, extremely dark room. Get a bedside fan so you can cool off if you get hot. Use gentle white noise to block out environmental noises. I have the Rain, Rain white noise app on my phone, which lets me mix my own perfect white noise ("City Rain" plus "Cat Purring").

Make your bedroom a beautiful, comfortable place to sleep.

Take melatonin

Since you already have high levels of melatonin, it would seem counterproductive to take *more* melatonin. Science is funny that way.

We don't know for sure why women with PCOS don't respond appropriately to the melatonin they naturally produce, but there may be a problem with melatonin receptors. One piece of evidence is that although we have high levels of melatonin in our blood, we have abnormally low levels in our ovary follicles, where melatonin promotes healthy eggs. Clearly, our cells aren't using all of the melatonin we are making.[31]

The good news is that we PCOS women respond really well to melatonin supplements.

Bedtime melatonin helps pretty much everyone, including PCOS women, fall asleep faster, sleep longer, and sleep better. It's worth taking just for that.[32,33]

But the benefits for PCOS women extend beyond sleep. Melatonin supplements improve the health of our ovaries and increase our estrogen levels, and this improves everything related to PCOS, including our fertility. In a recent study, PCOS women who took 2 mg of melatonin at bedtime for six months menstruated more regularly, had improved egg quality, and experienced a marked reduction in testosterone levels.[34,35,36]

To get the best benefits, take melatonin twice per night — a tiny dose in the early evening and a slightly larger dose at bedtime.

Take a low dose about two hours before bedtime to trigger your body's transition into sleep mode. I recommend 0.5 mg at 8PM. I give my patients Pure Encapsulations Melatonin 0.5 mg. This low dose mimics your natural melatonin cycle. It's the safest, least habit-forming, and most effective way to give your melatonin cycle a little nudge to get things going.[37]

It will make you really tired around 10PM (assuming you don't counteract it with bright light from light bulbs and screens). Low-dose, pre-bedtime melatonin facilitates going to bed, falling asleep, and staying asleep.

Additionally, you should take another slightly larger dose at bedtime. I recommend 1 to 2 mg, and I like Douglas Laboratories Melatonin. The 1 mg tablets are chewable, so you can keep them by your bed and grab an extra for those nights when you need a little more help falling asleep.

Despite the exciting studies about melatonin, I do not recommend taking higher doses. Melatonin is a hormone and health benefits come from having the right amount. More is not better. In fact, too much melatonin, especially at the wrong time, will disrupt your melatonin cycle.

In the store, you'll see dosages up to 10 mg. This is a lot of melatonin. If you were to take that much at bedtime for several nights in a row, you would mess up your melatonin cycle. You might start waking up too early in the morning, or more likely, you would feel extremely sleepy at wake up time. You would run the risk of developing melatonin resistance where your melatonin receptors would stop responding to melatonin.

Additionally, the melatonin would flip from being a fertility aid to being a contraceptive. High doses of melatonin actually stop ovulation.[38]

Weird, huh? So stick with small, properly-timed doses.

I never thought I had sleep problems. Then, I took melatonin for the first time.

I woke up and thought, "Oh my goodness, I never knew sleep could feel that deep and luxurious."

I felt profoundly calm and energetic all at once. It was the most restorative sleep I'd ever had.

Even if you think you are sleeping fine, you should try melatonin. The biggest risk is that you could feel a little sleepy first thing when you wake up. Get a dose of sunshine to wash that away.

You might discover, as I did, that there is a whole universe of incredible sleep that you never dreamed of.

Relax

Once you get melatonin functioning properly, the next step is to tackle cortisol. You need some cortisol. You just need less of it, and you need it to follow its proper rhythm.

The best way to do this is to incorporate a wide variety of relaxation practices into your day. Each of these tips is a small, beautiful gift to yourself that will help you feel good, reduce stress, and sleep better.

Aromatherapy

At its most basic, aromatherapy is the use of fragrance to moderate emotion and improve health.

Your sense of smell is directly connected to the amygdala, a part of your brain that registers stress and triggers cortisol production. So, you can significantly lower your cortisol level through your sense of smell.[39,40]

Aromatherapy is so effective that it is popping up all over hospitals — in waiting rooms, surgical wards, and labor and delivery rooms — as a low-cost, low-risk strategy to help patients manage stress, fear, and pain.

And if you use it in your bedroom, it will lower your cortisol levels and improve your sleep.[41]

All you need are a diffuser and essential oils. The essential oils should be pure and highly concentrated; you'll only use a few drops at a time. I recommend Simplers Botanicals brand.

For relaxation, my favorite oils are lavender, sweet orange, and bergamot.

Do not substitute commercial air fresheners and scented candles. They contain artificial fragrances made in a laboratory, and they release all sorts of toxic chemicals into the air such as phthalates, benzene, and even lead. Besides, studies show that they don't work to reduce stress and cortisol. You need to get the real thing.[42,43]

Ashwagandha

Ashwagandha is one most effective supplements for lowering blood serum cortisol levels. In a recent study, people who took ashwagandha daily for 60 days experienced a 28% drop in cortisol. This corresponded to a 44% decrease in stress and a 70% reduction in anxiety and insomnia.[44]

I recommend that my patients take 1 capsule daily of the Pure Encapsulations Ashwagandha, 500 mg.

> Just a heads up that if you take ashwagandha frequently and you have thyroid issues, you should monitor your thyroid levels. Remember, nothing ever does just one thing. Ashwagandha can mildly stimulate your thyroid to produce more thyroid hormone, and in fact, it may be a future treatment for mild hypothyroidism.[45]

Hot bath

A warm bath before bed is incredible for sleep. This is true for men and women of all ages. In one study, when people took a one-hour bath at 90 degrees fahrenheit, their cortisol levels dropped by 34%. When people take a warm bath before bed, they fall asleep faster. They experience more slow-wave, deep sleep. And they wake in the morning feeling refreshed.[46,47]

Meditation

I love meditation. If you meditate consistently over time, your brain actually changes. The amygdala is the part of your brain that originates stress, anxiety, and fear and triggers the hypothalamus to produce more cortisol. Meditation causes the amygdala to physically shrink. Simultaneously, the parts of your brain involved in learning, memory, and emotional regulation get denser. These structural brain changes correlate exactly to how people feel — smarter, calmer, happier, and less stressed out.[48,49]

So I recommend meditation to everyone, but especially for people who have trouble sleeping because they can't turn off their minds. Just five minutes a day will give you wonderful benefits. If you don't know where to start, check out meditation apps. I love Headspace, but you should find what works for you.

Tea

I don't think I can explain how much I adore tea. I have a whole cabinet full of mugs, most of which are like soup bowls with handles. In the evenings, drink teas that reduce stress and anxiety. I particularly like chamomile, passionflower, and lemon balm. Chamomile and passionflower are mild sedatives, so they will help you fall asleep faster. You can also drink ashwagandha tea, although it's not nearly as strong ashwagandha in capsule form.

Drink coffee only in the morning

Coffee contains caffeine, which is a stimulant. It wakes you up and gets the neurons in your brain firing. This is great in the morning. In fact, most studies show that a morning cup of coffee is good for mood and cognition, may protect against chronic health diseases, and has very few side effects.[50]

If you are more of a tea drinker, both black and green tea provide a great morning caffeine wake-up, with the added benefits of being antioxidant and anti-inflammatory.

But caffeine stays active in your blood for at least six hours. So, an afternoon cup of coffee is not such a good thing.

Caffeine keeps you awake by blocking a neurotransmitter called adenosine. This chemical builds up in your brain over the course of the day and it makes you feel sleepy, creating what we call sleep pressure. A good dose of sleep pressure is necessary for falling asleep at night.

Just to be safe, cut the caffeine after about 1PM. No coffee. No black or green tea. No soda. No energy drinks.

Treat your obstructive sleep apnea

As many as 75% of women with PCOS have sleep apnea. As I mentioned before, sleep apnea is when, with or without snoring, you momentarily stop breathing in your sleep. In the short term, sleep apnea makes you feel tired and crummy, which is reason enough to treat it. But because it reduces your sleep quantity and quality, it is also an independent risk factor for all of the chronic diseases that PCOS already increases your risk for.[51]

If you feel tired during the day, if you get headaches or wake up with a dry mouth, if you ever wake up gasping, if you feel like you are in a mental fog, or if you know you snore, you should get assessed for sleep apnea.

Your doctor will set you up to do a sleep study, and if you get diagnosed, she will likely prescribe that you sleep with a Continuous Positive Airway Pressure (CPAP) device. This is the gold-standard treatment.

One of the most common frustrations women have with CPAP is that the device is annoying. It's fairly medical and definitely not sexy. But you should use it anyway.

In addition to all of the health benefits I've already mentioned that come with sleeping better, women who are diagnosed with sleep apnea and use a CPAP actually have better sex than those who don't. The main reason is that sleep apnea crushes your libido and causes sexual dysfunction.[52]

People who sleep better generally have more fulfilling sex lives. Also, if you snore, a CPAP device will quiet you down and make you a much better bedmate. Bonus: This is good for your partner's libido, too! And sleep apnea often drives couples into separate bedrooms, so if you can avoid that, people who sleep together have more sex.

Long story short, if you need a CPAP, get one and use it. You'll feel happier, healthier, and weirdly enough, sexier.

Here are a few extra suggestions to help with sleep apnea.

Avoid smoking, drinking, and sleeping pills

If you are a smoker, sleep apnea is just one more reason you should quit. Smoking causes airway inflammation and smokers have three times more sleep apnea than non-smokers. Alcohol and sleeping pills exacerbate sleep apnea by changing your sleep cycles and by relaxing and collapsing muscles in your neck even more than normal. In fact, heavy drinking can trigger sleep apnea in someone who doesn't otherwise have the condition.[53,54]

Myo-inositol

Take 4 grams of myo-inositol every day. This is one of my core PCOS supplement recommendations. Myo-inositol improves insulin resistance and studies show that insulin resistance is an important risk factor for sleep apnea.[55]

Oral mouth guard

These don't work as well as a CPAP, but they work a lot better than nothing. So if you can't manage the CPAP for whatever reason, try this option.

Sleep position

Most people's sleep apnea is worst when they lie flat on their backs. You can reduce airway constriction by propping yourself up with pillows and by sleeping on your side.

Weight loss

The heavier you are, the more pressure there is on your airway. Even moderate weight loss should improve sleep apnea. One of the best ways to jumpstart weight loss is by going on a light diet (see Chapter 5 on page 67). Another great trick is timed eating, which we'll explore in Chapter 7 on page 117. Oh, and when you finally do get some sleep, that will make future weight loss easier.

Treat GERD and other pain conditions

Any medical condition that causes physical, mental, or emotional discomfort can disrupt your sleep. If you leave these conditions untreated, you'll quickly end up in a terrible feedback loop — pain makes it hard to sleep and lack of sleep increases your sensitivity to pain.[56]

Gastroesophageal Reflux Disease (GERD)

GERD, or acid reflux, is one of the leading causes of sleep disturbances. We've known for some time that it's related to stress and to lack of sleep. So, again, GERD exacerbates sleep problems and sleep problems exacerbate GERD.

GERD is, at least in part, a circadian rhythm dysfunction of the gastrointestinal tract. 80% of GERD sufferers have nighttime heartburn. This is really weird if you think about it. Why is your stomach producing so much stomach acid in the middle of the night when there is nothing to digest? Your stomach is off the beat.[57]

Maybe it's not surprising that a promising treatment for GERD is melatonin. In one study, when GERD patients took melatonin for eight weeks, nearly all of them experienced a total remission of their GERD symptoms. Patients took 3 mg at bedtime, so if you wanted to try that for eight weeks, that would be fine and safe. After eight weeks, reduce the dosage to 2 mg at bedtime for maintenance.[58]

Pain

If you have pain, sleep can be very difficult and you need to treat it. The exact treatment depends on why you have pain. This is definitely a time when you need to work with your doctor.

Most pain has an inflammatory component so the 750 to 1500 mg of curcumin that I recommend as part of the core supplements may help.[59]

Troubleshooting

Sleep is a natural but extremely delicate and fragile process. A lot can go wrong. Even after you implement all of my suggestions, you may experience some challenges. Here's what to do (and what not to do!).

I feel sleepy in the morning.

Are you getting seven to eight hours of sleep? If not, then nothing will make you want to wake up in the morning.

If you get your seven to eight hours and you still wake up feeling tired, it may be that you haven't quite hit the end of your sleep cycle. When people (like campers) live without electrical lighting, melatonin plummets and cortisol rises an hour before they wake up. The rest of us generally experience this hormonal shift one hour after wake up.

Sunlight and a cup of coffee, black tea, or green tea can speed this shift along.

However, if you are doing everything right and you are still slogging through your morning or even your entire day, you need to make an appointment with your doctor. There are a variety of medical conditions that can cause fatigue, including hypothyroidism, depression, and anemia.

I get tired during the day.

Most people have an afternoon energy lull sometime after lunch. This seems to be a natural part of a normal human circadian rhythm. One theory is that ancient people napped to avoid the hottest part of the day. In many parts of the world, afternoon naps are still standard for healthy adults.

A short nap of five to twenty minutes will increase your alertness for the next one to three hours. And a nap will not make it harder to sleep at night. Longer naps may make you groggy upon awakening, but then you should feel alert for much longer.[60]

So, if you are tired and you can nap, feel free to nap away.

Otherwise, a brisk walk or a blast of bright sunshine should wake you up.

And again, if this is a chronic problem, make an appointment with your doctor.

I sleep a lot.

In this book, I focus on sleep deprivation because that is the common problem. According to a U.S. Gallup poll, 40% of Americans get less than seven hours of sleep per night, while only 5% get nine or more. For women with PCOS who trend towards being night owls, the number of long sleepers is even fewer.[61]

But, and this is a big "but," if you are one of those people who sleep a lot, you need to know that this is not healthy. Chronically getting more than eight hours of sleep every night is as bad for you as getting less than seven. It is associated with all of the same risks as sleep deprivation, including increased mortality rates.

If you commonly need more than eight hours of sleep to feel rested, you should see your doctor.

I can't sleep.

Challenges with falling asleep or middle-of-the-night awakenings can leave you staring at the ceiling. If this is a frequent problem, really focus on all of the relaxation tools earlier in this chapter to reduce cortisol and promote deeper, sounder sleep.

For the occasional bout of insomnia, I keep a bottle of the Douglas Laboratories Melatonin 1 mg by my bedside and if it's before 3AM, I'll take one or two chewable tablets and see if that does the trick.

While you wait for sleep, it's important that you don't stare at the clock. If there's a clock in your bedroom, turn it around.

Make sure you are comfortable. If you are hot, turn on a bedside fan. If you are thirsty, get a drink. If you have to pee, go do that, but don't turn on the bathroom light.

Some people enjoy listening to guided imagery or sleep hypnosis. There are all sorts of free and affordable apps that you can try. My patients are often happy with Health Journeys (www.HealthJourneys.com).

If you try everything and you just can't fall asleep, get up. As painful as that sounds, you do not want to lie in bed awake for long periods of time. You will train your body to associate your bed with wakefulness. Find a comfortable place with dim lighting to read a book or listen to music. Go back to bed and try again when you feel sleepy.

I travel.

When you travel across time zones, you cause abrupt circadian rhythm dysfunction. I get this all of the time because I lecture around the world.

This is the one situation where I recommend a very short, higher dose of melatonin.

On your first evening in a new time zone, take 5 mg of melatonin at your normal bedtime (between 10PM and 11PM in the new time zone). Do this for three nights in a row. You want to make sure you take a supplement that is instant release, not timed release or sustained release. This will reset your clock quickly. I recommend Thorne Melaton-5.[62]

Repeat this process when you return home as well.

I take sleeping pills.

Sleeping pills, also known as hypnotics, disrupt your natural sleep cycles and your circadian rhythm. They give you medicated sleep, which is not the same as natural, restorative sleep. And they can be extremely habit-forming. They are associated with an increased risk of cancer, accidents, infections, and overdoses. People take these drugs for years and years, but no one has studied their safety beyond twelve months.[63,64,65]

If you've already been taking sleeping pills on a regular basis, you should work with your doctor to develop a plan to wean off of them slowly. Most people do this by very incrementally lowering their dose to minimize withdrawal symptoms, especially withdrawal insomnia and sometime seizures.

There are very few situations where sleeping pills are appropriate. Every once in awhile, if you are in pain, if you need to sleep on a plane, or if you have a terrible head cold that's keeping you up, then taking a sleeping pill could be okay. But you should consider the risks, and sleeping pills should definitely not be your go-to sleep solution.

If you follow my recommendations, you should be able to sleep without resorting to hypnotics.

I take birth control pills.

Studies show that women who take oral contraceptives sleep differently than naturally cycling women. They have less slow wave non-REM sleep and their body temperature doesn't drop the way you'd expect. We don't yet understand the implications of these findings. But if you are taking hormonal birth control, you should know that they are changing your sleep.[66]

A quick summary

Good sleep is essential for good health.

PCOS sets you up for poor sleep by dysregulating your melatonin and cortisol levels and your entire circadian rhythm. Poor sleep is one of the driving causes of all the scary chronic health conditions associated with PCOS. Conversely, you can lower your risk for these conditions and improve your overall health by improving your sleep.

- Schedule your sleep so you follow the same sleep routine every day.
- Make your bedroom a fabulous place to sleep.
- Take melatonin before bed.
- Relax, starting a good two hours before bedtime.
- Limit caffeine to mornings only.
- Treat your sleep apnea.
- Treat your GERD and other pain conditions.

Healthy habits to get you started

☐ Use your phone's bedtime function or another program to set a daily alarm at your get-ready-for-bed time.

☐ Program your morning alarm to go off between 6AM and 7AM every day, even on the weekends. Have your alarm play a melody instead of loud beeping to avoid startling awake.

☐ Use a fitness tracker, like a Fitbit, to track your sleep and verify that you are getting seven to eight hours every night.

☐ Get a small bedside fan so you can cool down in the middle of the night.

☐ Download a white noise app that you can run on your phone. Bonus: You'll have it to use in hotel rooms.

☐ Get 0.5 mg, 1 mg, and 2 mg melatonin supplements. This allows you to take the lowest dose necessary at all times.

☐ Keep a bottle of chewable 1 mg melatonin by your bed so you can grab one if you can't sleep.

☐ Keep a bottle of 0.5 mg melatonin by your kitchen sink. Take one every night as you are cleaning up dinner.

☐ Keep a bottle of 2 mg melatonin by your toothbrush to take at bedtime.

☐ Subscribe to a guided meditation app or podcast.

☐ After dinner is cleaned up, relax with a warm cup of chamomile, passionflower, lemon balm, or ashwagandha tea.

☐ Take 500 mg of ashwagandha at bedtime each day .

☐ Take a warm bath before bed.

☐ Outfit your bedroom with an essential oil diffuser and essential oils. Lavender, sweet orange, and bergamot are great for sleep.

☐ Set up a sleep study to get tested for sleep apnea.

☐ Make a doctor's appointment if you are suffering from ongoing fatigue to rule out more serious conditions.

☐ If you are taking sleeping pills, make an appointment with your doctor to discuss weaning off of them.

☐ Assemble a travel kit that includes a sleep mask and a bottle of 5 mg melatonin.

CHAPTER 7

———

STEP 3:
Eat to the beat

The main reason your circadian rhythm is off the beat is that without properly timed light and plentiful estrogen, the master clock drifts off the 24-hour day. If that were all that happened, then your circadian rhythm might not be cued to the sun, but your master clock would keep all the organs and cells in your body synced to each other.

But that is not all that happens. Your body actually gets out of sync *with itself* because you have a second powerful timekeeper — your gut microbiome — that creates a second and often misaligned rhythm in your body.

Your gut microbiome is comprised of the microorganisms living inside your intestines. It sets the clocks in the liver, pancreas, and other gastrointestinal organs almost completely independently of the master clock.

Of course, your gut microbiome doesn't know when it's light or dark; it's inside your intestines. Instead, it knows when food comes in.

Historically, the clocks in our ancestors' bodies stayed aligned because meals and daylight went together, so their master clocks and gut clocks followed the same rhythm.

Today, nothing could be further from the truth. We have 24-hour diners, 24/7 grocery stores, and we all have stocked kitchens with electrical lighting, so we can eat whenever and as often as we'd like. And we do.

Most Americans start eating shortly after they wake up and they stop eating a bit before bedtime, averaging a 15-hour "eating window." An eating window is the time span that a person eats within, and it is marked by the first and last calories consumed over the course of a day. Digestion extends beyond the eating window to take care of that final evening snack.[1]

Your digestive tract needs to sleep, ideally for at least 12 hours every night.

Eating around the clock keeps your digestive system awake and working around the clock, and it stresses those organs because they never get time to rest and rejuvenate. Simultaneously, the circadian rhythm of your digestive system gets out of sync with the other circadian rhythms in your body, dysregulating your metabolism, hormone levels, and immune system and causing chronic, systemic inflammation.[2]

Hello, gut microbiome

Your gut microbiome is the most complex ecosystem ever discovered. Made of up thousands of microscopic species and trillions of organisms, your gut microbiome is a complex civilization of mostly bacteria, some fungi, and a few viruses. The more we learn about the gut microbiome, the more we discover that it's way more complicated than whatever we thought before.

The microbiome is critical to human digestion. Different bacteria perform different functions. Some digest complex carbohydrates and release short-chain fatty acids. Some break down fats and proteins and extract amino acids. Some break down polyphenols from plants. Some synthesize vitamins. Our gut microbiome produces nutrients essential for human health that we cannot make on our own.[3]

As impressive as this is, your gut microbiome does way more than help you digest food. It communicates with all of the other systems in your body, and it sends out circadian signals.

This is incredible, when you stop to think about it. These microorganisms that were not created by your body send signals to your gastrointestinal tract, your immune system, and even your brain. They produce short-chain fatty acids that set the peripheral clocks in your digestive organs. They help produce your immune system's T-cells, which seek out and destroy foreign pathogens. They produce human neurotransmitters like norepinephrine, dopamine, and serotonin.[4,5,6]

In fact, the gut microbiome is so critical to normal human hormonal functioning that many scientists now categorize the gut microbiome as a virtual endocrine organ.[7]

Of course, the gut microbiome is timed. Every single one of the 30 trillion or so microbes has its own clock genes, and each behaves totally differently during the day and the night.[8]

They set their clocks by food. When you eat, your gut microbiome says, "Day!" and when food stops, it says, "Night!" And it projects these signals out to the rest of your body. In particular, this gut signal sets the clock in your liver, which is the metabolic workhorse in your body.

Hello, liver

The microbiome sends circadian signals from the intestinal tract through the portal vein directly to the liver.[9]

Many people love their liver for its role in processing alcohol, but that's only a tiny fraction of what it does. It's really one of the most incredible and possibly underappreciated organs in the human body.

To date we know of over 500 critical tasks that the liver performs daily that cover detoxification, nutrient metabolism, fat production and storage, blood sugar control, blood cell recycling, and metabolic homeostasis. It actually grows by as much as 40% during the day and then it shrinks again at night while you sleep. Or at least, that's what it does when it's on the right timing.[10,11]

Metabolism, done right

Your metabolism is a complex and highly coordinated dance of hormones, nutrients, energy consumption, and energy production that is highly dependent upon circadian rhythm.

When you wake up, your low melatonin and high cortisol levels get you ready for a big breakfast. In anticipation of breakfast, your pancreas pumps out insulin and your insulin sensitivity is high. Your body is primed to metabolize food.

So, you eat breakfast. As the sugars and fats from your meal enter your bloodstream, the insulin in your blood opens your cells to receive sugar to burn as energy. Your cells always use sugar first and store fat.

Right after you eat, there are so many circulating fats and sugars that the liver processes most of them. It converts sugars into a compound called glycogen (GLY-koh-jen), which it temporarily stores inside itself. It converts fatty acids into triglycerides to be stored in fat cells.

While your body is digesting your meal, you are totally in sugar- and fat-storage mode.

When all of the sugars and fats from your meal have been stored, your liver senses a drop in blood sugar and a corresponding drop in insulin. This triggers the next stage in metabolism, glycogenolysis (gly-ko-jen-ALL-eh-sis).

Your body's cells love sugar, especially your brain cells and your red blood cells. It is their favorite, most efficient source of fuel. So, your liver triggers the pancreas to release less insulin and instead release glucagon (GLOO-ka-gon), a hormone responsible for stabilizing blood sugar. It tells the liver to release its stored glycogen as sugar slowly back into the bloodstream.

You are now in sugar-burning mode.

As the liver's glycogen stores decrease, you enter the next phase of metabolism, gluconeogenesis (gloo-koh-nee-eh-JEN-eh-sis), where the liver turns a variety of non-sugar compounds, including certain amino acids, into sugar and releases that sugar into the blood to maintain a stable blood sugar level. And, for the first time in this metabolic process, your fat cells release fatty acids back into the bloodstream for your body's cells to use as energy.[12]

You are now in sugar- and fat-burning mode.

If you are exercising and burning energy, you pass through these metabolic phases quickly. If you are sitting, it can take ten hours to get to gluconeogenesis. And that's only if you stop eating. The minute you put more food in your mouth, your whole metabolism stops whatever it's doing and jumps back to the beginning of the process. Your body goes back to sugar- and fat-storage mode.

Metabolism, done the American way

Your body is supposed to cycle through these phases several times throughout the day, basically once per meal. By the end of the day, a healthy liver has expanded considerably, storing glycogen, bile, and other compounds, and it requires a nighttime fast to return to its original size. When the liver doesn't get this time off, it remains large and becomes inflamed.[13]

So, if you really wanted to break this incredible metabolic cycle, the first thing you would do is live in the modern day United States (or any other Westernized country of your choice). And then you would do what most Americans do: You would eat a lot, mostly sugars and fats, and critically, you would eat *all of the time.*

This "all of the time" part is especially detrimental because when you eat around the clock, your body stays in storage mode. It is constantly taking in sugars and fats. It can never burn them. The pancreas is constantly producing insulin to keep your cells absorbing sugars because no matter how much sugar you eat, your body cannot allow your blood sugar to get too high. The sugar must be stored.

Constantly high insulin levels lead to insulin resistance, which leads to more insulin, which eventually leads to diabetes.

High insulin is supposed to block your fat cells from releasing fatty acids into your bloodstream. But insulin resistance breaks this checks and balances system. Your fat cells, specifically the ones in your arms and legs, start releasing fatty acids into your blood. Where do they go? Your body's other cells are still burning sugar. They won't take fatty acids. So your liver and your other organs start absorbing these fats.[14]

The result is a fatty liver. Once the liver is fatty and inflamed, it stops responding to circadian and metabolic rhythms. It enters a state of uncontrolled gluconeogenesis, incessantly releasing fats and sugars into the bloodstream. This also keeps your body in storage mode.

Your liver isn't the only organ that gets fat. You also get fatty heart, fatty arteries, fatty muscles, and fatty pancreas. All this fat further increases inflammation and insulin resistance.

Oh, and remember leptin? It's your I-feel-full hormone and it gets released by your fat cells. So as you get more fat cells, you get more leptin, and that's supposed to make you eat less so you return to your healthy weight. Well, inflammation breaks this checks and balances system as well, and you get leptin resistance. You stay hungry so you actually eat more.[15]

Regardless of what you eat, eating around the clock contributes to fatty liver, heart disease, diabetes, and weight gain.

It's all connected

A poorly timed gut circadian rhythm impacts more than metabolism because the gut microbiome communicates directly with the master clock. The master clock has nutrient sensors that "see" the rise and fall of nutrients in the blood. When these signals are off rhythm, they confuse its master circadian signal. Consequently, eating late at night impedes falling asleep and worsens sleep apnea. It is associated with depression. Meal timing even influences fertility.[16,17,18,19]

PCOS amplifies the effects of constant eating because we are already predisposed to:

- inflammation
- obesity
- nonalcoholic fatty liver disease
- heart disease
- diabetes
- circadian rhythm dysfunction

We are primed for the cascade of broken checks and balances caused by irregular, around the clock eating.

The good news is that this is a relatively simple lifestyle change to make: Eat your meals over fewer hours during the day. And the health benefits are enormous — improved metabolism, lower inflammation, reduced risk for all chronic diseases, and improved fertility.[20]

A path forward

To get your gut clock back on the beat, you need to eat to the beat. And just as with light and sleep, you have to be stricter than the average woman because low estrogen means that none of your signaling works quite as well.

It's absolutely not fair. I'm with you on this. But it is what it is.

I recommend a simple strategy called "time-restricted eating" — eating and not eating within specified time windows. Use meals and fasts to set a strong circadian rhythm in your gut microbiome that aligns with the strong circadian rhythm you impose on your master clock. Simply put, eating goes with light and fasting goes with dark.

When I say "fast," I am referring to any period of time when you stop eating. A fast could be for a few hours (or even a few days!). Because humans evolved with fasting, our bodies need periods without food to rejuvenate and heal.

With timed-restricted eating, you establish a clear digestive circadian rhythm and a healthy metabolism. By transitioning between periods of fasting and eating every day, your metabolism adapts to switch seamlessly between sugar-burning and fat-burning modes. This, in turn, lowers blood sugar, improves insulin levels and insulin resistance, reduces inflammation, encourages your body to burn more fat, and helps you lose weight. It also improves sleep, immune system function, and fertility.

You can do this by simply changing *when* you eat.

Eat during the day, not at night

Create a daytime eating window that is 10 to 12 hours long and a nighttime fasting window that is 12 to 14 hours long. Fasting for 13 hours every night is ideal.[21]

The nighttime fast must be long enough for your liver to use up all of its glycogen stores so your metabolism transitions into fat-burning mode. Here's a schedule I recommend:

Breakfast: between 7AM and 8AM, shortly after you wake up.

Lunch: between noon and 1PM.

Dinner: between 5PM and 6PM.

Then, and this is the important part, at 7PM (or earlier) your eating window closes.

You can drink herbal tea or decaf coffee, but you should not consume anything with calories. No dessert. No after-dinner glass of wine. No late-night snacks.

You are done eating until breakfast the next day.

> This is not a calorie restricted plan. Eat the same quantity of food you normally would for breakfast, lunch, and dinner. If you get hungry and need to add a meal during day, you can do that. The point isn't to reduce the number of calories you consume — although you may naturally consume fewer calories by cutting out evening food and drinks — but rather to create a smaller eating window and a longer fasting window.

Aim for at least a 12-hour overnight fast every night. This is a safe time span for virtually everyone, unless perhaps you are pregnant or have a health condition that requires more frequent eating. But if you are reasonably healthy, start with a 12-hour overnight fast and see how you feel.

If after one month, your energy levels are good and you're not struggling with evening hunger, shrink your eating window by an hour. A 13-hour fast is where studies start really showing improved health outcomes like lower cancer risk, improved blood sugar, and reduced inflammation. If after another month all is still well, reduce your eating window by another hour for a 14-hour fasting window. In general, so long as you feel good, longer overnight fasts are better.

When people confine eating to daytime hours but otherwise don't change their diets, they improve their insulin sensitivity and other metabolic markers and usually lose weight. Another surprising benefit of daytime-only eating is a healthier gut microbiome. People who only eat during the day tend to have a "lean" microbiome, which means their microbiome doesn't extract as much sugar and fat from the foods they are eating. In contrast, nighttime eating and around the clock eating are associated with "obese" microbiomes that extract every last calorie from every bite of food you eat.

If you do only one thing from this chapter, this should be it. Eat during the day. Fast at night.

Eat breakfast like a queen and dinner like a pauper

Another easy way to eat with your circadian rhythm is to eat most of your calories earlier in the day. It's called "caloric timing." In the United States, most people eat a small breakfast or skip it altogether, a big lunch, and an even bigger dinner. This is totally backward from how our bodies are designed to eat. Breakfast should be your biggest meal-of-the-day, and dinner should be your smallest.

There was an incredible study done recently where researchers took two groups of obese women and fed them exactly the same diet. But, in one group, the women ate half of their calories for breakfast, a third of their calories for lunch, and then a very light dinner. In the other group, the participants flipped this caloric schedule. They ate a very light breakfast, a third of their calories for lunch, and half of their calories for dinner. They ate exactly the same foods, just swapped breakfast and dinner between the two groups.

Both groups lost weight, but the women who ate half of their calories for breakfast lost 2.5 times more weight just by eating their biggest meal in the morning instead of at night. And a ton of it was visceral belly fat. Additionally, the big breakfast group had better insulin levels, lower triglyceride levels (which is good), no post-meal glucose spikes (also good), and they felt less hungry all day because they had lower levels of ghrelin (the hunger hormone, also good).[22]

This same team of researchers did another nearly identical study with PCOS women. After 90 days of following a big-breakfast-small-dinner schedule, women with PCOS experienced a 56% decrease in insulin resistance, a 50% decrease in testosterone, and a 50% *increase* in ovulation.[23]

The big-breakfast-small-dinner schedule also lowers systemic inflammation and reduces breast cancer risk. And, because nighttime eating disrupts sleep, nixing late night snacks improves sleep quality.[24]

These benefits occur when you eat with your body's clocks. To shift your calories to earlier in the day without upsetting your stomach, take a week or two and slowly begin eating more for breakfast and less for dinner.

One way to do it this is to actually swap your meals. Eat what you'd normally eat for dinner at breakfast time and eat your breakfast for dinner. Yep, I mean eating chicken, roasted veggies, and a sweet potato for breakfast and a small veggie omelet with fruit for dinner.

Another benefit to this plan: constipation relief. Consistently eating a big breakfast stimulates the colon. So in addition to having a nice breakfast, you also get a nice morning poop. It's the little things in life, you know?

Eat dessert for breakfast

Eating dinner for breakfast includes eating dessert. Of course most desserts aren't good for you. But, and this is a huge "but," people are more successful sticking to a meal plan when they don't cut out their favorite foods. Even though I haven't told you to change what you eat, changing your caloric timing is enough to throw some people for a loop. There are rules, and that can make it feel like a diet.

So my advice is: If you like dessert, you should keep eating dessert.

Just eat it in the morning. That's when your insulin and your insulin sensitivity are already high. The morning is when your body is best adapted to handle a high-sugar, high-fat treat.

And science is totally on your side for this one. In another study, two groups of obese dieters were given calorically restrictive and identical daily food allotments, but one group dedicated some of their calories to a morning dessert, namely chocolate. After 16 weeks, both groups had lost an average of 33 pounds per person. That's great, but it's the second half of the study that's really interesting because around this point, people in the no-dessert group began to cheat. During the next 16 weeks, people in the no-dessert group *regained*, on average, 22 pounds per person, but people who ate dessert for breakfast continued to lose weight. By the end of 32 weeks, dieters who ate dessert for breakfast lost an average of 40 more pounds per person than dieters who tried to give up dessert.[25]

Is dessert good for you? No. But this is definitely a case where being not-perfect but successful is way better than trying for perfection and setting yourself up to fail.

So, be kind to yourself. Eat chocolate! I love dark chocolate, and I eat it almost every day, usually for breakfast.

Science also shows that chocolate makes people happy. Just sayin'.[26]

Eat meals, not snacks

Part of the problem with snacks is our definition of the word "snack." Most people distinguish snacks from meals based on size, time spent eating, location for eating (standing versus sitting, alone or with others), and nutritional quality. For many of us, when we think of grabbing a snack, we think of something saltier, fattier, sweeter, and more processed than something we would eat for a meal.[27]

Also, weirdly, if two people eat the same food but one thinks of it as a snack and one thinks of it as a meal, the person who thought "meal" will feel full longer and will overall eat less.[28]

Instead of eating snacks, I challenge you to eat meals. Here are a few excellent mini-meals to eat instead of snacks:

- Salad, any type that is primarily veggies, fruit, and/or nuts
- Fruit and peanut butter
- Turkey, avocado, and veggies wrapped in lettuce
- Veggie soup
- Refried beans and a fried egg
- Sushi
- Hummus and veggies
- Beef jerky, popcorn, nuts, seeds, and dried fruit for when you are on-the-go

If you are hungry and it's not a regular meal time but it's within your eating window, add another meal to your day. But between meals, try not to graze.

And don't sip calorie-packed drinks all day long either. Feel free to nurse black coffee, unsweetened tea, and water to your heart's content. But if a drink has calories, it should be consumed with a meal, or your body will experience that as snacking.

Chew gum

If you get hungry between meals, you can also alleviate the feeling by chewing xylitol (ZY-li-tall) gum.

Chewing gum, even after it's lost its flavor, reduces appetite and can help prevent impulsive eating.[29]

I specifically recommend xylitol gum because xylitol is the only non-caloric sweetener that is actually good for you. It protects your teeth by reducing the gingivitis-causing bacteria, mutans streptococci, without killing any beneficial bacteria in your oral or gut microbiomes. And chewing xylitol gum increases a special hormone called glucagon-like peptide-1 (GLP-1) that improves insulin function and is linked to weight loss in women with PCOS.[30,31]

Other sugar and sugar-free sweeteners are toxic to your microbiome, so stick to xylitol.[32,33]

I recommend Spry gum because this company uses an all-natural gum base derived from tree sap. Virtually every other gum out there uses a gum base made from a combination of plastic, rubber, and wax. Really.[34]

So if you need a little help getting from one meal to the next, or if you just enjoy chewing gum, I strongly recommend chewing sugar-free xylitol gum. It's actually good for you. Just don't substitute anything else. And go easy while you get your jaw muscles in shape. If you overdo it, you can give yourself a headache.[35]

Fast longer

Once you are comfortable with timed eating and caloric timing, try a longer fast. Humans evolved with fasting out of necessity, and even though our ancestors may not have enjoyed it, if their fasts were relatively brief, they gained pretty significant health benefits.

Fasting triggers a process called autophagy (aw-TAW-fah-jee).

"Auto" means "self," and "phagy" means "eating." Eating yourself? It sounds terrible, but that's what we are designed to do.

When no food comes in, eventually your body will burn the fat it's been storing. That is one of the first steps in triggering autophagy, but it's not autophagy itself.

Autophagy happens on the cellular level. When an individual cell stops receiving sugar as energy for an extended time, the cell looks for other sources of energy. It finds this energy within its own organelles, tiny organ-like structures. It breaks down old, diseased, and broken organelles into their foundational building blocks, such as amino acids and fatty acids, and uses those building blocks to create new, rejuvenated organelles.

In autophagy, our cells cannibalize and regenerate themselves without dying.

This extends their life and can help you stay younger longer.

Every cell in your body has a telomere (TELL-ah-meer), a tail-like structure that literally represents its finite life. Every time a cell dies completely and replaces itself in a different process called apoptosis (ay-POP-toe-sis), it consumes a piece of its telomere. Eventually, your telomeres are used up, and that's a big part of aging. Your organs get old because your cells can no longer replace themselves.

Autophagy extends the life of your cells and the organs they comprise because it enables them to renew and rejuvenate without using up any of their telomeres.

But it's not just about living longer. It's about living healthier. Healthy cells give you healthy organs and a healthy body.

So you want to trigger autophagy, but not all of the time. That's called starvation. Your cells can't recycle themselves endlessly. They need food.

You want your cells to get a tiny bit of autophagy every night. On top of that, periodic longer fasts will trigger more extensive autophagy. There are many different approaches to extended fasting. These are the ones I recommend.

Overnight fast

A 12- to 14-hour fast each night will trigger some degree of autophagy. After 12 hours without food, some of your cells will begin the process, but autophagy slows back down as soon as you break your fast, so you stop almost as soon as you start.[36]

Once or twice per week, you should eat an especially early dinner or skip dinner altogether so that your overnight fast lasts 16 to 18 hours. For every additional hour of fasting, your cells will identify and begin recycling more broken-down organelles. This is a great way to frequently experience more autophagy without significantly impacting your daily activities.

By the way, I don't recommend that you fast longer than 14 hours every single night because some studies show that female hormones are sensitive to fasting, and you can induce menstrual irregularity by long, daily fasts. Twice per week is perfect.[37,38]

5:2 fast

If you are up for a more serious twice-per-week fast, you can do the 5:2 fast instead. This is a popular form of fasting where you severely restrict your calories on two non-consecutive days of the week and then eat normally on the other five. So, for example, on Tuesdays and Thursdays, you only eat 500 calories, and on the other five days you eat normally, without binging to make up for the missed calories.

A stricter form of this fast is called Eat-Stop-Eat. Once or twice each week, you do a water fast for a full 24 hours.

Both of these fasts lead to weight loss. They improve the health of your gut microbiome. And they trigger longer periods of autophagy.[39,40]

I don't personally enjoy this type of fasting because it feels too consistently disruptive, and anyway, I prefer the fasting mimicking diet that I'm about to explain. But if you like it, it's a healthy and reasonable way to incorporate longer fasts into your life.

> If you have a history of eating disorders, be careful with fasting. There is no evidence that purposeful fasting can trigger disordered eating. In fact, in one study, obese women who participated in fasting reported less binge eating and depression. Even so, be careful and work with your doctor if you have any concerns.[41]

Fasting mimicking diet

Humans evolved to survive periods of famine. And to survive, humans needed to hunt and farm, plan and strategize, all without food. So our bodies have mechanisms that help us thrive while fasting.

During a prolonged fast, your body goes through powerful changes that can improve your metabolic health, sharpen your cognition, dramatically lower your risk for cancer, reverse some autoimmune diseases, improve blood sugar control, lower hypertension, and reduce your risk of Alzheimer's disease. Prolonged fasting can stimulate stem cells to produce brand new cells with long telomeres. It's an incredible process that we are just beginning to understand.

First, I want to tell you what happens to your body when you undergo a prolonged fast. Then I'm going to tell you how I *mimic* fasting for five days, so it's not miserable or stressful.

After one to three days of fasting, your liver uses up all of its glycogen stores and can no longer release sugar into the bloodstream. The only fuel left in your body is fat. So your body transitions into a fasting metabolic state called ketosis (kee-TOE-sis).

During ketosis, the liver converts fats into acids called ketones (KEE-tones) that your cells can use for food. At the same time, your insulin level drops dramatically because there is virtually no sugar in your blood. You enter full fat-burning mode.

On days three, four, and five, your cells have to start deciding which cells should be fed and which ones should starve. There simply isn't enough food. Cells that are healthy go through autophagy to recycle themselves and scavenge available energy. Cells that are sick or malfunctioning go through apoptosis and die. Critically, cancerous and precancerous cells are often dependent on sugar for energy and cannot metabolize ketones well, so they are particularly vulnerable to starvation during fasting and ketosis.[42]

During a prolonged fast, many of your organs physically shrink. Your kidneys and heart shrink by about 10%. Your liver shrinks by 30%. Your brain, however, is protected.[43]

By the end of your fast, you have gotten all of the benefits of a shorter fast — increased autophagy, lowered inflammation, and improved insulin resistance. Plus, you've burned days worth of fat and you've gotten rid of a significant percentage of your damaged cells. But the benefits don't end here.

On day six, you start eating again, and your organs jump into overdrive to rebuild their lost cells. They do this by turning on stem cells. People travel all over the world to get stem cells, but you have them in your own body and they can be stimulated into action by fasting. These stem cells make brand new cells with full-length telomeres. This means that your organs that shrunk during fasting regrow as younger versions of themselves.[44]

You can only get these benefits from a prolonged fast.

Or you can do what I do: the fasting mimicking diet, because nobody really wants to fast for days.

The fasting mimicking diet was developed by Dr. Valter Longo and his team of scientists at USC. It is five days of carefully selected and portioned food that allows you to eat very small meals without tipping your body out of its fasted state. It accomplishes this by including specific fats and carbohydrates that don't move the liver back to sugar- and fat-storage mode.

I get my fasting mimicking diet food from Dr. Longo's company, ProLon.

It's kind of pricey, especially since you get so little food (which is the point). But I think of this food as medicine, not as groceries. A benefit of using the ProLon meals is that they have been extensively tested and refined to maintain your fasting state while containing enough calories and nutrients that you don't stress your kidneys or lose lean muscle mass. This makes prolonged fasting safer and accessible to more people than a water fast or some kind of a do-it-yourself hack.[45,46]

According to Dr. Longo, a person with a perfect diet would benefit from doing the fasting mimicking diet twice per year. Most people should try to do an extended fast like this three to four times per year. This is the schedule that I am now on and I feel great. If you are trying to reverse metabolic or autoimmune problems, you may benefit from fasting 6 to 12 times per year, at least in the beginning. Every prolonged fast is beneficial, and the benefits of several rounds of prolonged fasting are cumulative.[47]

Prolonged fasting is like a total body reboot. Your circadian rhythm gets back in sync. Your gut microbiome gets fixed. Your inflammation goes down. Your metabolic health improves. You reduce your risk of dementia and cancer. Your immune system gets a reboot so you can reverse autoimmune diseases like multiple sclerosis and rheumatoid arthritis. If you are obese, you can safely lose a lot of weight without drugs or dangerous surgery.[48,49]

For many people, prolonged fasting can literally change their life.

The first time I did the five-day fasting mimicking diet, I worried that I would feel crappy. I couldn't take a week off of work, so I needed to be able to function normally.

The first two days were okay, but not great. I was a little hungry, but not overpoweringly so. I stayed busy so at least those days passed quickly, and I went to bed early because my husband wasn't fasting with me. Eating a tiny bowl of soup and then watching someone eat salmon just isn't that fun.

On day three, my body entered ketosis, and suddenly, I felt wonderful. I could feel my brain switch to using ketone bodies for energy. My mind was alert and my body felt strong and energetic. That feeling lasted for the rest of the fast.

Since that first fast, I have done twelve additional fasts, and counting. All of my metabolic markers are excellent, and over the past few years, my health has gotten better, even as I've gotten older.

The biggest improvement has been with my Hashimoto's thyroiditis. I have had autoimmune thyroid disease for over a decade. Last year, I had my thyroid bloodwork done and I had zero thyroid antibodies. Zero! My Hashimoto's has gone into remission.

Hashimoto's is a progressive autoimmune disease. Even with treatment, the thyroid is slowly destroyed. For many people, the disease eventually progresses to complete thyroid failure. In my body, this process has stopped.

I credit ProLon's fasting mimicking diet because it is the only treatment protocol I follow that has evidence of reversing autoimmunity.

And just so you know, I pay full price for my ProLon meals and I get no kickbacks. ProLon doesn't offer a doctor's discount, at least not that I know of. I use this fasting product because I trust the science and I believe the benefits far outweigh the cost.

Troubleshooting

Time-restricted eating can be a big change if you are used to eating around the clock like most people. Here are some challenges you might encounter and some tips for how to deal with them.

I'm hungry!

First off, recognize that hunger isn't dangerous or even bad for you. The problem with hunger is that it's uncomfortable and it drains your willpower over time. So, you don't want to be chronically hungry.

For mild hunger between meals, chew xylitol gum.

You may also be able to curb your appetite with water, green tea, or black coffee.

If that's not enough, eat a small meal.

But if you are frequently starving, the best thing to do is make sure you are eating a big breakfast. I wasn't kidding about actually eating your dinner for breakfast. The average American breakfast is all processed carbs, maybe with a splash of milk. If you are hungry, you need to eat more real food — the kind with fiber and protein. My favorite breakfast is two poached eggs on a big bed of sauteed greens with a side of asparagus, some walnuts, and one or two pieces of melon. After a meal like that, it takes a while to get hungry again.

I get non-diabetic low blood sugar.

Low blood sugar, also called hypoglycemia (hy-poe-gly-SEE-mee-ah) is a sign of insulin resistance. When your cells don't see insulin well, your pancreas produces ever-increasing amounts of insulin to move the sugar out of your bloodstream and into your cells. Sometimes, it overshoots. It releases too much insulin and that insulin shuttles too much sugar into the cells too quickly. When your blood sugar drops, you can feel weak, dizzy, shaky, nauseous, and have a hard time focusing. It's a terrible feeling that can leave you fatigued for hours afterwards.[50]

The answer is *not* to keep eating.

I know some people feel like they need to eat every two hours or so to keep their blood sugar stable. But I've got to tell you, you do *not* have to eat every two hours. If humans had to eat this often, our ancestors would have gone extinct a long time ago. They didn't go extinct because we all have biological mechanisms that allow us to fast and maintain stable blood sugar.

When you feel hypoglycemic, in the short term, eat a tiny snack so you feel better. Ideally something with a little sugar but mostly fat or protein, like some beef jerky, olives, avocado, or a handful of nuts, so you don't trigger an insulin spike.

In the long term, you need to even out your blood sugar levels by increasing insulin sensitivity so your pancreas doesn't work so hard. Eat a big breakfast and a small, early dinner. Fast overnight so your body relearns how to transition smoothly between all of the metabolic phases. Exercise a few times per week. And start reducing the amount of sugar you eat because sugar spikes lead to insulin spikes.

I have diabetes.

If you have diabetes, you should work with your physician to create a time-restricted eating plan. Any degree of fasting can increase your chances of hypoglycemia, which in a diabetic can lead to coma and death. Make sure you know what to do if your blood sugar gets too low. Fortunately, patients who work with their physician to monitor their blood sugar and possibly adjust their medication dosages while fasting have lower rates of hypoglycemia.[51]

Timed eating and fasting are generally safe and highly beneficial for people with diabetes.[52]

Start with overnight fasting. After an extended overnight fast, eat a dinner-sized, high-energy breakfast that includes mostly fruits and vegetables with a small source of protein such as eggs, fish, or beans. Diabetics who eat a healthy, big breakfast and then a smaller lunch and dinner have more stable blood sugar overall and can often reduce insulin usage over the course of the day. In contrast, diabetics who skip breakfast experience poor insulin response and impaired blood sugar regulation all day long.[53,54]

Researchers have tested longer fasts, up to a week in length, on diabetics with promising results. Fasting seems to be safe and leads to belly fat loss and improved metabolic markers such as lower blood pressure. Look into getting a continuous glucose monitor, a medical device that attaches to you skin and tracks your blood sugar level around the clock (see page 323), and be sure to do everything under the supervision of your doctor.[55]

I'm already skinny.

The benefits of timed eating and fasting extend well beyond weight loss. You still need to eat with your circadian rhythm, stimulate autophagy, and periodically rejuvenate your organs.

If your BMI is above 18.5 and you are not malnourished, then you should be safe to try all of the recommendations in this chapter.

A 12- to 14-hour overnight fast will maintain the circadian rhythm of your gut microbiome and liver, improve insulin resistance, and reduce systemic inflammation. Periodic 16- to 24-hour fasts will enhance autophagy. And you can do two to four rounds of ProLon each year to reduce your risk of long-term chronic diseases.

I'm an athlete.

So long as you are not underweight or malnourished, everything in this chapter is good for you. Many athletes practice intermittent fasting because it helps burn fat and build lean muscle.[56]

I'm pregnant or breastfeeding.

Congratulations! That's wonderful. This is a unique and important phase in your life and there's a lot that you can do to improve your health and the health of your baby.

But fasting is not one of them. If you are pregnant or breastfeeding, do not fast. Of course you should do some kind of overnight fast because that's called sleeping and you should eat your calories during the day to keep your circadian rhythm on the beat. But this is not a time to be obsessively rigid about caloric timing. Listen to your body. Be good, not perfect. Focus on other circadian strategies like light and sleep. Check out the section in Chapter 11 on pregnancy (page 288) .

Fasting made me stop menstruating.

For the vast majority of women, the fasting strategies in this chapter will improve your hormonal regulation and your metabolic profile, and consequently, most women will menstruate more regularly.

But, if you overdo it and your body thinks you are in a famine, it may turn off menstruation as a way of preventing pregnancy during a food shortage. If this is you, back off a little bit and take it slowly. Stick to 12 hours of overnight fasting. That will keep your circadian rhythm on the beat and give you enormous benefits. Allow your body time to adapt before trying a longer fast. And if longer fasts really mess with your system, don't do them.

I heard about this other diet ...

Oh my gosh, there are so many diets and cleanses out there. I can't possibly go into all of them. Here are a few of the diets that I see frequently in my practice and what I think about them.

- **Keto diet:** This is a high-fat, low-carb diet that induces ketosis. It's fine for short-term weight loss. I don't like when people do it longterm and stay in a state of perpetual ketosis. I'll talk about this more in Chapter 9 on page 167, but your microbiome needs a lot of fruits and vegetables to be healthy. I greatly prefer the fasting mimicking diet that gets you into ketosis for a few days and then returns you to normal, so you get all of the additional benefits like stimulated stem cells and rejuvenated organs.

- **Juice cleanses:** Usually, these are simply low-calorie diets. Most juices have too much sugar to induce a fasting state. Additionally, I am generally not a big fan of juicing because chewing is a critical part of the digestive process. When you chew, you mix your food with the digestive enzymes in saliva and you give your brain and stomach a heads-up that you're eating. That being said, if you want to drink only vegetable juice for a few days, it won't harm you. If you buy a commercial juice cleanse product, be careful that it doesn't include anything toxic, and don't go for longer than four to five days.[57]

- **Caloric restriction:** This is any diet where you reduce your caloric intake to 30% to 40% of your normal diet for an extended period of time. Consistent caloric restriction can trigger many of the same benefits as fasting. But I don't recommend caloric restriction because most people have a hard time maintaining it. And if you are successful, there is a very fine line between extended caloric restriction and anorexia. Actually, it's not even clear that that line exists. If you follow all of my guidelines and get your body on a strong circadian rhythm, you may find that you are less hungry and you need to eat less. That's healthy. But if you consistently eat less than your body wants and needs, you could end up with a dangerous eating disorder.[58,59]

A quick summary

You have a second, powerful circadian clock, your gut microbiome, that sets its time off of your eating and fasting schedule. You need to keep your gut clock and master clock on the same beat to avoid circadian rhythm and metabolic dysfunction.

- Eat during the day. Fast at night.
- Eat a big breakfast, a modest lunch, and a small dinner.
- Eat dessert with breakfast.
- Eat meals, not snacks.
- Chew xylitol gum.
- Try longer fasts.

Healthy habits to get you started

- ☐ Establish your 12-hour eating window and your 12-hour fasting window.

- ☐ At the end of your eating window, stop eating. Be very rigid on this one thing.

- ☐ Prepare a large breakfast the night before to quickly cook or reheat in the morning.

- ☐ Indulge in dessert for breakfast.

- ☐ Add a large plate of cut veggies or a salad to dinner so you can eat a light dinner without having it feel skimpy.

- ☐ Make a list of mini-meals you would enjoy and grocery shop for the ingredients.

- ☐ Throw out traditional snack foods like chips, granola bars, cookies, and crackers (or put them on a very high shelf where it's a pain to get them).

- ☐ Get a stainless steel thermos and sip on your favorite tea all day long. Green tea has caffeine and is great in the morning. Spearmint lowers testosterone and is wonderful in the afternoon. Ashwagandha lowers cortisol and is a perfect way to end your day.

☐ Buy xylitol gum and keep it with you during the day.

☐ Try an extended 16- to 18-hour overnight fast.

☐ Order the ProLon kit, pick a week, and embark on the fasting mimicking diet.

CHAPTER 8

STEP 4: Exercise any time you can

*E*xercise plays a unique and surprising role in your body, and my take on exercise is a bit unusual. Everyone knows that exercise builds strong, healthy muscles. And moderate exercise improves practically every single disease condition known to mankind — diabetes, heart disease, dementia, depression, *and* PCOS.

How does it do that? In terms of PCOS, the biggest benefit of exercise is a healthy gut microbiome.

Yes, you heard that right. You should exercise for your gut microbiome.

Your gut microbiome is your body's second timekeeper. You set your gut clock with timed eating, but your microbiome can only function properly if it is healthy.

When we think about nurturing our gut microbiome, it's easy to jump right to food, and we will talk about food in Chapter 9 on page 167. But, and I know this sounds crazy, irrespective of what you eat, exercise promotes the growth of beneficial microbes that support circadian and metabolic health.

Isn't that wild? When you exercise, you change your gut microbiome. And, importantly, exercise changes your microbiome in a way that nothing else can. There is no substitute. You can't eat extra kale or take probiotics to make up for a lack of exercise.

In fact, these changes to the gut microbiome are so critical that they may be the primary reason exercise makes people healthier.

In women with PCOS, aerobic exercise (the kind that raises your heart rate, like running and zumba) improves insulin sensitivity, lowers blood pressure, reduces the appearance of extra ovarian follicles (the "cysts" in in polycystic ovarian syndrome), improves anxiety and depression, lowers inflammation, and reduces hyperandrogenism. It protects against heart disease, Alzheimer's disease, and colon cancer. And, listen to this, aerobic exercise is twice as effective as dieting in increasing ovulation rates and decreasing testosterone levels.[1,2,3,4]

It creates all of these benefits, even if you don't lose weight. Actually, exercise generally is not the most effective way to lose a ton of weight. So we know that the benefits of exercise are not simply a side effect of weight loss.

Microbiome diversity

A healthy gut microbiome is a diverse microbiome. You want lots and lots of different types of microbes living in your gut. Science is still in the early stages of exploring this intricate microscopic world living within each of us, but what's clear is that when all of these little guys interact and compete with each other, something magical happens that keeps us healthy.

When we look at microbes, there are definitely good guys and bad guys, and you want lots of good guys and just a few bad guys. Even more than that, you want lots and lots of different species of microbes. There is no singular healthy gut microbiome. Some healthy people have more of this, some have more of that. There is enormous variability, which relates to age, gender, geography, and of course diet. But the one thing all healthy gut microbiomes share is diversity.

Within a healthy microbiome, there are several dominant beneficial bacteria populations that form the backbone of the microscopic community, and there are thousands of smaller populations of rarer bacteria, pathogens, viruses, and fungi. All these little guys move. They eat. Sometimes they eat each other. They help each other and compete with each other for resources. And they interact to create a dynamic, resilient ecosystem, which in turn makes you healthy.[5]

Unfortunately, women with PCOS have a less diverse gut microbiome than women without PCOS. There is something about PCOS that hurts our microbiome. It seems to be tied to hyperandrogenism because in women, more testosterone corresponds to less gut diversity. And for women who are obese, obesity also reduces diversity.[6,7,8]

This lack of diversity is called gut dysbiosis. It is linked to virtually every modern day disease, including diabetes, heart disease, colon cancer, irritable bowel syndrome, allergies, asthma, autism, anxiety, and depression. And, as I've mentioned, gut dysbiosis is a key feature of PCOS and obesity.[9]

Now, there is something of a chicken and the egg debate going on around this. Does gut dysbiosis cause disease or does disease cause gut dysbiosis? Probably, it's both. Gut dysbiosis gets triggered, either by disease, diet, or antibiotics, and once you have gut dysbiosis, you get diseases.

But either way, the fact remains that because you have PCOS, you have a less diverse gut microbiome and it hurts your health.

Exercise is like a party in your gut

Exercise is one of the best ways to counteract this. When you move your body, it's like there's a party in your gut and everyone is invited. Regardless of your diet, exercise builds gut microbiome diversity. On top of that, this diversity changes the gut ecosystem to favor the success of microbes that are especially beneficial to you, their human host.

In a recent study, a group of generally sedentary people were put on an exercise routine and then taken back off of it. Throughout the process, researchers analyzed stool (poop) samples to see how exercise impacted the participants' microbiomes.

When the participants started exercising, their microbiomes became more prolific and diverse, and they started producing more short-chain fatty acids. Short-chain fatty acids set the circadian clocks in the liver. They are absolutely essential for maintaining circadian health throughout your body, and more is always better.

When the participants stopped exercising, their microbiomes reverted to their less diverse states and short-chain fatty acid levels went back down.

In the study, people did 30 to 60 minutes of cardio three times per week. So they didn't exercise a ton, but they were consistent, and that seems to be essential.

Another cool thing that this study revealed is that not all short-chain fatty acid levels go up by the same amount when you exercise. The exercised microbiome produces more butyrate (BYOO-teh-rate), a particularly beneficial short-chain fatty acid that moderates inflammation. People with higher levels of butyrate are more resistant to inflammatory diseases and they are less likely to suffer from allergies.[10,11]

I know I keep saying this, but nothing in the body does just one thing. Butyrate is a great example. It is a critical circadian rhythm messenger, and it is the primary food for the cells that line your intestines and keep your poop away from your bloodstream. If you don't have enough butyrate, the cells in your intestinal lining starve. They start to pull apart and no longer provide a robust barrier between the fecal matter inside your intestines and the entire rest of your body. You don't want toxins, pathogens, and foreign molecules migrating through your intestinal wall into your bloodstream. They cause inflammation and autoimmune disease and contribute to a host of other health conditions.[12,13]

We call this leaky gut, and it is really bad for you. Butyrate is really good for you. Exercise is one of the best ways to get your gut microbiome to produce more butyrate.

Your PCOS body was designed for exercise

A lot of this book has been pretty gloom and doom about PCOS because modern day PCOS comes with a lot of pretty bad health symptoms and risks. "Modern day" is the critical phrase here. Remember, historically, having PCOS was an *advantage*. And one reason our grandmothers did so well is that PCOS increases your capacity to build muscle mass. PCOS makes you strong!

Testosterone is a performance enhancing drug. Athletes are banned from taking it. But, you naturally have an extra supply. When scientists looked at female Olympians, they discovered that around 40% of them have PCOS. That is four times higher than PCOS rates in the general population. Rates of PCOS were even higher when they looked at sports that require explosive power, like hockey and wrestling. PCOS women make incredible athletes.[14]

When matched for body composition, every PCOS woman, athlete or not, including you, is stronger than a non-PCOS woman. That means that right now, you are stronger than a non-PCOS woman who looks just like you.[15]

Not only that, when you increase your physical activity, you can build strength and oxygen capacity faster than the average woman. No matter what shape you are in today, if you have PCOS, that means you have a body that was designed to move!

When is the best time to exercise?

Now, since I talk so much about circadian rhythm, it's reasonable to ask, "Is there a best time to exercise?" The answer is a resounding, "Sort of."

Your body changes throughout the day so exercising at different times can do different things. Morning is better for weight loss. Afternoon and evening are better for strengthening. But, honestly, there isn't a bad time to exercise.[16,17]

The best time to exercise is any time you do it.

A path forward

Exercise is critical for good health. I'm sure that's not telling you anything new. But if you aren't exercising, I hope that you will start. Whether you are overweight or lean, PCOS has disrupted your gut microbiome and regular, moderate exercise is a fabulous way to heal it.

Just be safe. Any time a person starts a new exercise program, she risks injuring herself. If you are overweight, generally sedentary, already injured, or worried about getting injured, I recommend that you work with a personal trainer that specializes in women with your body type, fitness level, and fitness goals.

Move every day

A solid exercise plan that I personally have great success with is this: Move every day and exercise more rigorously for one hour, three times per week.

Moving is basically anything that is the opposite of sitting. Sitting as a daily activity is really terrible for you, so get up.[18]

Whenever you can, go for a walk. Garden. Go shopping in an actual store. Clean your house. Carry heavy things like groceries and children. Take the stairs.

When you are at work, if you have a desk job where you sit a lot, do "dynamic sitting." Sit on an exercise ball or a wobble stool instead of a chair or get an under-table fidget bar. Yes, this is a real thing and it can approximate walking at 2 mph! Take hourly stretching breaks. Get up frequently, even if it's just to grab a glass of water or use the bathroom. And when you can, opt for walking meetings.[19,20]

Move as much as you can. In all cases, any activity is better than none. Even fidgeting.

One powerful way to increase your daily movement is to wear an electronic fitness tracker, like a Fitbit. When people start a new exercise routine and wear a Fitbit, they move more than people who wear a simple pedometer or no tracking device.[21]

So move, move, move, and track your progress.

Take a walk after meals

A cool thing about exercise is that it's cumulative. You can do it all at once or you can sprinkle it throughout the day.

Probably the most successful advice I give to patients is, "Go for a 10-minute walk after every meal." It's a relatively easy thing to add to your day, and it gets you 30 minutes of daily movement.

Walking is really incredible for you. It's cheap, generally accessible, and is safe for pretty much everyone. And walking after meals improves your blood sugar levels and reduces insulin spikes more than resting or strenuous exercise, which is a huge bonus for us insulin resistant PCOS ladies.[22]

Plus, since you're not going to the gym or working up a sweat, you don't have to spend all of that extra time driving to and from the gym, changing clothes, and showering.

Working out can be kind of a production. Going for a walk is lovely.

Do something fun

Now, I've got to ask, "How do you feel about the gym?"

Because once you've figured out how to move every day, you still need to do more vigorous exercise for about one hour, three times per week.

Some people really like the gym. They put on headphones and work up a sweat. At the gym, you can focus and you can work out in exactly the way you want to.

Other people hate the gym. As in, they loathe it.

Personally, I'm sort of in the middle. If given a choice, I'll always choose the non-gym exercise option. Obviously, if you like the gym, knock yourself out. If you don't, then don't go to the gym.

Newsflash: You do not have to go to the gym to get fit.

You just need to move your body and you don't need the gym to do that. Trust me, our ancestors were in much better shape than most of us are today, and they didn't even have gyms.

So, my advice is to find something active that feels fun and you can enjoy doing a few times per week.

Here are some non-gym things to try.

- **Biking:** This is a non-weight bearing sport that can be great for people with injuries, especially joint problems. In many communities, you can also use your bike as a meaningful form of transportation.

- **Dancing:** Dance is a great way to get a full-body cardio workout that also includes balance and flexibility. Work with the teacher to adjust movements for your fitness and ability level. If you dance, there are so many different types — ballet, zumba, pole dancing, jazzercise — you will never get bored.

- **Golfing:** This is a skills sport enjoyed by people of all ages. There's something of a steep learning curve, but once you can hit the ball a moderate distance, you'll have a sport you can play for practically the rest of your life. The average golfer who walks an 18-hole course instead of using a golf cart will walk over five miles so this really is great exercise![23]

- **Hiking:** It's like walking, but in nature. Hiking is great because you can cover longer distances, and the natural, uneven trails are wonderful for balance.

- **Intramural sports:** Most communities have teams for adults to play a wide range of fun sports, including ultimate frisbee, flag football, broomball, soccer, softball, and dodgeball. The scheduled practices and games and the social support of being on a team make it easier to stick with it than a lot of other activities.

- **Rock climbing:** This sport is incredible for building balance and full body strength, with a focus on arm strength. Don't be intimidated by the gear. It's really not that hard to learn, and lots of women climb these days.

- **Running:** Running is popular because you can probably step out of your front door to do it and all you need is a pair of running shoes. However, be careful here. Novice runners, and particularly overweight novice runners, have very high injury rates. So if you want to start running, start *slowly.* [24]

- **Stand up paddle boarding:** SUPing builds balance and upper body strength. And if you go out on a lake in the morning when it's still and quiet, it's extremely meditative.

- **Swimming:** This sport is great for everyone, but it's especially helpful for anyone who has an injury because it's non-weight bearing. A bonus is that if the pool temperature is cool, it will rev up your metabolism.[25]

- **Yoga:** Yoga builds strength, flexibility, and balance, and the meditative aspect lowers stress. In a recent study of PCOS women, women who practiced yoga improved their hormonal profiles and menstrual regularity more than women who did comparable other exercises. Plus, yoga is an activity that you can do for your whole life.[26]

I can't mention everything here because there are so many fun ways to get your move on! I left out tennis, tai chi, CrossFit, racketball, gymnastics, and karate, to name a few. And by the way, I don't care how old you are. You are never too old to learn a new sport.

In fact, physical activity is one of the best things you can do to prevent physical and mental aging. So if you want to stay young, move![27]

One reason I listed a bunch of activities here is that I also want you to mix it up so you are doing different things. You want to use your body in a lot of ways so you build all of your muscles. You also want to weatherproof your workout so you can go outside on nice days and stay inside on hot, rainy, or snowy days.

All of this variety creates physical resiliency.

Focus on functional fitness

When I talk about physical fitness with my patients, I focus on "functional fitness," which means getting your body in shape so that you can comfortably perform the activities that make your life wonderful. This is important for non-athletes and athletes alike.

It's about walking distances that allow you to enjoy your community. It's about maintaining your home and participating in activities with friends and family. It's about having the confidence to try something new without worrying about hurting yourself. It's about having a body that is fit in the right ways to enable a life that feels good. And you get to decide what that means for you.

On a practical level, this means exercising in ways that promote strength, cardiovascular fitness, flexibility, and balance.

Very few activities cover all four areas of functional fitness, which is another reason I recommend mixing things up. You can pair zumba with yoga, or SUPing with swimming. Keep it fun. Keep it interesting. And keep it new!

Exercise whenever you can

Every organ in your body has its own clocks, including your muscles. So it makes sense that there is a circadian rhythm to exercise. It's true that there are benefits to exercising at different times of the day, but that being said, no one has ever found a really bad time to exercise, except maybe in the middle of the night when you should be asleep.

If you are able to exercise in the morning before breakfast, you will maximize weight loss. When you wake up, you are in a fasted state. Your glycogen stores are gone, and, assuming you had an early dinner the night before, your metabolism has already shifted to fat burning. If you exercise in this fasting state, you will burn even more fat and lose weight.[28]

The optimal weight-loss schedule is to wake up and exercise first thing. After your workout, wait another 30 minutes before eating to take full advantage of your post exercise fat-burning capacity. Maybe take a shower and get ready. And then eat a large, healthy breakfast.

As an added bonus, morning exercise seems to inhibit food cravings later in the day so it may make your time-restricted eating routine easier.[29]

If afternoon or evening activities are better for you, you should work out with confidence knowing that this is when your muscles perform the best. If you are hoping to improve strength or flexibility, you'll see more gains if you exercise later in the day. Afternoon activity also has the greatest impact on regulating your circadian rhythm.[30]

So if you have the freedom to schedule your workouts, focus on the mornings for weight loss and the afternoons and evenings for building strength and flexibility. But don't sweat it. Squeeze in movement whenever you can.

Troubleshooting

Starting and then sticking to a new exercise routine is notoriously hard. Every year, a kazillion people make a new year's resolution to get in shape, and maybe three of them succeed. We are busy. We have our daily habits and they are hard to change. Here are some of my best tips for how to make exercise a positive and consistent part of your life.

I don't like exercise.
If you are obese, your obesity may cause you to move less and tire quickly. Hating exercise can actually be a symptom of obesity. This is because obesity causes inflammation and inflammation causes fatigue.

You are *not* lazy. Your body is fighting an incessant battle with inflammation and so your body doesn't want to exercise.[31]

Be kind to yourself and have faith that this feeling will go away as you bring your inflammation under control. You come from a long line of strong women. That strength is in you. It's literally in your genes.

Also, remember that you are in this for the long run, as in, for your whole life. Start slowly and find something that you enjoy. Not to be trite, but, just do it!

I don't have any time.
I know! It's so hard to make time for exercise. I don't have any time either.

My best advice is to prioritize non-athletic daily movement. Add physical activities like walking, lifting, carrying, and taking stairs, into your regular day in every single way you can. Tiny bits of movement, done frequently, add up.

Then, find an activity you love. Find something that you love so much that you will compromise on something else in your life to fit this activity into your schedule. And then put it on your schedule. No excuses.

I love stand up paddle boarding. There are a couple of beautiful lakes near my house, and I go out early in the morning. It's cool and quiet and I can hear the paddle dipping in and out of the water. Sometimes I see cranes hunting along the banks or fish rising and forming ripples across the surface of the water.

It's not the most vigorous exercise in the world, but paddling is good for my arms and back. It quiets my mind. And if my balance is off, I fall in, and then I've mixed things up by adding swimming!

I keep "forgetting."

If you somehow keep getting to the end of your day and discovering that despite the best of intentions, you did not exercise again, here are some tips for turning intentions into action.

- Do something you can look forward to. If you find something that you enjoy, it will be easier to prioritize it.

- Start small. If your proposed exercise routine overwhelms you, go smaller. Every movement you add to your life is an improvement. So do what you can do, and then slowly add more.

- Get an electronic fitness tracker, like a Fitbit. When people frequently check in on their progress, they make more progress.

- Hire a personal trainer. If you develop a good relationship with a trainer, you are more likely to stick with your exercise program and see great results.[32]

- Go to scheduled classes and pay ahead of time. It's much easier to follow through on a plan when the plan is concrete and specific. Also, if you go to the same class every week, you will build relationships, which brings me to my next tip.[33]

- Get a fitness buddy. Social support is one of those things that consistently helps everyone stick to a new habit or goal. Find a friend to exercise with or at least find someone to check up on your progress every so often.[34]

I'm ill, injured, or disabled.

If you face physical challenges when it comes to exercise, I highly recommend that you work with a trainer who specializes in women of your age, weight, ability, and fitness level.

If you are able to walk, start with walking. Most people can walk safely and this is a great way to begin building strength. There are also some fabulous water fitness classes and yoga classes that cater to people with mobility challenges.

If you live in a metro area, seek out an adaptive fitness center. They specialize in training people with a wide array of disabilities and injuries. Unfortunately, not every community has one of these incredible centers, but if you are lucky enough to live near one, you should definitely take advantage of this amazing resource.

Exercise makes me hungry.

Different people respond differently to exercise. For most people, exercise is an appetite suppressant. Those lucky ducks will exercise and then feel less hungry all day so it becomes easier to stick to their timed eating regimen. Other people end up feeling famished. It's impossible to predict how any one person will react, but if you are in the "I am starving!" camp, you might be worried that exercise will make you *gain* weight.[35]

First off, exercise is good for you, no matter what you weigh. So please don't quit. Keep it up!

My advice is to eat what you need to eat in order to feel good. Remember, I do not recommend calorie restriction. Just stick to your time-restricted eating schedule. Eat within your eating window. Focus on having a big, healthy breakfast. If exercise makes you crave sweets, have your dessert with your breakfast when your insulin is most effective.

Also, make sure you get your bright morning light. Light therapy helps treat binge eating and other eating disorders.[36]

I really want to lose weight.

When people exercise, they always improve their body composition. They add muscle. They may lose some belly fat. But in general, when they lose weight, it's moderate at best. That being said, there are some ways to really target weight loss.

One way is to exercise in a fasted state. Often, people do this in the morning before breakfast. If you do moderate exercise after fasting for 10 to 12 hours, your body will be in fat-burning mode and you will use your fat stores for energy.

You also may want to try HIIT. It's hot!

HIIT stands for high-intensity interval training, and it is the best exercise routine for most people who want to lose body fat, with a few caveats. Basically, in a HIIT routine, you work out at peak intensity for short bursts of time, followed by short rest periods. One of the benefits of HIIT is that you can get a serious workout done in 30 minutes.

However, be really careful. HIIT is strenuous, so even beginner routines require a base level of fitness. Most women need to train to get ready for it. Also, it is not comfortable. It's really hard to push yourself to your limits. Most people do best when they take a class or use a trainer because it's hard to do something that feels crappy. Be safe. Anytime you are working at your limit, you run the risk of injury. Again, working with a knowledgeable trainer can make HIIT safer.

But, if you are careful and safe and you do a HIIT routine that makes sense for you, it really is an incredible way to lose weight, increase strength, and build overall health. A recent study compared HIIT to moderate intensity sustained exercise, and women who did HIIT were able to exercise for half the time of the sustained exercise group and saw as good or better results.[37]

A quick summary

Gut microbiome diversity is critical for maintaining circadian rhythm and supporting overall health. Unfortunately, women with PCOS have less gut microbiome diversity. Fortunately, exercise increases gut microbiome diversity and promotes the growth of especially helpful bacteria. We all need to exercise to stay healthy.

- Move every day.
- Take a walk after meals.
- Do something fun and strenuous three times per week.
- Focus on functional fitness.
- Time your workouts to your fitness goals.

Healthy habits to get you started

- [ ] Wear a fitness tracker like a Fitbit.

- [ ] Always take the farthest parking spot and always take the stairs.

- [ ] Whenever you can do so safely, carry your groceries to your car instead of wheeling them in the grocery cart.

- [ ] Any time it's appropriate, sit on the ground. Getting up and down off the ground is a skill you never want to lose.

- [ ] Stretch your muscles while watching TV.

- [ ] Take a walk after dinner. Or after breakfast. Or after lunch. Or all three!

- [ ] Make an appointment with a fitness trainer. You can find one at a local gym where you feel comfortable working out.

- [ ] Sign up for a recurring exercise class and prepay.

- [ ] Find an exercise buddy.

- [ ] Try a new sport or fitness activity.

- [ ] Block off fitness time on your calendar.

CHAPTER 9

STEP 5:
Feed your gut

*O*ur bacterial cells outnumber our human cells 10:1 and our bacterial DNA outnumber our human DNA 100:1. You really are more bacteria than human.[1]

These microbes live in communities on your skin and in your mouth, vagina, and gastrointestinal tract, or gut. Your gut microbiome is a collection of around 100 trillion microbes found mostly in your large intestine, or colon.

Your gut microbiome is essential for maintaining circadian rhythm because it is the primary timesetter for your liver, which then orchestrates metabolism. Circadian rhythm and metabolism are two reasons a healthy gut microbiome is essential for healing PCOS.

There are three additional jobs that the gut microbiome performs that help determine the severity of your PCOS — digestion, immune system programming, and hormonal regulation.

Your gut and digestion

It's not surprising that a healthy gut microbiome promotes healthy digestion, both nutritionally and functionally.

Specific microbes digest all sorts of food molecules that humans otherwise cannot, converting them to compounds essential for good nutrition. Specific bacteria deconstruct proteins into amino acids. Other bacteria synthesize vitamin K and many B vitamins. Several bacterial populations work together to break down polyphenols, powerful nutrients from plants. When people have less diverse, unhealthy microbiomes, they are not able to extract the anti-inflammatory, antioxidant, and anti-cancer nutrients found in many foods.[2]

There are also certain bacteria that turn our food into harmful compounds. Meat, fish, dairy, and eggs contain choline and carnitine. If you eat a lot of meat, your microbiome develops a large population of bacteria that metabolise choline and carnitine into trimethylamine, which the liver then converts to trimethylamine-N-oxide (TMAO). A high TMAO level strongly predicts atherosclerosis, heart disease, kidney disease, and stroke, and it is likely one of the biggest reasons that eating a lot of meat is bad for you.[3,4]

While your gut microbiome digests your food, it orchestrates the food's movement through your digestive tract. Bacteria release gas and neurotransmitters that stimulate colonic movement. When all goes well, everything moves at a comfortable speed, never too fast, never too slow, and always in the right direction.[5]

For the 40% of PCOS women with irritable bowel syndrome, digestion is not this simple. Women with irritable bowel syndrome have an altered gut microbiome that changes their gut function. They may regularly experience constipation, diarrhea, bloating, cramping, and excessive gas, often accompanied by severe pain.[6,7]

Surprisingly, even gastrointestinal pain is impacted by the microbiome. In a healthy microbiome, certain bacteria desensitize intestinal nerve endings and pain receptors so the digestive tract can expand and move pain-free. Gut dysbiosis prevents these bacteria from doing their job and causes hypersensitivity in the nerves surrounding the digestive tract, increasing the perception of pain.[8]

In terms of digestion, a healthy gut microbiome improves your nutrition and maintains digestive comfort. A dysbiotic gut gives you cardiovascular disease and irritable bowel syndrome, two conditions that are common among PCOS women.

Your gut and your immune system

The gut is home to 70% of your immune system because eating is the most dangerous thing you do. Your digestive tract handles more toxins and pathogens than any other part of your body.

Your immune system and your gut microbiome have an amazing, delicately balanced relationship that is fine-tuned for mutual survival. You and your microbiome both benefit when pathogenic bacteria are controlled so your microbiome trains your immune cells to recognize and quickly destroy these bacteria. Simultaneously, your microbiome triggers your immune system to release Treg (TEE-reg) immune cells that down-regulate your immune and inflammatory responses to benign cells and molecules, reducing autoimmunity and allergies.

An unhealthy gut microbiome does not properly moderate and program your immune system. It doesn't control pathogens. It doesn't target inflammation towards infections and away from your own cells. Consequently, gut dysbiosis contributes to run-away inflammation and increases your risk of autoimmune disease, two more factors that make PCOS much worse.[9,10]

Your gut and your hormones

Additionally, your gut microbiome balances the levels, rhythms, and availability of several important messenger molecules. Your gut produces 90% of your body's serotonin, a feel-good neurotransmitter that stabilizes your mood and the nerves throughout your body. Serotonin is a primary building block of melatonin, an antioxidant hormone that regulates your sleep-wake cycle. So a healthy gut microbiome improves mood, sleep, and the overall functioning of your central nervous system.[11,12,13,14,15]

Your gut also plays a critical role in the activation and metabolism of estrogen. In the female body, everything eventually ties back to estrogen, and gut health is no different.

A subset of the bacteria living in your gut are called the "estrobolome" (ess-TRAWB-oh-lome) and they recycle your estrogen. When naturally circulating estrogen in your bloodstream gets to your liver, your liver binds the estrogen into larger molecules that can be excreted through your urine or stool. In your gut, certain bacteria contain a special enzyme that frees your estrogen and puts it back into circulation in your body.[16]

Women with a healthy gut microbiome have a healthy estrobolome and higher levels of recirculating estrogens. In contrast, women with PCOS seem to have higher levels of recirculating androgens and lower levels of recirculating estrogens. It's as if our bodies are conserving testosterone and giving away the small, precious amounts of estrogen that we have![17,18]

A tantalizing new study suggests that fixing the PCOS microbiome can increase estrogen and decrease testosterone levels. In the study, PCOS rats received a fecal microbiota transplantation (FMT). Basically, scientists took poop from healthy, non-PCOS rats and inserted it into the colons of PCOS rats so that the bacteria from the healthy rats could colonize the intestines of PCOS rats. After the FMT, PCOS rats had increased cycling estrogen, lower testosterone, and their previously polycystic ovaries healed into normally functioning ovaries. By healing the estrobolome, scientists reversed PCOS.[19]

It's premature to recommend fecal transplants for PCOS women, but it's pretty clear that healing the gut microbiome is essential to healing PCOS. A healthy gut microbiome synchronizes your circadian rhythm, normalizes your metabolism, promotes healthy digestion, programs your immune system, and balances your hormones. It is likely even a source of free estrogen.

Nurturing a healthy microbiome

There are two key characteristics of a healthy, happy gut microbiome. One we talked about in the last chapter, diversity. The other is balance.

A diverse gut microbiome is exactly what it sounds like: a microbiome populated with lots and lots of different types of microbes. The more variety the better. This creates stability and resilience in the microbial community.

A balanced gut microbiome is a little harder to quantify. It primarily contains microbes that best align with your health. You need lots of bacteria that produce nutrients, serotonin, and short-chain fatty acids, especially butyrate. You need bacteria that can properly program your immune system. You need a robust estrobolome. A balanced microbiome produces hundreds of essential compounds and performs hundreds of different jobs in the body. We need the right numbers of all the right microbes to get these jobs done.

At the same time, we want to limit the microbes that produce toxins. Some bacteria, such as e-coli, produce endotoxins that cause inflammation and are linked to diabetes and heart disease. Others produce TMAO, which also causes heart disease. Certain bacteria are associated with higher rates of cancer, mental health disorders, irritable bowel syndrome, asthma, and allergies. In fact, researchers right now are exploring whether Parkinson's and other neurodegenerative diseases start in the gut. Everyone has some bad bacteria in their guts, but you really, really, really don't want a lot of them.[20,21,22,23]

So how do we create a diverse, resilient gut microbiome that has more good bacteria than bad bacteria and can perform all of the functions that we need it to? This ecosystem is too complex to simply take a probiotic capsule or otherwise artificially manufacture a perfect microbiome. At least today, we have to do this the old fashioned way.

Exercise is the first half of the equation. Good bacteria love exercise.

The second half is food. Good bacteria and bad bacteria eat totally different diets. Good bacteria love fruits and vegetables. Bad bacteria love sugar, fat, and processed foods.

This makes complete sense when you think about it. We all know that fruits and vegetables are good for us. But why? Part of the reason is that they are full of nutrients, which our human cells need. But the other part of it is that they are full of fiber. Humans for the most part cannot digest fiber. But guess who can? The beneficial bacteria in your gut.

They *need* fiber. It is absolutely essential to their survival. The more high-fiber foods you eat, the more beneficial bacteria you will have in your gut microbiome. It really is that simple.

In contrast, bad bacteria love junk food. And perhaps more than that, they love all of the free space that your good bacteria leave behind when they starve to death from lack of fiber in your diet.

As complex as our microbiome is, to make it healthy and get the full benefits of a balanced and diverse gut microbiome, all you need is exercise and plant fiber.

Your hunter-gatherer ancestors ate 100 to 150 grams of fiber every day. So even though PCOS predisposed your female ancestors to gut dysbiosis, they had plenty of beneficial gut microbes to offset this risk because they ate tons of fiber. A high-fiber diet was another lifestyle condition that kept ancient PCOS mild.[24]

Compare the fiber content of an ancient diet to today's standard diet.

Most Americans eat between 5 and 14 grams of fiber per day. The USDA recommends 28 grams per day for someone eating a 2000 calorie diet. This is about as much fiber as most people who are trying to eat healthy take in. The only people who eat more fiber are vegetarians, who average 32 grams per day, and vegans, who eat about 40 grams per day.[25,26]

It is extremely hard to eat enough fiber because most of us eat some variation of the Standard American Diet. Heavy in sugar, fat, and white flour, this diet primarily feeds the bad bacteria and may be one of the worst diets ever created for gut microbiome health and for the overall health of PCOS women.

To heal your PCOS, you need to eat differently. You need to eat for your gut microbiome.

A path forward

So here's the plan: Feed the good guys and starve the bad guys.

Think of your gut microbiome as a pet bunny. Really, there are more accurate analogies — a garden, a rainforest, a society — but because we are so connected to our microbiome, it's helpful to imagine it as a personal pet that goes everywhere with you. Like a pet bunny, your microbiome is a living thing that depends on you for its survival. It needs you to feed it, to nurture it, to give it exercise, and, obviously, to not abuse or poison it.

Just like a real pet bunny, this microbiome pet bunny really likes to eat plants. The more, the better.

Eat mostly plants

The diet I recommend is simple. Eat mostly foods that come from plants — fruits, vegetables, beans, nuts, and whole grains. You can eat them fresh or cook them however you want. You can use spices and sauces. You can get them canned, jarred, and frozen.

Of course there are more and less healthy ways to eat your plants and I'll explain that in a bit. But at the end of the day, the most important thing is to eat lots and lots of plants so that you support a large microbiome of beneficial, plant-eating bacteria.

There are several ways to approach this:

- If you look at your plate, at every meal and at every mini-meal (a.k.a. snack), at least three-quarters of your plate should be plants.

- If you break your meal into courses, the first course should be one to two cups of fruit or veggies. I like to start every meal, including breakfast, with a big salad made from at least two cups of greens with nuts and veggies on top.

- Aim for six to nine cups of plant-based foods every day. That's two to three full cups of plants at breakfast, lunch, and dinner.

The rest of your diet can include meat, fish, poultry, and eggs. You can have your favorite foods. You can have dessert, especially at breakfast.

The thing is, if you focus on eating a lot of plants, almost everything else dietary-wise will fall into place because you just won't have room in your stomach for significant quantities of unhealthy foods. You'll naturally eat less bread, pasta, French fries, burgers, granola bars, and ice cream, because, seriously, where are you going to put them?

Eat as much fiber as you can

When you select plant-based foods, make sure that some of them are exceptionally high-fiber. Your microbiome bunny needs a large quantity and variety of fiber to stay healthy. More fiber is always better.

Try to eat at least 30 grams of fiber every day. It's less than our ancestors ate but at least three times as much as the average American.

Below is an example of how to eat 30 grams of fiber. I suggest you use this as a template because it provides a good range of fibers and nutrients.

1 cup of beans (any type)	15 grams (You're halfway there!)
1 apple with skin	4 grams
1 tablespoon of flaxseed	3 grams
3 cups of salad greens	3 grams (This gets you to 25 grams!)
¼ cup of nuts/seeds	3 grams
½ cup of any fruit or veggie	2 grams (That's 30 grams!)

I eat beans or lentils almost every day because they are one of the highest fiber foods out there, averaging a whopping 15 grams per cup.

Most fruits, vegetables, and grains average three to five grams of fiber per cup. Salad greens are generally one gram of fiber per cup.

High-fiber foods form the backbone of a high-fiber diet. Here are some of my favorites:

- Beans and lentils: 10 to 16 grams per cup; most are 15 grams per cup
- Raspberries and blackberries: 8 grams per cup
- Artichokes: 10 grams per medium artichoke
- Green peas: 9 grams per cup
- Avocado: 9 grams per medium avocado
- Chia seeds: 5.5 grams per tablespoon[27,28,29]

Even when you include at least one of these foods in your daily diet, you still need about six cups of plant-based foods to reach 30 grams of fiber. Two cups per meal is a great rule of thumb. And remember, 30 grams is the minimum. There is no maximum.

If you are worried about the effect of all this fiber on your digestion, you can increase your serving over the course of several weeks.

In a study about beans and gas (yes, scientists study this), participants ate ½ cup of beans every day for eight weeks. At the end of the first week, 35% felt gassy, but this number dropped rapidly. After four weeks, only 11% were gassy, and by the end of eight weeks, only 3% of participants were still experiencing increased flatulence. Note that a full 65% of people experienced no noticeable change in flatulence, and in all cases, the flatulence was tolerable enough that no participants dropped out of the study.[30]

So, don't be afraid of fiber. Change your diet slowly and see how you feel.

I recommend increasing your daily fiber by about 5 grams per week, and even in the beginning, eat half a cup of beans every day. If you feel gassy or uncomfortable, stay at your current fiber intake level until your microbiome adjusts and you feel better. Then add more fiber until you get to 30 grams per day.

Homemade beans taste better than canned beans, are much cheaper, and don't come in containers that may be lined with toxic chemicals (more about that in the next chapter!). But, making your own beans from scratch is time consuming ... unless you have an Instant Pot. The Instant Pot is a bean game-changer. You can go from a bag of rock-hard dry beans to a pot of ready-to-eat deliciousness in under an hour.

It's also great for brown rice, stews, and homemade broth.

If you can afford it and have a spot in your kitchen to store it, I highly recommend that everybody get an Instant Pot.

Eat the rainbow

Your body needs hundreds of different nutrients, and your microbiome bunny needs dozens of types of fibers to stay healthy. It's impossible to plan a diet that systematically includes them all, so instead, think about eating colors. The pigments in plants are created by various phytochemicals that each have unique health benefits. If you eat plant-based foods that naturally come in all of the colors of the rainbow, you'll get a wide range of nutrients for you and your microbiome bunny.

Only naturally occurring food colors count. Artificial food colors are chemicals made in a lab and have been linked to cancer, neurotoxicity, and behavior problems.[31]

Try to eat at least three natural plant colors at every meal, and make sure that you eat one fruit or vegetable of every color of the rainbow at least every other day. By mixing up the color palate on your plate, you'll have a healthy, well-rounded diet and a healthy, well-rounded microbiome.

Eat organic

To whatever degree your budget will allow, eat organic. I know, I know, I know. Organic food is so expensive. And sometimes, you can't even get it. But eating organic is really important.

Organic foods are healthier than their conventional counterparts. Organic fruits and vegetables have more antioxidants and nutrients than conventional produce. Organic meats and dairy have more omega-3s. And on top of that, organic foods have fewer pesticide residues.[32,33]

Here's why you should care about pesticides. While scientists and lobbyists debate the impacts that these chemicals have on human cells, we have clear scientific data showing that these chemicals harm your gut microbiome bunny.

Exposure to one of the most widely used types of insecticides, organophosphates, causes insulin resistance by changing short-chain fatty acid production and impairing the gut's ability to regulate the liver, leading to uncontrolled gluconeogenesis (release of sugars and fats into the bloodstream) and eventually diabetes.[34,35]

Additionally, the world's most commonly used herbicide, glyphosate, known by its trade name Roundup, kills off several beneficial microbiome bacteria and seems to favor pathogenic bacteria that produce neurotoxins.[36]

When you eat organic foods, you protect your fragile microbiome from poisons that selectively kill some of your most critical bacteria.

If you can't afford to go 100% organic, choose organic when you buy the "dirty dozen," the most pesticide-laden produce according Environment Working Group (www.ewg.org/foodnews/dirty-dozen.php):

1. Strawberries
2. Spinach
3. Nectarines
4. Apples
5. Grapes
6. Peaches
7. Cherries
8. Pears
9. Tomatoes
10. Celery
11. Potatoes
12. Sweet bell peppers

Also choose organic for any foods that are a staple of your diet. That will go a long way toward reducing your pesticide exposure.

To date, we really don't know what level of exposure to pesticides is safe for our microbiome and consequently, for us. But, honestly, it's probably pretty darn close to zero.

Eat raw and minimally processed foods

A raw food is anything that hasn't been cooked. Raw fruits and vegetables are a critical part of a healthy diet because certain essential nutrients like vitamin C, carotenoids, and some antioxidants are destroyed by heat. A diet rich in raw fruits and vegetables lowers blood pressure and protects against heart disease. People who eat more raw fruits and veggies have better mental health and lower levels of depression and anxiety. Additionally, raw plant-based foods are covered in many bacteria colonies that can help populate your gut microbiome and improve your immune system.[37,38,39]

So eat lots of salads, fresh fruit, raw nuts, and carrot sticks.

It is also critical to eat minimally processed foods.

When we think about "processed foods," most people imagine sweet and salty snacks that come wrapped in bright cellophane packages. "Processed food" is often synonymous with "bad for you." But that's not fair or accurate.

Cooking, fermenting, canning, and whatever is done to corn to make cheese puffs are all forms of food processing. Food processing is any method of changing food after its harvest, so technically, everything we eat except whole, raw fruits and vegetables are processed foods.

Some forms of minimal food processing actually make food safer and *more* nutritious.

Cooking, the most ancient method of processing food, increases the availability of calories and specific nutrients in plants. It kills pathogens and makes meat safe. It softens food and makes tubers and grains edible. Cooking shaped our evolution as humans by expanding our potential food sources and allowing us to get more energy from less food in less time, freeing our ancestors to develop art, culture, and technology. Cooking is great. Without cooking, we wouldn't be human.[40,41]

Fermentation is another ancient form of food processing that employs bacteria or yeast to convert sugars to lactic acid. Historically used to preserve foods before the invention of refrigeration, fermentation increases foods' nutritional quality and, importantly, supplies your gut with a huge dose of healthy microbes. Fermented foods are alive with trillions of bacteria that can survive the journey through your digestive tract and improve the health of your microbiome.[42]

When buying fermented foods such as sauerkraut, kimchi, and kombucha, look for products that are still alive. These can be hard to find because live, fermented foods release bubbles and constantly expand. Left on a shelf in a jar for long enough, they explode. So, most companies heat pasteurize them, preserving the taste but killing the microbes, which means no explosions and no bacteria.

Your best bet is to check your grocery store's refrigerated section (that's where my local shop keeps a few varieties of live sauerkraut), or try a local health food store or farmer's market. If you're adventurous, you can make your own, and then you'll know you're getting a microbe-rich product.

Fermenting may be a bit outside your kitchen comfort zone at first, but you can make a fresh batch of sauerkraut in minutes. It's simple, fun, and practically foolproof. All you need is fresh cabbage, iodine-free salt, a tamper (to smoosh down the cabbage), and some jars. I really like *Fermented Vegetables* by Kirsten and Christopher Shockey as an intro.

A small, four-ounce serving of homemade sauerkraut has as many beneficial bacteria as 200 probiotic capsules from the supplements section of your local store. If you can ferment, your microbiome will thank you![43]

Canning and freezing are also excellent processing methods, preserving foods, often at the peak of freshness, and increasing the convenience and availability of nutritious foods year round.

Minimally processed foods are foods that have been cooked, fermented, canned, or frozen. So long as they aren't doctored up with lots of food additives like sugar, salt, and artificial ingredients, you should eat as much of these foods as you can.

Avoid highly processed foods

"Highly processed foods" are a totally different story. These are foods that have been processed in such a way that they no longer deliver the nutrition of natural foods, and they often contain unnatural ingredients that are bad for you.

In many of these foods, the nutritious parts are deliberately removed to enhance appearance and flavor. White rice and white flour lack their nutritious but firm brown bran. Potato chips lack potato skins. Applesauce doesn't include apple skins. Juice is missing the whole fruit.

Often, these food products are combined with food additives, colors, and flavors to make them look and taste good and last pretty much forever. This includes almost the entire snack aisle of the grocery store and covers most products that come in a box or a bag. It also includes most ready-to-eat convenience foods like microwave dinners, canned soups, and boxed mixes.

Some of these foods have undergone such a significant shift in form that they no longer resemble whatever they were when they were harvested. They have been ground up, separated into tiny components, mixed with fillers, and reformed into fun, novel shapes like hot dogs, chips, crackers, and any cereal that looks like balls, stars, or inner tubes.

Highly processed foods deliver a double whammy to your health. First of all, they usually contain chemicals and high levels of sugar, fat, and salt that are downright bad for you. These ingredients make you sick.

Secondly, these foods take the place of nutritious food in your diet. You are only going to eat so much during the day. If you fill up on junk food, how are you going to eat six to nine cups of fruits, vegetables, and whole grains? Every time you eat something bad for you, it's a missed opportunity to eat something healing and wholesome.

The simplest way to avoid highly processed foods is to buy fresh food and prepare it yourself. In most grocery stores, this means doing the vast majority of your shopping along the outer perimeter of the store where you'll usually find fruits, vegetables, meat, and eggs.

I only buy a couple of minimally processed items from the inner aisles of my grocery store. These are grains like quinoa and buckwheat; dried foods like beans, raisins, dates, and nuts; cooking essentials like oil, salt, and spices; hot drink items like tea, coffee, and almond milk; jarred basics like stewed tomatoes, olives, and pickles; and simple condiments like vinegar and mustard. Everything else that I buy and eat is a fruit, a vegetable, or a protein.

Limit sugar, fat, and salt

When you buy processed food, you need to read the label.

This is another reason I try to avoid processed foods — I hate reading labels. But for most people, including me, it's not feasible to make everything from scratch. So, I try to buy the healthiest products available without making myself too crazy.

One rule is to limit sugar, fat, and salt.

Sugar

Here, I mean added sugars — cane sugar, high fructose corn syrup, fruit juice concentrate, maple syrup, honey, agave nectar — not the sugars that occur naturally in fruits and vegetables. Check the ingredients. If any sweetener is one of the first three to five ingredients, look for a less sweetened option.

Even if you don't have diabetes, you should eat like you do because women with PCOS have quadruple the risk of developing type 2 diabetes compared to non-PCOS women, and we develop it years earlier. Reducing your sugar intake will dramatically reduce your risk of type 2 diabetes.[44]

All women with PCOS are insulin resistant. No matter how good we are with circadian rhythm and exercise, no matter how many supplements and how much fiber we consume, our bodies are always just a little bit insulin resistant.

This has likely been true for PCOS women throughout history. Our ancestors weren't diabetic, but they didn't handle sugar well. Of course, it didn't matter because who was eating tons of sugar back then? It didn't exist.

But now sugar is in *everything!*

Here's a fun fact: There are 4 grams of sugar in a teaspoon. Keep that in mind next time you look at a food label. It's pretty rare to find a processed food item with less than 2 teaspoons (8 grams) of sugar per serving!

The average American consumes about 65 pounds of sugar a year (almost 20 teaspoons every single day). And it is linked to virtually every chronic health condition, not just diabetes.[45]

Sugar causes obesity. It causes non-alcoholic fatty liver disease and heart disease. It impacts mental health and is linked to depression, mood disorders, and Alzheimer's disease. Sugar increases your risk of endometrial cancer and not only that, it feeds cancer cells so they grow more quickly.[46,47,48,49,50,51]

A high-sugar diet is really terrible for you because sugar is inflammatory. Every time you eat sugar, you trigger your body's immune system to create inflammation. The more sugar you eat, the more inflammation you create. Guess what your PCOS body doesn't need more of? Inflammation.[52]

So stick to a low-sugar diet.

Fat

Keep your eye on your fat intake. There is nothing wrong with reasonable amounts of fat in your diet. Fat contains and facilitates the absorption of critical fat-soluble vitamins — vitamins A, E, and K. You need fat, just not a lot. An ideal diet is moderate- to low-fat, where 25% to 30% of your calories come from fat. Anything higher or lower leads to poorer health outcomes.[53]

Most people don't struggle with eating enough fat, but many people eat too much. A high-fat diet is toxic to your microbiome and causes inflammation.[54,55]

Specifically, fats reshape your microbiome into an "obesity microbiome" that is especially good at extracting calories from food. Several studies in rodents show that a high-fat diet causes obesity and leads to an altered microbiome. This obesity microbiome can be transferred via a fecal microbiota transplantation to non-obese mice, who then become obese, even when they eat a normal rodent diet. The obesity microbiome extracts and stores more energy from the same amount of food.[56,57]

We see an identical pattern in humans. If a person eats a high fat diet, she will get a dysbiotic, obesity microbiome. At that point, even when she eats healthy foods, she absorbs significantly more calories than someone with a non-obese microbiome and she stores more of those calories as fat.[58]

The best way to convert an obesity microbiome into a lean microbiome is to eat lots of plants and eat less fat.

So what does a diet look like where only 25% to 30% of calories come from fat? This is really hard to quantify because fat is calorie-dense and tends to be inside of other foods. We don't see the fat we eat. Also, some fats are better than others, and this can get really complicated really fast. So, here are a few simple guidelines to help you create a healthy, low- to moderate-fat diet.

So long as you don't go overboard, don't worry about:

- Fat found in fruits and vegetables, like avocados and nuts. In general, even though these are high-fat foods, they fill you up so well that you probably won't gorge on them. An avocado and a handful of nuts every day is a healthy, filling addition to almost any diet.

- Fat found in fatty fish like salmon and sardines. These are primarily omega-3 fatty acids and they are actually anti-inflammatory.

- Fat found in eggs and lean cuts of meat and poultry. This includes all chicken and turkey cuts, so long as you remove the skin, and most cuts of beef and pork that don't have significant visible fat.

Just stick to a 3 oz serving, which is about the size of a deck of cards or bar of soap.

- Fat of any type used for sautéing, so long as it's just a tablespoon or two.

If you get most of your fat from plant-based foods; moderate servings of fish, eggs, and lean meats; and a bit of cooking oil here and there, you'll be eating the right amount of fat.

In contrast, these are the foods that will push your diet into the high-fat zone. These foods are the biggest sources of dietary fat for most Americans, and they are also the most inflammatory types of fat. Try to limit or avoid:

- Fatty meats like bacon, sausage, hamburger, and baby back ribs.

- Processed meats like pepperoni and hot dogs.

- Dairy fat, especially anything with cream or cheese, including pizza, nachos, alfredo sauce, and dips.

- Fast food, especially deep-fried foods like French fries and fried chicken.

- Desserts, especially ice cream and baked goods like cookies and cakes.[59]

Get your dietary fat from plants, lean meats, and small amounts of fat used in cooking. Cut back on or cut out fatty meat, dairy, fast food, and dessert.

And then don't worry about it. Don't go fat free because you need some fats in your diet. Definitely don't choose low-fat processed foods over full-fat regular versions because low-fat items almost always have more sugar, and sugar is generally worse for you than fat. Just aim for moderation.[60]

Artificial trans fats are 100% bad for you and no amounts are safe. Fortunately, artificial trans fats, which are found in partially hydrogenated oils, were banned from American foods in June, 2018, with very few extensions. If you are outside the United States, you should check labels, and if you see any amount of partially hydrogenated oil, put the item back.[61]

Salt

Salt, like fat, is a necessary component of a healthy diet. As with fat, a lot of salt is not good for you.

Doctors have long recommended that patients with high blood pressure limit their salt intake because salt can cause strokes, cardiovascular disease, and heart attacks. Recent studies also show that salt stimulates specific immune cells called pathogenic TH17 cells, which cause a variety of autoimmune diseases.[62]

As with fat, too little salt is also bad for you and may actually increase your risk of heart disease.[63]

Consequently, most people should eat 1500 mg to 2300 mg of sodium per day, which is about a half teaspoon to just under one teaspoon of salt. Any more or any less will put your health at risk.

Today, most people eat much more than the recommended daily amount of salt. And most of this salt comes from fast food and processed food, not the little salt shaker on your table. So, yet again, my advice is to eat raw or minimally processed foods, and then just add the amount of salt that tastes good.[64]

Some sugars, fats, and salts are better than others. I am wary of delving too deeply into "choose this, not that" discussions because when eating plans become complicated, they become harder to stick to. But, if you are curious, here are the best choices for:

- **Sugar:** Choose honey and maple syrup because they contain nutrients and antioxidants. When purchasing honey, buy it from a farmers market or buy it organic. Otherwise, it may be thinned with corn syrup and contaminated with illegal antibiotics. For maple syrup, make sure it's actual maple syrup made from the sap of a maple tree. It should be watery, not thick and viscous. Grade B is darker than grade A and contains more nutrients. Pancake syrup, the kind that you get at a diner or in a woman-shaped bottle, is flavored corn syrup with caramel coloring and has no health benefits.[65,66,67]

- **Fat, for cooking:** Animal fats, such as lard or bacon grease, and coconut oil are more heat-stable than vegetable oils such as olive oil, canola oil, or sunflower oil. When liquid oils are heated to high temperatures, they go through a process called oxidation where they accumulate carcinogenic compounds. If you must cook with a liquid oil, choose olive oil because it's more heat stable than other oils.[68]

- **Fat, for salads:** If you are making a salad dressing, dip, or sauce that won't be heated, extra virgin olive oil is the clear winner. Its well-researched benefits include lowering inflammation, lowering your risk of cardiovascular disease, and lowering your risk of diabetes. Store your oil in a cool, dark place to keep it from going bad, and use it up within a year.[69,70]

- **Salt:** Choose sea salt or pink Himalayan salt because they are less likely to contribute to hypertension and they provide trace minerals that improve your health.

Avoid the "big six"

Some things we eat impede the healing process for PCOS women and undermine much of the good work we do in other areas of our lives. Even in moderation, they hurt you and your microbiome bunny. These are the six things you should not eat: alcohol, artificial sweeteners, antibiotics from agriculture, dairy, emulsifiers, and gluten.

Alcohol

Women with PCOS have double the risk of getting non-alcoholic fatty liver disease compared to women without PCOS. And although obesity is a significant risk factor, even lean PCOS women can develop fatty liver. PCOS is an enormous independent risk factor for fatty liver disease.[71]

If allowed to progress, this disease can lead to liver failure, liver cancer, and either a liver transplant or death. Non-alcoholic fatty liver disease is currently the fastest growing cause of liver transplants, especially among young adults.

There are two things you can do to lower your risk.

First, if you are overweight, you should lose weight. A whopping 80% of obese PCOS women have fatty liver. This book should help you do this.[72]

The other thing you should do is avoid alcohol like the plague.

I hate giving this advice because I love a nice glass of wine with dinner. Giving up alcohol entirely made me sad, but the science is what it is, whether we like it or not. And it's clear.

For all PCOS women at all body weights, even a very small amount of alcohol consumption, even one drink per week, is associated with a dramatic increase in fatty liver disease. Additionally, alcohol increases hyperandrogenism, and it increases your risk of many types of cancer.[73,74]

Alcohol isn't good for anyone, and it really isn't good for PCOS women. For some reason, our livers do not process alcohol as well as the livers of non-PCOS women do. They just don't.

And do you know what's worse than forgoing a glass of wine? A liver transplant.

Antibiotics from agriculture

Antibiotics are commonly found in milk, eggs, meat, chicken, and fish, but you won't see them in the ingredients list. To avoid them, look for products that are antibiotic-free.

It's crazy, but 80% of the antibiotics used in the United States every year are fed to meat and poultry raised for human consumption. There is so much to say about this: how it decimates the human gut microbiome, how it promotes obesity and contributes to antibiotic resistance, how it supports factory farming and environmental degradation. It's terrible.[75]

Antibiotics' job is to kill bacteria and they remain active even after they are consumed by animals. The antibiotics are metabolized into a food animal's muscles and you get a dose when you eat that animal. Those antibiotics are still potent when they make their way into your intestines where they then proceed to kill your microbiome bunny.

The best way to avoid eating antibiotics is to buy organic or antibiotic-free meat, eggs, and dairy. And buy wild caught fish because farmed fish are loaded with antibiotics.

Artificial sweeteners

Artificial sweeteners have been around for almost 100 years and they have long been marketed as a no-calorie way for dieters to have sweets. The problem is that people who favor artificial sweeteners gain weight and develop diabetes just like people who eat sugar. And for the longest time, no one could figure out how something without calories could contribute to obesity.

The answer is the microbiome. Studies show that all three of the most common artificial sweeteners — aspartame, sucralose, and saccharin — create gut dysbiosis that leads directly to weight gain and glucose intolerance.[76]

Sugar is bad for you. So are fake sugars. At the end of the day, the best solution is to wean yourself off sweeteners, artificial and natural. Eventually, your tastes will change and you won't crave sweets nearly as much. And when you do have a sweet treat, you'll be satisfied with much less.

Dairy

Dairy is a highly inflammatory food group filled with hormones. It is particularly problematic for women with PCOS.

Milk is the food that a mama cow makes for her baby cow. It is full of the nutrients and hormones that a baby cow needs to grow big and strong. Women with PCOS already have hormonal irregularities. Guess what we don't need — cow hormones!

We used to call people who couldn't digest the lactose in milk "lactose intolerant." Then we discovered that lactose intolerance was normal for humans, and the ability to digest milk into adulthood was a weird genetic adaptation of small populations of Europeans. So now, we call people who can drink milk "lactase persistent" and everyone else is just normal.

In fact, consuming dairy is an independent risk factor for developing PCOS. The more milk, yogurt, and cheese a young girl eats, the more likely it is she will develop PCOS when she becomes a woman.[77]

Dairy also makes some of the symptoms of PCOS much worse.

In humans, cow growth hormones and cow growth factors contribute significantly to acne. Most women with PCOS continue to have acne long after their teenage years due to high testosterone levels. Well, one side effect of the growth hormones in dairy is that they sensitize androgen receptors. In a woman with PCOS, this is devastating. You already have too much testosterone. Dairy makes your body extra responsive to all of that testosterone. This leads to skin oil overproduction, inflammation, and an altered skin microbiome that can trigger horrible cystic acne that is virtually impossible to treat.[78,79]

As if that wasn't enough, dairy also contributes to infertility, especially in the later reproductive years. The problem here is a little known dairy sugar called galactose, which just so happens to be toxic to human ovarian germ cells. These cells are critical to the maturation of viable eggs in your ovaries. The more milk a woman consumes, the more likely she is to experience a steep and early decline in fertility as she ages.[80]

So, for the sake of your skin, your fertility, your hormones, and your health, wean yourself off of cow's milk. Opt for an organic, non-dairy milk alternative such as soy milk, coconut milk, or my favorite, almond milk.

Emulsifiers

Emulsifiers allow unblendable ingredients in foods (think oil and water) to be evenly blended, and they are used practically everywhere in packaged foods to improve texture and consistency. They also cause intestinal inflammation. In fact, a common emulsifier, carrageenan, is used in scientific labs to induce intestinal inflammation in rodents so that scientists can study gastrointestinal diseases.[81]

Your intestines are coated in a mucosal lining that protects it from pathogens and prevents leaky gut. Emulsifiers dissolve this lining. They emulsify it, really. At the same time, they disrupt your microbiome and stimulate inflammation.[82]

You can find carrageenan in conventional and organic foods such as almond milk, ice cream, infant formula, coffee creamer, and even some pet foods. Read labels to find carrageenan-free products.

Other more natural emulsifiers like guar gum and xanthan gum have a better safety profile, but you probably shouldn't eat too much of them either.

Gluten

Gluten is a protein found in wheat, barley, rye, and products made from those grains, such as pasta, cereals, crackers, breads, and other baked goods. It's also in soy sauce, salad dressings, soups, candy bars, French fries, beer, and, oh my gosh, it's in everything. Everything processed, that is.

Going gluten free means reading lots and lots of labels. Remember, when you choose unprocessed foods, there are no labels!

The problem with gluten is that many people do not tolerate it well. And even for people who seem okay, gluten contributes to leaky gut, which then causes inflammation and increases your susceptibility to autoimmune diseases, allergies, heart disease, cancer, and diabetes — conditions you are already at risk for.

When all people eat gluten, they produce a protein called zonulin. This metabolite breaks down the mucosal lining of the intestines to cause leaky gut. Consequently, gluten is bad for everyone, and it is especially bad for people with celiac disease, non-celiac gluten sensitivity, and other conditions on the autoimmune spectrum.[83]

About 1% of the population has celiac disease. This is double historical rates and seems to be rising. People with celiac disease have an autoimmune response to gluten that leads to intestinal destruction. This is diagnosed with bloodwork and an intestinal biopsy. Celiac disease is an extremely serious autoimmune disease and people with celiac disease need to be 100% vigilant in avoiding all exposure to gluten.[84]

One important thing to know is that at least half of all celiac patients do not have gastrointestinal symptoms. Some have anemia, headaches, infertility, and osteoporosis. Some are completely asymptomatic. The true rate of celiac disease may be five times higher than the current estimate.[85]

Beyond this group, a much larger population of people are gluten sensitive. They do not have gluten antibodies but they experience a wide range of symptoms when they eat gluten, including irritable bowel syndrome, muscle and joint pain, headaches, and eczema. These patients have non-celiac gluten sensitivity. Even though non-celiac gluten sensitivity isn't officially an autoimmune disease, there is likely an immune component to this condition.[86]

Recently, there has been something of a backlash against gluten-free diets and people who have non-celiac gluten sensitivity, with some people even claiming that the condition doesn't exist. Gluten sensitivity is real, and zonulin can now be used to identify this condition.

In a recent study, researchers analysed the zonulin levels in four groups of participants — those with celiac disease, those with gluten sensitivity, those with irritable bowel syndrome with diarrhea, and those with healthy gastrointestinal functioning. Participants with celiac disease and with gluten sensitivity had very high levels of zonulin. Those with irritable bowel syndrome also had high levels, but only half as much as the celiac and gluten sensitive participants. Participants without gastrointestinal problems had the lowest zonulin levels.[87]

In normal digestion, zonulin is part of the intestinal response to food poisoning. It opens gaps in the intestinal walls to allow more water to enter the intestines and flush dangerous food out of the body as diarrhea.

Gluten triggers this same response in everybody. In some people, it is mild and unnoticeable. In others, it makes them sick and vulnerable to long-term, chronic diseases.

Autoimmune diseases tend to cluster. People with one autoimmune disease frequently have several. Celiac disease often goes hand in hand with type 1 diabetes, liver autoimmune diseases, thyroid autoimmune diseases, and peripheral neuropathy. Non-celiac gluten sensitivity is often seen in patients with Hashimoto's thyroiditis, dermatitis herpetiformis, psoriasis, and rheumatologic diseases.

You should care about this because scientists are now questioning whether PCOS itself is an autoimmune disorder. Virtually all PCOS women have autoantibodies, antibodies targeted at your own cells. And once you have autoantibodies, you are at risk of developing a wide range of autoimmune diseases.[88]

Women with PCOS have much higher rates of Hashimoto's, Graves' disease, and Lupus than non-PCOS women. So, you should do everything you can to reduce your risk of autoimmune disease. And that includes removing gluten from your diet.

Take a daily probiotic

A probiotic is a product containing live, beneficial bacteria.

Strangely enough, most probiotic bacteria don't actually stay and colonize your gut microbiome, but they confer beneficial changes. On their way through your digestive tract, probiotic bacteria kill pathogenic bacteria. They increase the mucosal lining of the intestine to protect against leaky gut. They lower inflammation. And they decrease gut pain sensitivity. And then you poop them out.[89,90]

That's why you need to take probiotics daily to get the most benefit.

I recommend that everyone take a good probiotic, one that has at least five different types of bacteria and at least five billion colony forming units (CFU). I often give my patients Ortho Molecular Products Ortho-biotic because each capsule has 20 billion CFU and the pills are shelf-stable. That means they don't need to be refrigerated, so you don't have to worry about the bacteria dying while being shipped. I also use Pure Encapsulations Probiotic-5 because it is particularly good at healing leaky gut.

Microbiome reboot: Go vegan for 6 months

If you are are willing and able, one of the best things you can do for your health is eat vegan for six months — no meat, no chicken, no fish, no eggs, no dairy. Just plants. This is the best way to reboot your microbiome. A plant-based diet will kill off an obesity microbiome and nurture a lean microbiome. It will kill the bacteria that turn meat into TMAO and promote heart disease. It will build microbiome diversity.[91]

Any amount of time eating a vegan diet will impact your microbiome but it takes several months for a new microbiome to get established and stable. When a person makes a short-term dietary change, her microbiome will revert back to its original state as soon as she reverts back to her original diet. So I recommend sticking with a vegan diet for six months.[92]

As long as you eat a wide variety of raw and minimally processed plants, eat the rainbow, and include whole grains, beans, lentils, and nuts, you don't need to worry about nutrition. You'll get enough protein and you'll get all of your vitamins and nutrients, with two important exceptions — vitamin B12 and omega-3. B12 is found almost exclusively in animal protein, and omega-3 comes mainly from fish.

Take a good multivitamin that has at least 6 mcg of B12 and supplement with at least a gram of omega-3 daily. I recommend Pure Encapsulations O.N.E. Omega, which contains exactly one gram.

After six months, you can decide whether you want to remain vegan or revert to a plant-heavy omnivore diet. What's best depends on your health, age, lifestyle, and, honestly, what makes you happy.

In general, vegans are healthier than most omnivores. Vegans maintain a healthier weight. They have a more diverse microbiome. They eat more fiber. They have less cancer, heart disease, diabetes, and autoimmune disease. Vegans have an overall 14% decrease in dying from all causes. Additionally, a vegan diet is better for the environment, especially when you buy local, organic, unprocessed agricultural products.[93]

As we age, we need more protein to protect our muscles from age-associated muscle loss. In general, it is easier to get enough protein when you eat an omnivore diet that includes lean, organic meat and eggs.

This is the diet I eat, a mostly plant-based omnivore menu. It's the perfect middle ground for me. I focus on eating a wide array of plants that span the colors of the rainbow, and I add in very small amounts of animal protein. My diet is fun, interesting, delicious, and healthy — all things that a diet should be. I can eat at restaurants and parties without much trouble. And I don't feel bogged down with lots of rigid rules.

Buy some great cookbooks

If you are cooking most of your meals at home, you need to have a few go-to cookbooks. Unfortunately, it's hard to find a great cookbook, especially one that is compatible with a plant-based, gluten-free, dairy-free, sugar-lite diet. If I were a great cook, I'd write one myself.

But let's be honest: I'm a much better doctor than chef. Fortunately, there are some great new cookbooks full of tasty recipes that align pretty well with my dietary recommendations.

Here are a few cookbooks that you should consider picking up to help you on your journey to a better diet and better health.

- *The Anti-Inflammatory Diet Cookbook* by Madeline Given, NC: These are simple, flavorful recipes, and most can be made and served in under an hour. Not all of the recipes fit with my dietary advice, but most do. And all of the recipes have dietary labels at the top, like "gluten free" and "dairy free", so it's easy to find the recipes that work for you.

- *Fermented Vegetables* by Kirsten and Christopher Shockey: This book is a great introduction to fermenting a huge array of vegetables. It covers all of the knowledge, materials, and techniques you'll need to make a wide array of beautiful, delicious fermentations, and it includes vibrant pictures to keep you inspired.

- *Eat to Live Quick and Easy Cookbook* by Joel Fuhrman, M.D.: If you are only going to own one of Dr. Fuhrman's excellent recipe books, this is the one to get. The recipes are quick, simple, nutrient-dense, and tasty. Most are vegan and gluten free. They all come with beautiful, full-page pictures.

- *Instant Loss Cookbook: Cook Your Way to a Healthy Weight with 125 Recipes for Your Instant Pot®, Pressure Cooker, and More* by Brittany Williams: This is an incredible cookbook, filled with 125 recipes that the author used to lose 125 pounds. The recipes are simple, delicious, and based on Williams' philosophy, JERF: Just eat real food. They are gluten-free, dairy-free, and meat-lite — exactly my recommendations.

Troubleshooting

It's always hard to change your diet. First, focus on adding more fruits and veggies to each meal rather than cutting things out. Let healthy foods naturally crowd out less healthy foods. Remember that at every meal, you need to feed your human cells and your microbiome bunny. Here are some tips for overcoming common challenges.

I simply can't eat that much fiber.

If six to nine cups of plant-based foods feels like a lot, focus on high-fiber foods so you get more fiber with less bulk. See my list of the highest fiber foods on page 176.

You can also take a fiber supplement, but make sure you find one that contains a wide variety of fibers and no additives. And be sure to drink lots of water.

Many name brand fiber supplements contain artificial colors and sweeteners, and most contain high quantities of a single type of fiber, such as inulin (sometimes listed as chicory root), psyllium husk, corn bran, or cellulose (sometimes from wood pulp).

For overall gut health plus fiber, I recommend Pure Encapsulations G.I. Fortify. It contains a blend of fibers, plus the amino acid L-Glutamine, and other soothing agents, called demulcents. I especially like that it contains Triphala for easing constipation. You can get it in powder or capsule form. Capsules are easier to take; the powder works better, but it's thick and some people don't like the taste.

An alternative diverse, prebiotic fiber supplement that will nurture your microbiome is Hyperbiotics Prebiotic Organic Proprietary Blend. And if you are constipated, I recommend Organic India Whole Husk Psyllium. These are two totally different products that confer totally different health benefits. You can actually take both of them if you want to.

Just remember, your body and microbiome need *hundreds* of different types of fibers and nutrients. Think of a fiber supplement as an insurance policy for days when your diet is a bit subpar. Fiber supplements can help ease constipation, improve metabolic markers, and enhance microbiome diversity, but they don't provide the same degree of benefits as a high-fiber, whole foods diet.[94,95,96]

I get food cravings.

Are you ready to have your mind blown? Your microbiome can cause food cravings. Remember how bacteria release hormones and other signaling agents? Well, your gut is directly connected to your brain by something called the vagus nerve. Bacteria send signals through this nerve and actually influence your thoughts to create food cravings.[97]

They do this for survival.

When you change your diet, some bacteria start starving. And because they don't want to starve, they send food craving signals to your brain to encourage you to eat what they need to survive.

So, if you feel cravings, especially for fatty and sugary foods, recognize that these are the dying cries of your bad bacteria. As intense as the cravings may be, if you can ignore them, they will go away. As soon as those bacteria are gone, the cravings will be, too.

I love dessert!

Me, too! Dessert is tough because it is so much more than food. Dessert can be a treat, a joyful moment shared among friends and family, a guilty pleasure, a reward, a sweet end to a tough day.

I have not given up dessert. I wouldn't want to give up dessert. I tried and it made me sad.

But I eat so little sugar these days that what feels like dessert has changed for me. My desserts tend to be smaller (just a few bites), more natural, and less sweet than traditional baked goods and ice cream. Here are my favorite guilty pleasures.

- **Dark chocolate:** I love dark chocolate so much. It is my favorite treat. It's easy to find dark chocolate that is low in sugar and dairy free. And as an added benefit, dark chocolate is high in polyphenols, which are powerful antioxidants and anti-inflammatories. For a decadent treat, melt some dark chocolate in your microwave. Dip dried fruits and nuts into it, roll in shredded coconut, and chill in your fridge. You can do this with fresh fruits, too, but then eat them right away because the warm chocolate cooks them a bit and they get mushy quickly.[98]

- **Dried fruit:** Dried fruits are filled with nutrients and fiber. They are easy to grab on the go and a handful does a great job of filling you up. Sweet and sticky dates are a luxurious, guilt-free end to a meal.

- **Berries with coconut whipped cream:** Did you know that you can make whipped cream from coconut cream? Chill a can of coconut cream (not coconut milk) in the fridge. Discard the runny water, place the cream in a mixing bowl, and whip. I make mine sugar-free but you could add a tiny bit of honey or maple syrup to give it a hint of sweetness. Berries are beautiful little fruits filled with antioxidants and fiber. Put a dollop of coconut whipped cream on a bowl of berries, shave some dark chocolate on top, and you'll have a healthy treat that doesn't feel healthy at all.

- **Smoothie popsicles:** For a cool treat on a hot day, make a fruit smoothie by blending fruits and berries with your favorite milk substitute. Add coconut cream or a frozen banana for creaminess, and freeze it in a popsicle mold. Even better, make a variety of different-colored smoothies and layer them into popsicle molds for beautiful rainbow frozen treats.

I have food allergies.

Up to 10% of U.S. adults have a food allergy. If that's you, depending on what you are allergic to, you may need to adjust this diet to fit your allergies. But it's possible that a high-fiber diet will improve your allergy symptoms.[99]

Leaky gut seems to play a critical role in the development of many food allergies, and scientists are currently exploring theories that a high-fiber diet, by healing leaky gut, may reduce or even reverse some food allergies.[100,101]

Promising new research shows that certain fiber-loving, short-chain fatty acid producing bacteria strains called Clostridia (not to be confused with the highly pathogenic *Clostridium difficile*) can reverse some food allergies in mice. In the study, scientists induced peanut allergies in mice by killing their gut microbiomes with antibiotics early in life. The scientists then inoculated the mice with several strains of Clostridia, and the mice lost their peanut allergies.[102]

It's all very exciting. Possible allergy reduction is just one more reason to eat lots of fiber.

I need antibiotics.

When you take antibiotics, you risk destroying your gut microbiome. Medically-necessary antibiotics are miracle drugs that save lives. But when used improperly, they foster antibiotic resistance, gut dysbiosis, and an increased susceptibility to infection and metabolic disease. Additionally, the more rounds of antibiotics you take, the higher your risk of developing diabetes. If you are prescribed an antibiotic, make sure that it is medically necessary and there is not a safe option to watch and wait. Many mild infections, such as ear infections, will resolve on their own without medication.[103]

If you do need to take antibiotics, take them properly, take the full dose, and do everything you can to nurture the regrowth of a diverse and healthy microbiome.

The problem with antibiotics is that they kill a lot of different species of microbes throughout your body. A stable microbiome ecosystem resists change because all of the ecological niches are filled. Antibiotics open up lots of space in your microbiome community and pathogenic bacteria often grow back first, creating gut dysbiosis.[104]

At least one-third of people who take antibiotics develop antibiotic-associated diarrhea (AAD). When people take probiotics, their risk of AAD decreases by 43%.[105,106]

Anytime you take antibiotics, take a daily probiotic and load up on fresh fruits and veggies and fermented foods to minimize the damage. Do this throughout your treatment and for several weeks afterward. You need to repopulate your microbiome with beneficial bacteria as quickly as possible and provide these good guys with lots of fiber to eat.

I have irritable bowel syndrome.

If you have irritable bowel syndrome, the advice in this chapter should help. Eat a high-fiber diet and try eating vegan to further improve your gut microbiome.

Take an IBS-targeted probiotic. There are dozens of studies showing that specific probiotics can alleviate irritable bowel symptoms. The complicated thing is that you have to use the right strains. Hyperbiotics PRO-15 Probiotics include many of the most promising bacterial strains: *B. infantis, B. breve, B. lactis, L. plantarum, L. rhamnosus, L. acidophilus, and L. casei.*

If you start taking probiotics and eating lots of plant-based foods and you develop severe, painful gas, you should set up an appointment with your gastroenterologist to see if you have Small Intestinal Bacterial Overgrowth (SIBO). Check out the section on SIBO on page 270.

I take medication for heartburn.

If you are taking proton pump inhibitors (PPIs) for heartburn, acid reflux, or gastroesophageal reflux disease (GERD), you should attempt to wean off of these drugs because they disrupt your gut microbiome and harm your health.

PPIs, which include brands such as Nexium, Prilosec, and Prevacid, have a long list of serious side effects.

They dramatically decrease your stomach acid production, which is why they make your heartburn feel better. However, stomach acid plays an important role in killing dangerous bacteria. Consequently, PPIs disrupt the balance in your gut microbiome and promote abnormally large populations of pathogenic microbes. They increase your risk of food poisoning and gastrointestinal infections, and specifically, they double your risk of acquiring a *Clostridium difficile* infection, which causes severe diarrhea.[107,108,109]

Stomach acid is part of the digestion process that makes several critical nutrients available. People taking PPIs can become deficient in vitamin B12, vitamin C, calcium, iron, and magnesium, and this leads to an increase in muscle spasms, heart palpitations, and bone fractures.[110]

PPIs also disrupt acid production in cells and organs outside the stomach. So people who take PPIs have an increased risk of heart attack, chronic kidney disease, and dementia.[111]

They even *increase* your risk of cancer, the very thing they are supposed to protect you against. Many people take PPIs because they are worried about Barrett's Esophagus, where esophageal tissue is damaged and becomes susceptible to esophageal cancer. Historically, people with Barrett's Esophagus were given PPIs to reduce acid in the esophagus to prevent cancer. Unfortunately, PPIs don't change your risk of esophageal cancer, but they do increase your risk of gastric cancer.[112,113]

It is completely appropriate to take PPIs short-term as part of the treatment to heal bleeding ulcers or severe hemorrhagic gastritis. But it is not a reasonable treatment for routine heartburn or GERD.

If you are taking a PPI, please make an appointment with your doctor to review your treatment plan and assess whether you can wean yourself off these powerful pharmaceuticals. PPIs can cause a condition called rebound hypersecretion, where your body begins to overproduce acid. Basically, the very act of stopping PPIs can cause GERD. Work with a knowledgeable doctor or other health care specialist to slowly wean off these drugs by splitting pills and/or increasing dosage intervals.

All of the recommendations in this book will help ease your heartburn or GERD by fixing your circadian rhythm, nurturing your gut microbiome, improving digestion, and facilitating weight loss. Pay attention to foods and emotions that trigger your heartburn and adjust accordingly. But if you still experience occasional symptoms, there are safer alternatives to PPIs that can relieve your pain and discomfort.

New research shows that GERD may actually be caused by circadian rhythm dysfunction. Consequently, melatonin is a promising new GERD treatment. Try taking 3 mg at bedtime for 8 weeks, with or without other GERD medications. Then slowly decrease your melatonin dose down to 0.5 to 1 mg per night.[114]

For periodic heartburn flare-ups, H2-receptor antagonists, also known as H2-blockers, temporarily decrease stomach acid and are sold under the brand names Pepcid and Zantac. The benefit of these drugs is that they beginning working almost immediately and they only work for up to twelve hours. Then your stomach acid production goes back to normal. If you use them occasionally, they don't carry anywhere near the same risks as PPIs. Just be careful because they can cause leaky gut if you use them regularly. They are cheap and available over-the-counter, and if you only use them on occasion, they are safe.[115]

A quick summary

You are the sole caretaker of your microbiome bunny, the 100 trillion microbes that call you home. To nurture a healthy microbiome, you have to feed it healthy foods — a variety of plants with lots of fiber. If you eat this way, virtually every other dietary recommendation will take care of itself. And the impact on your health will be dramatic.

- Eat mostly plants.
- Eat lots of fiber. Fiber, fiber, fiber!
- Eat organic, raw and minimally processed foods that span all of the colors of the rainbow.
- Limit sugar, fat, and salt.
- Avoid alcohol, antibiotics from agriculture, artificial sweeteners, dairy, emulsifiers, and gluten.
- Take a daily probiotic.
- Reboot your microbiome by eating vegan for six months.
- Invest in some great cookbooks that support a mostly vegan, gluten free diet.

Healthy habits to get you started

- ☐ Every week, buy and eat (per person in your household): ½ lb of dried beans, 1 lb of leafy greens, 7 pieces of fruit, 1 melon, 2 lbs of any type of vegetables, ½ lb of dried whole grains, and ½ lb of nuts or seeds. This is a good starter shopping list.

- ☐ Every time you go grocery shopping, buy at least one produce item from every color of the rainbow.

- ☐ Shop the perimeter of your grocery store and buy primarily raw and minimally processed foods.

- ☐ Print out a copy of the "dirty dozen" (see page 178) and buy those items organic.

- ☐ Read food labels. Watch for added fat, salt, sugar, and artificial ingredients. Only buy antibiotic-free animal products.

- ☐ Eat something from a plant at every meal.

- ☐ Plants first! Start every meal with one cup of plant-based food.

- ☐ Cook vegetables in the evening so you can reheat them for breakfast.

- ☐ Buy an Instant Pot, an Instant Pot cookbook, and a variety of organic, dried beans.

☐ Cook a huge pot of beans on Sunday and eat them throughout the week.

☐ Plan your meals so you don't get to dinner time and discover your fridge is empty.

☐ Limit restaurant meals to once per week.

☐ Eat a salad for dinner every day.

☐ Keep a bowl of fruit on your table.

☐ Keep flaxseeds on your kitchen table and sprinkle them on anything that seems good. They spruce up salads, oatmeal, and steamed broccoli.

☐ Join a Community Supported Agriculture (CSA) program to receive a box of farm-fresh produce every week.

☐ Invest in some fun, new cookbooks.

CHAPTER 10

STEP 6:
Live clean and pure

*T*oxins and toxic substances are everywhere.

Of course this has always been true. Many living creatures such as rattlesnakes, black widows, bees, jellyfish, mushrooms, oleander trees, rhubarb, and hemlock plants create toxins to protect themselves. Heavy metals such mercury and lead are poisonous. Other natural toxic compounds include arsenic, cyanide, and chlorine gas.

The natural environment is full of poisons. In fact, the most toxic substance in the world, botulinum, produced by a bacteria called *Clostridium botulinum* and the cause of botulism, is such a potent neurotoxin that an adult human can be killed by just 70 micrograms, which is less than the size of a common pinhead. And it is totally natural.

Our ancestors were exposed daily to hundreds of natural toxic chemicals and toxins. We evolved with these compounds. Many of them, like snake venom and poisonous mushrooms, our ancestors learned to avoid. But for a number of these substances, our ancestors encountered them so frequently and in such small quantities that their bodies adapted.

Many of the healthy, plant-based foods we eat actually contain toxins. Broccoli, cabbage, strawberries, mustard, rice, beans, and nuts — to varying degrees, they are all toxic, and yet we are able to eat them. Humans evolved enzymes that can break down common foodborne toxins and make them safe, and in many cases, our gut microbiome developed enzymes to do it for us. Then, our internal detoxification system, primarily our liver and kidneys, filters them out. Our ability to safely metabolize a wide array of toxins is the primary reason humans can eat so many different types of food. No other creatures can survive on as varied a diet as we humans can.[1,2]

Today, however, our modern environment is chemically toxic in a way that our ancestral environments were not. We daily encounter hundreds of new, synthetic chemicals that we have not evolved to safely metabolize.

In the United States, there are more than 80,000 registered industrial chemicals that can be used in home, garden, and personal care products. Virtually all of these chemicals go into our bodies and environments without safety testing. Chemicals operate under a premise of innocent until proven guilty. And the burden of proof is very high and very costly.[3]

Because these chemicals haven't been tested, we don't know which ones are safe and which ones are dangerous. And even if we did, it's virtually impossible to cherry pick which chemicals to avoid and which to use because companies often hide their products' ingredients under the guise of protecting trade secrets.

Endocrine disruptors

One group of particularly dangerous chemicals, especially for women with PCOS, are endocrine disruptors.

Your endocrine system is the system of hormones that your body's organs use to communicate with each other. When your master clock sets the daily circadian rhythm and broadcasts it out to the rest of your body, it uses the endocrine system. Your metabolism depends on hormones. When you are sick or injured, hormones upregulate your immune system to protect your body and downregulate it when the threat has passed. Your endocrine system controls your emotions and orchestrates your menstrual cycle. It coordinates all bodily functions and maintains balance throughout your whole body.

Endocrine disruptors do exactly what their name suggests: disrupt your body's hormone communication pathways and the systems that depend on them.

There are thousands of known endocrine-disrupting chemicals. Some of them are so ubiquitous that they are practically household names: BPA, phthalates, dioxin, perchlorate, and PFCs, to name a few.

PCOS is an endocrine disorder. Hormonal imbalance is a defining feature of this condition. Our hormones are already struggling to do their jobs. Flooding our bodies with fake estrogens, thyroid blockers, and androgen enhancers will only make our PCOS worse.

BPA and PCOS

The story of one chemical, bisphenol A (BPA), and PCOS is a great example of how an endocrine disruptor can play an ongoing role in human disease.

BPA is special because it is everywhere. You find it in hard, clear plastics. It's in the lining of cans. It's in receipts from stores and restaurants. It is even in dental sealants. And, according to the Centers for Disease Control and Prevention (CDC), it's in the bodies of 95% of Americans. It is in the uteruses of pregnant women and in the breast milk of nursing mothers.[4,5,6]

BPA is also highly researched, in part because it started out as a pharmaceutical.

It was first synthesized in 1891 and later studied in the 1930's as a synthetic estrogen for women experiencing premenstrual syndrome, menopause, and other female medical conditions. It eventually lost out to diethylstilbestrol (DES), a stronger synthetic estrogen that was given to millions of pregnant women to prevent miscarriage and was later pulled off the market for causing birth defects and previously rare vaginal cancers in baby girls.

BPA was never marketed as a drug, but in the 1950s, it became a key ingredient in clear, hard polycarbonate plastic. We've been finding new uses for it ever since. Today, in the U.S. alone, we produce over 2.5 billion pounds (that's billion, with a 'b') of BPA every year, earning it the dubious classification, "high production volume chemical."[7,8]

Because of its unique history, we know a lot about BPA.

Its estrogenic properties likely play a role in the development of PCOS and in the severity of today's PCOS symptoms, starting with fetal exposure in the mother's womb. BPA crosses the placenta into the uterus and triggers something called altered fetal programming. When a fetus is developing and her organ systems are forming, endocrine disruptors cause physiological and metabolic errors that can persist throughout a person's life, setting the stage for adult chronic diseases (like PCOS!) even before a child has drawn her first breath.[9,10]

We know that high levels of testosterone in the womb can trigger PCOS. It now seems that high levels of BPA do the same thing. In fact, in rodents we can induce PCOS by exposing fetuses to environmentally relevant levels of BPA.[11,12]

Once a fetus has been exposed to high levels of BPA, those levels stay high for the rest of her life. Women with PCOS, as adults, still have higher levels of BPA in their blood than women without PCOS. And the difference is dramatic. Even though we live in the same places as non-PCOS women and eat the same food, we seem to store BPA in our bodies in a way that other women don't.[13]

So we know that women with PCOS have high levels of BPA. These levels remain high when PCOS women get pregnant so their fetuses are also exposed to high levels of BPA. And fetal exposure to BPA causes hyperandrogenism and polycystic ovaries. These children grow up to have PCOS and high levels of BPA.

But, the story doesn't end there. A collection of studies also show that in addition to possibly causing PCOS, BPA makes PCOS worse.

BPA is linked to higher testosterone levels in women. The more BPA, the more testosterone, the more severe the PCOS. Basically, BPA exacerbates acne, hirsutism, and thinning hair.[14]

BPA goes hand-in-hand with obesity. The more BPA found in your urine, the more you weigh. We used to think this was coincidental. BPA is found in packaged foods, which overweight people theoretically eat more of. But new evidence points to a causal relationship. When we are exposed to BPA, our body metabolizes it into a compound called BPA-glucuronide, which circulates throughout our bodies and reprograms cell DNA so they store more fat. BPA exposure triggers fat accumulation and prevents fat burning by altering your metabolism.[15,16]

Remember how PCOS women are prone to fatty liver disease? Well, newborn exposure to BPA (via formula or breast milk) reprograms an infant's liver genes to make her more susceptible to fatty liver disease later in life. Adults with non-alcoholic fatty liver disease have higher blood levels of BPA than those without fatty liver disease but who otherwise share similar risk profiles.[17,18,19]

Recall how women with PCOS have a dysbiotic gut microbiome, and 40% of us have irritable bowel syndrome? Well, BPA kills beneficial gut bacteria and favors a dysbiotic gut microbiome that mirrors the high-fat, high-sugar, Standard American Diet microbiome. On top of that, we can now give bunnies irritable bowel syndrome simply by feeding them BPA at clinically relevant levels to disrupt their microbiomes.[20,21]

Lastly, remember how women with PCOS have a dysregulated circadian rhythm? Well, BPA actually changes the expression of clock genes throughout your body, and it seems to do so in a way that promotes inflammation and obesity.[22]

And on and on! BPA plays an undeniable role in the widespread severity of modern PCOS.

And there are thousands of endocrine disruptors

By now, you may be wondering how to avoid BPA. Great, you should definitely avoid BPA. It's in hard plastics, canned food, dental sealants, and cash register receipts.

But here's the kicker: There are thousands of endocrine-disrupting chemicals. BPA is just one that we happen to have a lot of research on, but other than that, it's not special.

The real question is: Do women with PCOS have higher levels of many common chemicals in our blood. The answer seems to be, yes.

We only know if a chemical is present if we go looking for it. There isn't a what-chemicals-are-here? test. There's just the is-this-specific-chemical-here? test. And when we run those tests on women with PCOS, the answer is almost always, yes, the chemical is here and at higher levels than average.

In our blood and urine, we PCOS women have higher levels of polychlorinated biphenyls (PCBs), organochlorine pesticides, and polycyclic aromatic hydrocarbons (PAHs). We have higher levels of perfluorooctanoate (PFOA) and perfluorooctane sulfonate (PFOS). These chemicals are *all* endocrine disruptors.[23,24]

We don't know exactly why PCOS women accumulate them, but it probably all comes down to the liver. Doesn't everything? It seems that, for whatever reason, women with PCOS are just less good at processing toxic chemicals and toxins than other women. And when we can't process them, we store them in our fat cells, which is the body's way of quarantining toxic substances and protecting itself. Then the fat cells slowly release these toxic substances at the speed at which we can process them. But for most of us, chemicals come in faster than we can get them out. So we accumulate more and more.

Because many of these chemicals can induce PCOS, one theory gaining traction is that varying exposure levels to various endocrine-disrupting chemicals, and specifically, exposure levels at critical moments of development, contribute to the wide variety of PCOS symptoms and severity that we see amongst PCOS women today.[25]

You have PCOS because you inherited PCOS genes from your mother. Your exact PCOS was shaped by the chemicals you and your mother were exposed to and the times and levels of those exposures.

A path forward

Clearly past exposure, especially fetal exposure, is a critical problem, and it's one that you cannot undo. This is true for me, too, and for my daughters, who were all born before BPA and phthalates and the rest were big news. There is no "undo" in life, but we can all be healthier going forward. And if you have children or are planning to have children, you can help them be healthier, too.

Toxic substances usually enter our bodies through one of three pathways — we eat them, we touch them, or we breathe them.

The vast majority of the toxic chemicals in our bodies enter through our mouth. Eating organic foods will reduce your exposure to pesticides, some of which are endocrine disruptors and all of which are poisons.

To get rid of the rest, you need to clean them out of your home, your body, and your life.

Eat less meat

Not only is this healthy diet advice, it's great clean-living advice.

Most endocrine disruptors are fat soluble. They accumulate in fats, first in the fat in your food and then in the fat in your body. Consequently, endocrine disruptors and other fat soluble toxins tend to concentrate in animals higher up the food chain. We see this in predator fish and birds as well as in humans.

People who eat lower on the food chain carry fewer toxic chemicals in their bodies, so eating primarily a plant-based diet is one of the best ways to avoid endocrine disruptors.[26]

Amongst animal products, processed meats, poultry, and cream-based dairy, like cheese and ice cream (Psst! Go dairy free!), are particularly high in endocrine disruptors like phthalates. In processed meats, the chemicals probably come from the plastics involved in processing and storing. In poultry, the culprit seems to be animal feed. In dairy, our best guess is that phthalates leach into milk fat from the plastic tubing that the milk is pumped through during processing. So, when you do eat meat and animal products, buy organic, pasture-raised, and minimally processed.[27]

Fish is another surprising source of endocrine disruptors. Fish routinely consume microplastics (tiny plastic particles floating in the water), which are then stored throughout their bodies. When we eat them, the microplastics are passed to us. Seafood may also be contaminated with antibiotics and mercury. Choosing safer fish can be complicated so I rely on the Monterey Bay Aquarium's Seafood Watch to identify healthy and sustainable seafood (www.seafoodwatch.org). And even so, I limit fish to wild-caught salmon twice per month.[28]

Eat at home

Restaurant food is another potent source of endocrine disruptors. People who eat at restaurants have phthalate levels that are on average 35% higher than people who eat their meals at home. As of yet, we don't know exactly why, but our best guess is that there is an accumulation of exposures from plastic in food shipping, storage, preparation, and cooking.[29]

So when you can, cook your own food. It's healthier and cheaper anyway. And when you eat out, consider eating vegan since we know that chemicals accumulate in fats and animal products.

Use less plastic

As a general rule, plastic + food = plastic chemicals in your food. And "plastic" includes soft plastic, hard plastic, acrylic, melamine, plastic wrap, plastic clamshells, and plastic bags. So do what you can to use less plastic.

Instead, buy and store your food in glass, ceramic, stainless steel, cloth, and paper. When you buy condiments like pasta sauce, salad dressing, mustard, and olives, choose the ones in glass jars. At home, store leftovers in glass or stainless steel containers, and pack lunches in glass or stainless steel containers as well. Swap your plastic wrap for aluminum foil, those cool beeswax wraps, or just a bowl with a plate on top.

Be extra careful with hot food. Plastic + food + heat = an extra dose of plastic chemicals.

In microwaves, use glass and ceramic only. If you have a microwavable dinner or frozen veggies in a bag and the packaging says microwave safe, do not believe them! All that means is that the packaging won't melt. Those containers are lined with plastic. If you heat the plastic, it will leach chemicals into your food, and then you will be eating plastic chemicals. Even most cardboard takeout boxes are lined with plastic. Basically, if it's shiny, it's probably plastic and it should not be heated.

There are a few other sources of plastic-food contact that are easy to overlook. On the stovetop, use wooden, silicon, or metal cooking utensils instead of nylon (It's plastic!). For cookware, go with enamel, stainless steel, or cast iron. The plasma perfluoroalkyl substances (PFASs) used in most nonstick cookware and other nonstick items are linked to metabolic disorders in women. Oh, and be on the lookout for kitchen appliances that might combine heat and plastic. Electric water kettles, coffee makers that use those little disposable cups, drip coffee makers, and yogurt makers come to mind, but I'm sure there are others.[30]

Swapping plastic for non-plastic alternatives in your kitchen can be time consuming and expensive, so take the time you need. Prioritize items that come in contact with hot food. Plates and serveware, microwave plate covers, food storage containers, and cooking utensils are great places to start.

Be wary of canned food

All cans are lined with some type of epoxy resin to keep the food from coming into contact with the metal. Most can linings on the shelf today still contain BPA, which we already know is terrible for you. Most of the BPA-free cans contain BPS instead, which is at least as bad as BPA but less well-known and less regulated.

If you are willing to do a lot of research, a few brands have replaced their can linings with bisphenol-free liners. Some are better than others. The Environmental Working Group's report on canned foods is a good place to start: www.ewg.org/research/bpa-canned-food.

I feel comfortable eating canned foods from Eden Foods and Amy's.

Chemical contaminant levels in canned foods vary dramatically. Foods that tend to accumulate BPA (or BPS or other plasticizers) are solid, high fat, highly acidic (like tomatoes), and sterilized at high heat. Canned soups and canned pastas have the highest levels of endocrine disruptors.[31]

Glass jars are an ideal, although often more expensive, alternative to cans. Tetra Pak boxes, which are cardboard boxes lined with polyethylene plastic and aluminum, are another option for soups, stewed tomatoes, and beans. They may not be perfect but they seem to be better than most cans.

The best solution is to eat foods that are fresh, frozen, or dried (such as beans or rice). When they are organic, these are the cleanest foods you can buy.

Ditto for drinks

What goes for food goes for drinks. Ditch your plastic water bottle and opt for glass or stainless steel. If you carry your coffee or tea in a thermos, it should also be stainless steel or heat resistant glass.

What about canned drinks? At this time, it seems that all of these cans are lined with BPA — beer, soda, sparkling water, coconut water — all of them. There have been very few studies on how much BPA leaches from these cans into the drinks.

In one study, canned soy milk, perhaps because of its fat content, raised the BPA level of participants' urine by 1600%! Canned soy milk is not a common drink in the U.S. but this study made me rethink canned coconut milk. I now recommend powdered coconut milk for cooking.[32]

Other canned drinks don't seem to leach BPA. I wish there were more data, but if your canned drink is fat free, it's probably safe.[33]

Filter your water

I recommend that you drink and cook with filtered tap water. If you live somewhere with particularly bad tap water, then bottled might be better.

How you should filter your water depends on the chemicals in your tap water. A good place to start is the Environmental Working Group's tap water database (www.ewg.org/tapwater). It's hard to know what filter you need if you don't know what's in your water. Investigating this can be eye opening. My daughter's water in Boulder, CO actually has testosterone in it. Just what a woman with PCOS needs to be drinking — more testosterone!

Contaminants, particularly lead and copper, can be introduced into your tap water as the water travels through pipes from the water treatment center or well to your home. In the United States, there are literally millions of lead water pipes that need to be replaced, plus millions more that are copper held together with lead solder. Plastic water pipes also seem to contaminate water with a wide array of toxic chemicals. Your water company can tell you what type of municipal pipes your water travels through, but the only way to really know your drinking water is safe is to have the water in your home tested by a state-certified lab.

Additionally, your tap water likely contains small amounts of chlorine that you'll want to filter out. Water chlorination is one of the greatest health achievements of the 20th century and has been critical to stopping the spread of waterborne diseases like typhoid. Even today, it kills pathogens like giardia and e-coli. And that's great.

But, by the time chlorine gets to your tap, it's done its job and is now a problem. That's because chlorine kills bacteria, and even in small amounts, it is deadly to your gut microbiome. Chlorinated drinking water is linked to gut dysbiosis and colorectal cancer.[34]

Now if you are thinking that bottled water is better, think again. For all its problems, tap water is more regulated than bottled water, and most bottled water is just filtered municipal water, anyway. It's cheaper and better to freshly filter your water yourself and store it in a non-plastic bottle.[35]

So, once you know what's in your water to the degree that you can, pick a filter based on your budget and space. I know it's overwhelming because there are approximately a kazillion options.

Right now, I have a Brita pitcher, which I used to love. But I am replacing it because I am concerned that the Tritan BPA-free plastic isn't safe. It's really hard to win with plastic because we keep discovering new dangerous chemicals in the "safer" alternatives. I'm considering switching to a Big Berkey stainless steel countertop water filter or a whole house water filter. At the end of the day, plastic-free is always safest.[36]

Clean your air

According to the Environmental Protection Agency, most American adults spend more than 90% of their time indoors, and indoor air quality (IAQ) can be significantly more polluted than the air right outside. Poor air can give you asthma and make you sick. Around the world, four million people die from indoor air pollution every year.[37,38,39]

Just about everything in your house and workspace are off-gassing, releasing tiny particles into the air that you may or may not be able to smell. You breathe in these particles and they enter your bloodstream through your lungs. Many of these airborne chemicals, including BPA, phthalates, brominated flame retardants, and PCBs, are endocrine disruptors.[40,41]

Here are some potent sources of indoor air pollution:

- Household cleaners
- Air fresheners
- Radon (get your home checked if it hasn't been)
- Building and furniture materials
- Paint
- Thirdhand tobacco smoke (the kind that clings to walls and upholstery)
- Mold

Any time you have a choice, choose natural products, or at least less toxic products. Solid wood is better than medium-density fibreboard (MDF) or plywood, which off-gas formaldehyde, a neurotoxin. Wool carpets are better than synthetic carpets, and avoid stain guards because they are made from perfluorochemicals (PFCs), which are neurotoxic and immunotoxic endocrine disrupting chemicals. Polyester shower curtains are better than vinyl, which offgasses phthalates. Choose low-VOC (volatile organic compounds) paints. Buy spring mattresses that don't contain fire retardants. Choose natural cleaners. If you like air fresheners, go with essential oils. Get your home checked for radon if you haven't, and obviously, don't smoke.

Basically, every time you bring a product into your home, make sure it is the safest product you can afford.

Beyond that, there are a few key things you can do to improve your indoor air quality.

Open the windows

In all but the world's most polluted cities, the air outside is cleaner than the air inside. Whenever the weather allows, open your windows. Open every window you can, and if there's no breeze, use a fan to create one. Fill your indoor space with outdoor air.

Get a HEPA air filter

An air filter is one of the best ways to clean indoor air when you can't open the windows.

A HEPA (high-efficiency particulate air) filter can remove 50% to 80% of airborne particles in a room and this can reduce your exposure to a wide range of chemicals. Indoor air pollution raises your risk of cardiovascular disease, diabetes, and cancer, and a HEPA filter counteracts that risk. Additionally, for adults and children with asthma and environmental allergies, HEPA filters reduce respiratory symptoms.[42]

A whole house HEPA filter attached to your central heating and cooling system is the most efficient way to do this, but portable HEPA filters work great, too. You just need to make sure you have one powerful enough to clean the space it's in.[43]

Run it day and night, even when you are not around.

Vacuum

Household dust is full of toxic chemicals and endocrine disruptors, including phthalates, flame retardants, and pesticides. Most of these chemicals (and the dirt they cling to) get tracked in from outside, so it's a good idea to take your shoes off at the door. Other toxic chemicals in dust are tiny particles that are shed from items in your home or office like paint, furniture foam, and carpet fibers. Get rid of them by vacuuming at least weekly with a HEPA filter vacuum cleaner.[44,45,46]

Use personal products that you could eat

It's a bit of an exaggeration, but it's a good rule of thumb: If it's poisonous to eat, you shouldn't put it on your skin, in your mouth, on your hair, on your nails, or in your vagina. Anything that you put on your body will end up in your bloodstream. Of course, your makeup and shampoo don't need to taste good because you aren't actually going to eat them, but if you did eat them, they shouldn't kill you.

The simplest way to do this is to actually use food products on your body. Coconut oil and shea butter are great moisturizers. Baking soda is an effective deodorant and toothpaste. Apple cider vinegar is a good hair conditioner. As an added bonus, these products are cheap compared to marketed beauty products.

Beyond your pantry, there is an entire universe of natural and organic beauty products that will help you look, feel, and smell great without poisoning you or our planet.

Ditto for home and garden products, within reason

The same philosophy holds true (or mostly true) for products we use in our homes and gardens.

You can clean almost anything in your house with vinegar, and if something needs a good scrubbing, try baking soda. Beyond that, again, look for all natural, organic, and eco-friendly products.

In your yard, use organic fertilizers (you definitely can't eat these, but your plants will love them). And do everything you can to avoid pesticides. If you do have a pest problem, try natural solutions first. Ladybugs eat aphids. You can get poison-free yellow jacket traps. Snails hate crushed eggshell, and ants hate cinnamon.

If you do use poisons, research eco-friendly pest control methods to find the safest options. The same goes for weed control. Oh, and just for a little perspective, a couple of weeds or slugs never killed anyone, but commercial weed killers and pesticides cause cancer.[47]

Troubleshooting

Aim for balance. We all live in the modern world and living in the modern world involves being exposed to modern chemicals.

The average woman uses 12 personal care products every day, which contain, on average, a sum of 168 unique ingredients. Between laundry soap, toilet bowl cleaner, glass cleaner, wood oil, and so on, most of us have another dozen or more household products that we use regularly. Then there are the garden chemicals, which all seem to contain a skull and crossbones. It's dizzying.[48]

As women with PCOS, we have to avoid what we can. Some of these chemicals cause PCOS. Some of these chemicals make PCOS worse.

Make smart choices to reduce your exposures when, where, and however you can.

I am overwhelmed and don't know what I should buy

I know, it seems like you need to be a chemist to figure out what's safe. Fortunately, there are scientists who have worked together to produce tools to make it easier for you to choose safer products.

One tool I like is the Healthy Living app by the Environmental Working Group. Get this app on your phone. It allows you to scan a product's barcode, and it will tell you how safe or dangerous that product is.

A good approach is to upgrade your products as they run out and need to be replaced. This allows you to focus on one or two products at a time so you don't get overwhelmed.

I know these chemicals can be scary, but focus on the things that you're buying today and let the rest go so you can live your life.

You don't have to be perfect. I'm certainly not. My glass tupperware have plastic lids. I dye my hair (shhh!). Sometimes I whiten my porcelain sink with Ajax because it works better than the natural products and I can't stand having a stained, ugly kitchen sink. Recently, we had termites and we had to fumigate the whole house. Stuff happens.

So, do what you can, when it makes sense. It's virtually impossible to be perfect, but we can all do better, myself included!

I don't know how to cook

Me, neither! Just ask my kids.

But it's extremely important to cook as many of your meals as you can. A couple of things have really helped me:

- I make simple food that tastes good roasted or steamed. It's not always fancy (ok, it's never fancy), but I like it and it makes me feel good.

- I have a couple of reliable cookbooks that I can use when I want to go above and beyond, like when my kids are visiting. Check out my cookbook recommendations on page 198.

- I bought an Instant Pot so I can make beans, stews, and chilis in a jiffy, which is important because I often get home late from work.

Oh, and I married someone who cooks much better than me. If this works out for you, I highly recommend this solution.

When I lose weight, I feel terrible

You're losing weight and that means you are getting healthier. But sometimes when people lose weight, they actually feel sick. If this is you, I'm sorry.

Remember how we all store toxins in our fat cells? Well, when you lose weight, your fat cells shrink and they release these toxins into your bloodstream, making you feel crummy. Some people describe this feeling as flu-like, with muscle aches, headache, and fatigue.[49,50]

A couple of things can help.

- Lose weight slowly. If you lose weight quickly, a lot of toxins get dumped into your bloodstream all at once. There is no way around this. Your body can more easily process them if it has more time to do so.

- Give your liver some extra detoxing power. I recommend my patients who are losing weight take a supplement by Pure Encapsulations called Liver-G.I. Detox. It has a combination of ingredients that support liver function and help it process toxins more efficiently.

- Eat a lot of fiber. When your liver processes toxins, it releases them into the intestines. There, they need to be sequestered with what we call binders, or they will just seep through the intestinal wall and back into your bloodstream. Insoluble fibers found in nuts and beans bind to toxic metals and chemicals so they can be pooped out.

- Minimize your exposure to new toxins and toxic chemicals. Your body will be better able to process the chemicals coming out of your fat cells if it isn't also processing new chemicals that you are absorbing from your food and environment.

Once your weight is stable, your toxic burden will decrease. Take extra good care of yourself while you are losing weight, and remember that it will get better.[51]

A quick summary

Do the best you can to reduce your exposure to endocrine-disrupting chemicals without making yourself too crazy. These chemicals are everywhere because they are cheap, convenient, and only minimally regulated. Take them out of your life as you can.

- Eat less meat and animal products.
- Use less plastic.
- Avoid cans.
- Eat mostly food that is fresh, frozen, or dried.
- Filter your water and your air.
- Use natural, organic products for your body, home, and garden.
- Strive for better. Don't make yourself crazy.

Healthy habits to get you started

- [ ] Swap your plastic water bottle for a stainless steel water bottle. Throw away or recycle all of your plastic water bottles and do not buy new ones.

- [ ] Buy a stainless steel or glass thermos for your coffee or tea.

- [ ] Every week, get two plastic items out of your kitchen and replace them with non-plastic alternatives.

- [ ] Find alternatives to foods that you usually buy in cans. Search for products in Tetra Pak boxes, glass jars, and the freezer section. For beans and soups, buy dried items that you can make in an Instant Pot.

- [ ] Replace your vinyl shower curtain with one that is polyester or nylon.

- [ ] Buy a water filter, and get an extra filter cartridge to keep on hand so you are ready when it comes time to replace it.

- [ ] Buy HEPA air filters for your living and sleeping spaces at home and at work.

- [ ] When the weather is nice, open all of the windows in your house and work space.

- [ ] Vacuum every week with a vacuum cleaner that has a HEPA filter.

☐ Take off your shoes inside.

☐ Every time a home or personal care product runs out, replace it with an organic or more natural product.

☐ Practice organic gardening.

CHAPTER 11

STEP 7:
Personalize your plan

$\mathcal{T}$here are as many variations of PCOS as there are women with PCOS. If you follow my protocol, you will get healthier. As you get healthier, your inflammation and testosterone levels will go down. Your insulin sensitivity and metabolic profile will improve. And all of your symptoms will get better. But they may not all heal completely.

Remember, some of your PCOS genes were programmed when you were a fetus in your mother's womb. Your estrogen receptors and possibly some of your other hormonal receptors were damaged. You don't aromatize testosterone into estrogen as efficiently as you need to. And although we can make everything better, that isn't always enough for a full recovery.

So in this chapter, I revisit many of the biggest PCOS symptoms and lay out additional, innovative ways to address them. Nothing in this chapter is as powerful as the protocol in the first part of this book. But if you follow the protocol and need a little extra love in a few areas, this will help a lot.

My advice here is brief, more of a jumping off point than a full treatment plan, because a complete discussion of each symptom could be a book unto itself.

Also, bear in mind that although I know a lot of stuff about a lot of stuff, I don't know everything about everything. I'm not a gastroenterologist. I'm not a cardiologist. I'm an Integrative OB-GYN. For many of my patients, I am their primary care physician, but I am only a part of their medical care team. Please treat this chapter (and this book) in the same way.

PCOS is a complicated medical condition. I hope you have a team of doctors that you trust to help you manage your most serious symptoms. I am sharing my knowledge so you can work with your doctors to create the best treatment plan possible.

As always, where it seems helpful, I'll mention the specific products that I use in my practice. This is to reduce the amount of research you need to do, not to hawk products. In most cases, I don't have a relationship with these products beyond that I've researched them and my patients like them. In Appendix C (page 331), I've included a full disclosure of the supplement and medical brands with which I do have a professional relationship.

I also mention a few pharmaceuticals that do a good job of addressing problems without creating a slew of even worse side effects. Obviously, these treatments are not do-it-yourself. You'll need a doctor to write your prescriptions and monitor your progress.

My hope is that these are the final tools you need to take full control of your health.

Follow the protocol and get your circadian rhythm back on the beat. Take the core supplements (page 19). Time your light and dark exposures. Get enough sleep at the right time. Eat during the day and stop eating at night. Exercise. Feed your gut microbiome. Avoid poisoning yourself with toxins and endocrine disruptors. And see how far that gets you.

Then use the tools here to get the rest of the way to the health and happiness you seek. Find what works for you.

Acne

Acne is a symptom of elevated testosterone and internal inflammation, specifically gut inflammation. It's tempting to treat it with skin creams and antibiotics, but trust me, that is not the most effective plan. To improve acne, you need to reduce systemic inflammation throughout your body, lower testosterone levels, and reestablish a healthy skin microbiome. Healing acne requires healing your whole body. It is slow going, so expect it to take six months to see full results.

Do-it-yourself options

Acne is a billion-dollar industry. With thousands of products available, figuring out what will work for you can be a time-consuming, expensive, and frustrating experience. Here are the products and strategies that have given my patients the best results.

Dairy-free
If you haven't cut out dairy yet, do that first. Dairy is inflammatory and exacerbates acne.

Over-the-counter skin care products
Oh boy, oh boy, there are a ton of acne skin creams. Most of them range from mildly effective to totally ineffective, but there are a few that provide great results.

Made from sugar cane, glycolic acid is a type of alpha hydroxy acid (AHA) that exfoliates dead skin cells, removes skin oil, and promotes collagen production. Just be aware that the results are cumulative and it can take several weeks to see a reduction in acne. In one study, participants applied a 10% glycolic acid serum daily. Participants noticed visible improvements at day 45 and continued to see improvements through day 90, with minimal side effects.[1]

Niacinamide (NY-ah-sin-ah-mide), a vitamin B3 compound, controls acne by reducing pathogenic bacteria populations and moderating skin oil production. I usually prescribe my patients a skin gel with 4% niacinamide, but because it's vitamin B3, you can also find dozens of over-the-counter skin creams with up to 5% niacinamide.[2]

Tea tree oil is a well-researched essential oil and broad-spectrum antimicrobial that targets acne-causing bacteria. One study compared the effectiveness of a 5% tea tree oil to a 5% benzoyl peroxide lotion. Both preparations effectively reduced acne severity, but patients using tea tree oil experienced significantly less burning, itching, and flaking. I recommend Simplers Botanicals Clear Skin, an organic essential oil with tea tree, lavender, and thyme. Apply it twice daily.[3,4,5]

Probiotic skin care products

Probiotics for your skin can help reestablish a healthy skin microbiome, reducing the presence of pathogenic, acne-causing bacteria. In my office, we carry the Glowbiotics skin care line.[6]

Spearmint Tea

Spearmint tea is a potent anti-androgen. It reduces your testosterone levels and helps prevent acne. You may be able to find Traditional Medicinals Organic Spearmint Herbal Tea in your local grocery store. Drink two cups per day to see results.[7]

Vitamin E and zinc supplements

People with acne generally have low levels of both vitamin E and zinc in their blood.[8,9]

Make sure you are taking a multivitamin that includes vitamin E. On top of that, I will give my patients Pure Encapsulations Vitamin E (with Mixed Tocopherols) — one capsule per day for six months. Each bottle has 90 capsules, so buy two bottles and when they are empty, stop. At this point, your vitamin E levels should have recovered and your skin will be clearer. You then start what we call the maintenance phase, and the vitamin E in your multivitamin should be plenty.

Additionally, make sure you are getting 30 mg of zinc. Otherwise, find a supplement to get to that level. Check your multivitamin first. Depending on what's already in it, you may want to take more. I usually give my patients Pure Encapsulations Zinc 15 or Zinc 30.

With zinc, be careful because taking more than 50 mg per day can cause copper deficiency. If you get bloodwork done that shows you are low in zinc and your doctor recommends taking a higher daily dosage, be sure to pair it with a copper supplement. I usually add 1 mg of copper.

With-your-doctor options

If the do-it-yourself options aren't enough, your doctor may prescribe pharmaceuticals to lower your testosterone and reduce the appearance of your acne. Be sure to use two forms of birth control if you take anything that may cause birth defects.

There are a wide array of cosmetic procedures that can reduce the appearance of acne scars. You should have all cosmetic procedures done by a board-certified dermatologist, plastic surgeon, or cosmetic surgeon. Make sure you fully understand the costs, risks, post treatment care, and any anticipated maintenance procedures.

Blue light LED therapy

Blue light therapy is one of the few cosmetic treatments that is excellent for women with active acne. Light treatment is FDA-approved to heal existing outbreaks and prevent new ones by killing the bacteria responsible for most acne lesions and by downregulating oil glands so they produce less oil.

It's fabulous. You lie down under a bright LED panel for about 30 minutes, take a nap if you want to, and then you go about your day with brighter skin. There is zero redness, zero pain, and it works on all skin types. A standard course of treatment is twice a week for four weeks, and the results last for several months.[10]

In my office, I use a professional light panel called Celluma. Most LED light therapy uses narrowband blue light, which really targets acne. Red light is better for reducing inflammation and promoting healing. The Celluma incorporates blue and red lights and provides my patients with spectacular results.

Although a professional treatment gives you the best coverage and most consistent results, you can also do this at home. I encourage my patients to buy the professional grade Celluma device I use in my office or a less-expensive consumer version. If you use it twice weekly for long enough, it eventually pays for itself.[11]

High-dose vitamin A and isotretinoin

High-dose vitamin A is similar to isotretinoin, which used to be called Accutane. I prefer Vitamin A over isotretinoin because it is a natural product, and the dosing can be finely adjusted to your individual needs.

PCOS women tend to respond pretty well to this treatment during the treatment phase, but we have higher relapse rates. For most women, high-dose vitamin A or isotretinoin treatment leads to a permanent reduction in acne. With PCOS women, acne tends to come back.[12,13]

Whether you go with high-dose vitamin A or isotretinoin, this treatment requires the supervision of a doctor. There are several serious side effects that you must be monitored for. Because it can cause birth defects, you must be very careful with birth control.

Laser treatments

Many women, after they get their acne under control, are left with significant scarring. Lasers are a great tool for reducing the appearance of scars (and wrinkles!).

There are two main types of laser treatments, ablative and non-ablative.

Ablative lasers remove the outer layers of skin and stimulate collagen formation in underlying skin. This is a serious skin treatment. Most women need to be sedated and you will leave the dermatologist's office with your face covered in bandages. It takes two to four weeks to heal. If you go this route, find a board certified cosmetic surgeon to perform your treatment and consider having it done in the fall because you'll need to stay out of the sun for several months.

Although many women get great results, I don't offer ablative laser resurfacing in my office because it carries a risk of infection, scarring, and skin pigmentation changes. Plus, most of my patients can't take two weeks off of work to hide in their homes while the skin on their face grows back.

In my office, I have the FRAXEL, a non-ablative laser. Instead of burning off your skin, this laser creates thousands of micro-wounds under the skin's surface. These tiny laser injuries induce the body to heal, replacing scar tissue with new, healthy skin cells and increasing collagen production. The results aren't quite as good as the results from an ablative laser, but the risk of side effects is much lower and there's no real downtime.

It takes about six FRAXEL sessions to fully repair severe acne scars. After each session, your skin may be pink, as if you had a mild sunburn. But this is the kind of treatment that most women can get on their lunch break and then, with a bit of makeup, go right back to work. It's a gradual, gentle, natural way to repair acne-scarred skin.

Microneedling

Microneedling is another treatment that can reduce the appear of acne scars. It sounds medieval, but in this treatment, your doctor uses a pen-like tool outfitted with needles to make thousands of pin-pricks in your skin. These tiny wounds encourage collagen production that fills in scars and wrinkles. Microneedling is similar to the FRAXEL, but much less expensive.

It takes several sessions to reach full effects.

You can buy do-it-yourself microneedle rollers, but there isn't any data showing that they do anything. The needles your doctor uses are 1mm to 3mm long. The home roller devices have needles that are only 0.25mm long. Anecdotally, many people like them, and you probably can't hurt yourself, but there isn't enough data for me to recommend them.

Platelet Rich Plasma (PRP)

Sometimes called a vampire facial, PRP is one of my favorite scar-reducing treatments. It combines microneedling, to injure and open the skin, with platelets to promote new skin cell growth.

Before your PRP facial begins, your blood will be drawn and centrifuged to separate the plasma that contains concentrated platelets. Platelets are special blood components that help your skin heal, and they activate when skin is damaged. By concentrating platelets in plasma, you can deliver more natural healing power to your skin cells than your body can do on its own.

Once your platelets are isolated, your doctor will microneedle your skin. The platelet rich plasma is then painted onto your skin where it seeps deep into the tiny wounds to promote new tissue growth, which naturally fills in the indented scars.

PRP is typically done monthly until you get your desired results. Some women need only three sessions.

Prescription topicals

I haven't been impressed with the data on most prescription creams. PCOS women tend to have severe acne or cystic acne. Most prescription topicals are better for mild to moderate acne and not for cystic. And at that point, you might as well use an over-the-counter topical like glycolic acid, niacinamide, or tea tree oil. So I generally don't prescribe these.

Spironolactone

Spironolactone (spy-roh-noh-LACK-tone) is an antiandrogen pharmaceutical. It's a diuretic used to treat high blood pressure and heart failure that, as a side effect, blocks testosterone receptors. For many women, it reduces the acne and hirsutism caused by PCOS. If you do use spironolactone, you can start with a low-dose therapy of 25 mg/day instead of the more typical 100 mg/day.[14,15]

I have also prescribed it as a topical cream with moderate success. Your doctor would need to order it from a compounding pharmacy.

This drug causes birth defects, so you must combine it with reliable birth control.

Alopecia

Alopecia is another sign of elevated testosterone levels, so many of the recommendations overlap with those for acne. With androgenic alopecia, testosterone shrinks your scalp hair follicles, causing the actual hair shafts to likewise shrink in diameter until normal scalp hairs fall out and are replaced by fine, peach fuzz hairs. To treat androgenic alopecia, you must reduce testosterone levels. Scalp treatments can protect the hair follicles from the effects of testosterone and stimulate the hair follicles to expand and grow thicker, longer hairs.

Do-it-yourself options

There are several treatments you can do on your own to lower testosterone and promote new hair growth.

Low Level Laser Therapy (LLLT) Helmet

For a couple hundred dollars, you can buy a light helmet that will regrow some of your hair. Through a process called photobiostimulation, the lasers stimulate the stem cells in each hair follicle to increase overall hair density and increase the strength and thickness of each individual hair. You'll need to reliably use it every other day for about half an hour, but it's just a helmet so you can do computer work or watch TV while you're wearing it. Look for a device that is FDA-cleared.[16]

Rogaine

Rogaine, the brand name for minoxidil (mi-NOX-i-dill), is the only topical product with FDA-approval to treat hair loss in women. On the plus side, it works pretty well for about a third of women and you can buy it over-the-counter at any drug store. On the down side, it can cause an increase in body hair growth (it gave me werewolf hands), and you have to use it forever because if you stop, any new hair regrowth will fall out.[17]

Rogaine sells a 2% minoxidil cream for women, but many women need to use the men's 5% concentration to see results, which is an off-label use of the product. If you try Rogaine, get the foam version because it is easier and more pleasant to apply and is less irritating to your scalp.[18]

Spearmint Tea

As with acne, spearmint tea can be helpful. It reduces your testosterone level and may minimize future hair loss. Drink two cups per day to see results.

Zinc supplements

Zinc improves the testosterone profile of women with PCOS and reduces hair loss (and acne and hirsutism). Take 30 mg of zinc daily. Remember to check your multivitamin zinc content make sure you don't take more than 50 mg total, or you can cause a copper deficiency.[19]

With-your-doctor options

There are a few other medical options that can help regrow your hair.

Platelet-rich plasma (PRP)

PRP therapy is a great option for treating androgenic alopecia. The platelet rich plasma is injected directly into the scalp into areas with thinning hair. It stimulates the stem cells in each hair follicle to regenerate and revert back to their youthful, healthy activity. I offer this treatment in my practice and many of my patients have seen great results.

I usually administer this treatment once a month for three months and then once every three months for maintenance. PRP consistently outperforms Rogaine. After three sessions, most women see significant hair regrowth, and the new hairs have nice, thick shafts.[20,21]

Spironolactone

Because spironolactone is an antiandrogen, it can help slow or even stop the progression of androgenic alopecia and may promote new hair growth. Studies show that spironolactone can be effectively combined with 5% minoxidil (Rogaine) to increase minoxidil's effectiveness. As with acne treatments, I prefer that patients start with a low-dose therapy of 25 mg/day instead of the more typical 100 to 200 mg/day to minimize side effects. This drug causes birth defects, so you must combine it with reliable birth control.[22,23]

Topical finasteride

Finasteride (fi-NAS-teh-ride), brand name Propecia, is a powerful prescription antiandrogen that can be taken in pill form or applied topically. Oral finasteride can cause depression and sexual dysfunction, so when I recommend it, I usually prescribe a 0.2% finasteride cream. Finasteride in any format can cause birth defects so use reliable birth control while using this pharmaceutical.

I often send my patients to our local compounding pharmacy to get a cream that combines finasteride and minoxidil with betamethasone diprorionate and tretinoin. This mix is more potent than any single pharmaceutical is on its own. You'll need a prescription and a compounding pharmacy that can fill it.

Autoimmune Disease

Autoimmunity occurs when your immune system can't differentiate between foreign molecules and self molecules and so it mistakenly attacks the cells of your own body. Three conditions that lead to autoimmunity are inflammation, overstimulation of your immune system, and the presence of foreign molecules in your bloodstream.

You'll need to address all of these issues to improve your autoimmune symptoms.

Do-it-yourself options

If you've been diagnosed with an autoimmune disease, work with your doctor to create a comprehensive treatment plan. Everything in this book should be done in conjunction with that plan, not in place of it. But as you go through this book, let your doctor know what you're doing because when you heal your circadian rhythm and your gut, you may reduce your autoimmune symptoms and need to adjust your medication.

Using the protocol in this book, I reversed my Hashimoto's thyroiditis. I hope you see similar results. So, keep your doctor in the loop, even with supplements and lifestyle changes.

Fasting mimicking diet

L-Nutra, the company that developed ProLon, is in the early stages of testing the effects of a fasting mimicking diet on autoimmune diseases. So far, the results are extremely promising. In several rodent models of multiple sclerosis, a fasting mimicking diet can reduce or even reverse symptoms of autoimmunity.[24]

When a person has an autoimmune disease, certain immune cells malfunction and become overactive. A fasting mimicking diet causes many immune cells throughout the body to go through apoptosis, programmed cell death. At the end of fasting, refeeding stimulates immune cell regeneration, but these new cells are "naive," meaning they don't exhibit autoimmune behavior. At the same time, the fasting mimicking diet increases anti-inflammatory and anti-autoimmune Treg cells.[25]

All of this implies that several rounds of a fasting mimicking diet should reprogram your immune system and reverse autoimmunity.

This is what I've seen in my own life and in my own patients. It took 13 rounds of the fasting mimicking diet, ProLon, but I have successfully reversed my Hashimoto's.

Fiber, fiber, fiber

There is a high correlation between leaky gut and autoimmune disease. When you have leaky gut, all sorts of foreign bodies pass through your intestinal wall into your bloodstream and trigger an immune reaction. A high-fiber diet, by increasing short-chain fatty acid production and decreasing leaky gut, is protective against a wide range of autoimmune diseases.[26,27]

A gluten free, dairy free, and low-salt diet

If you haven't already, now is the time to go gluten free and dairy free. Gluten, along with several other proteins found in wheat and dairy, increases leaky gut and can induce autoimmunity through a process called molecular mimicry. Wheat and dairy proteins are so similar to proteins in our own body tissues that when we make antigens against them, the antigens attack our own tissues as well, simply because our bodies can't tell the difference. Get rid of those foreign proteins and your body should stop making antigens. So, stop eating gluten and dairy.[28]

And eat less salt. A high-salt diet activates your immune system, increases inflammation, and makes you more susceptible to autoimmune diseases.[2]

Omega-3s

If you haven't started taking omega-3's, now is a good time. These fatty acids reduce inflammation and down-regulate inflammatory cytokines that are involved in autoimmune diseases. They also directly protect against certain autoimmune diseases like Lupus.[30,31]

Because any fish you eat may contain toxic chemicals, I prefer to eat fish only once or twice per month and take a high quality omega-3 supplement that contains 600 mg of EPA and 400 mg of DHA, two essential omega-3s. Look for a supplement that is free from environmental toxins. I give my patients Pure Encapsulations O.N.E. Omega. I trust Pure Encapsulations because they stringently test for all impurities, not just mercury.

If you are following a vegan diet, you can find vegan omega-3 supplements made from algae. You can also eat a tablespoon of flaxseeds, which contain ALA, a third type of omega-3 that your body can somewhat inefficiently convert to EPA and DHA.

Protection for your skin, mouth, vagina

Most autoimmune-inducing foreign molecules enter your body through your intestinal wall. That's why we spend so much time talking about leaky gut. But your body has other interfaces with the outside world that can allow autoimmune-inducing molecules into your bloodstream.

Your skin is the next biggest, so I recommend all-natural, organic skin care products. In particular, make sure you are using a very gentle soap that does not contain sodium lauryl sulfate (SLS). Harsh chemicals like SLS disrupt the skin barrier function, increase skin inflammation, and make the skin less able to keep out pathogens and foreign molecules.[32]

For your mouth, it may seem obvious, but don't put anything in there that's toxic. Make sure you are using a natural toothpaste that does not contain triclosan, an antibacterial. And avoid mouthwash.

And don't forget about your vagina. It is really incredible how many chemicals we women are willing to put in our vaginas. Everything you put in there gets absorbed into your bloodstream and also changes the delicate vaginal microbiome. For menstruation, I recommend organic tampons, menstrual cups, period panties, and sanitary pads. And for lubrication, I recommend coconut oil (but not with condoms!) and aloe vera, which is water based and condom safe.

With-your-doctor options

If you have an autoimmune disease, you should work with your doctor to decide what pharmaceuticals will best treat your specific condition. Consider adding low-dose naltrexone to your treatment plan.

Low-dose naltrexone (LDN)

Naltrexone is a prescription pharmaceutical that blocks opioid receptors and is most commonly used to treat opioid addiction. In low doses, naltrexone is anti-autoimmune and is also a powerful anti-inflammatory. Doctors have been using LDN for 30 years to successfully treat a wide range of immune disorders, including many autoimmune diseases.[33,34]

A normal dose of naltrexone for opioid addiction is usually 50-100 mg. With LDN, your doctor will prescribe a tiny dose of 3 to 4 mg per day. This low dose blocks opioid receptors for just 1 to 2 hours in the middle of the night and stimulates the body to produce more endorphins and endorphin-related peptides, which are critical to proper immune system function. This is an off-label use, but naltrexone is an affordable generic drug, and at low doses, it has a strong safety profile. You would need your doctor to prescribe it and get it through a compounding pharmacy.

To begin a patient on LDN, I start with a tiny dose of 1.5 mg at bedtime and increase the dose to 3 mg and then to a maximum of 4.5 mg, depending on response and tolerability. LDN is not a fast miracle cure, and may require many months of use to see the benefits.

Cardiovascular Disease

Cardiovascular disease and hypertension are part of the metabolic dysfunction that is practically a calling card of PCOS. All of the recommendations in this book will ameliorate this chronic condition and reduce your risk of a heart attack or stroke. Get your circadian rhythm under control so that you stop storing visceral fat, which is a major risk factor for cardiovascular events. Make sure you are taking curcumin because it is particularly beneficial for cardiovascular health.[35]

Do-it-yourself options

Anything that improves your overall health will improve your cardiovascular health. On top of all of the great ideas in this book, here are a few more things you can try to lower your blood pressure and increase the health of your circulatory system.

Magnesium

Magnesium is an essential macromineral that plays a role in over 300 body-wide functions. Especially vital to heart health, it lowers blood pressure, reduces atherosclerosis, and increases blood flow. After a heart attack, many patients are given magnesium to reduce mortality from arrhythmia, an irregular heart beat. Additionally, magnesium regulates blood sugar, promotes better sleep, lowers anxiety, and reduces constipation.[36]

It's hard to overestimate how important magnesium is, and most Americans don't get enough through their diets. In fact, at least half of Americans are magnesium deficient and many more may have subclinical magnesium deficiency.[37]

If you eat the high-fiber, plant-based diet I recommend, you'll definitely increase your magnesium levels. Beans, almonds, and pumpkin seeds are particularly good sources of magnesium.

If you have any cardiovascular risk factors, you should take 400 mg of magnesium citrate or glycinate to protect your heart and blood vessels. I recommend Pure Encapsulations Magnesium Glycinate. Take 3 to 4 capsules daily with food.

Nitric oxide

Nitric oxide is a molecular messenger and vasodilator. It keeps blood vessels soft, flexible, and open, and it decreases blood pressure. Women with PCOS often have low levels of nitric oxide.[38]

Your body makes nitric oxide from nitrates in green, leafy vegetables and other foods, such as beets. The process starts in your mouth when you chew your food and mix it with the microbes and enzymes in your saliva. This converts the nitrates into nitrites. Then, in your stomach, your stomach acid converts the nitrites into nitric oxide, which goes straight into your bloodstream and maintains cardiovascular health.

For this process to work, you must have a healthy oral microbiome that can produce all of the enzymes needed to convert nitrates to nitrites. Our human cells can't produce these enzymes. So avoid toothpaste that contains triclosan, a powerful antimicrobial. Colgate toothpaste seems to be the last holdout that contains triclosan. Also, do not use mouthwash. These products kill everything, including our good bacteria.

When people use mouthwash, specifically, their capacity to create oral nitrites decreases by 90% and their blood pressure increases.[39]

Support your oral microbiome, and eat lots of nitrate-rich leafy green vegetables.

There are also nitric oxide supplements which increase your body's production of nitric oxide. I encourage all of my PCOS patients with vascular challenges to take either Pure Encapsulations Nitric Oxide Ultra or HumanN Neo40. Take either supplement twice daily, 20 minutes before a meal.

With-your-doctor options

As always, work with your doctor to determine the best plan for managing your cardiovascular health. As you adopt the protocol in this book, monitor your blood pressure, your cholesterol levels, and your triglyceride level. If you are taking pharmaceuticals such as statins or blood pressure medications, I hope that you can reduce your dosage and eventually get off of them.

Wean off of proton pump inhibitors (PPIs), if possible

Unless you have very specific and severe gastrointestinal conditions, such as bleeding ulcers, if you are taking a PPI, you should wean yourself off of these powerful drugs under the supervision of your doctor. For people with cardiovascular disease, PPIs increase your chances of suffering a heart attack. PPIs reduce stomach acid dramatically, and stomach acid is essential to creating nitric oxide. Without nitric oxide, your arteries harden and you develop high blood pressure and cardiovascular disease.[40]

For alternative treatments, see the section on heartburn and PPIs on page 204.

Contraception

Contraception is a problem. There is nothing on the market that I completely love.

As I've mentioned before, I'm not a fan of synthetic hormonal contraceptives. That covers all forms of birth control pills, patches, injections, rings, and most intrauterine devices (IUDs). They are endocrine disruptors that increase your risk of breast cancer, cervical cancer, depression, and suicide. They raise your triglyceride levels and are never recommended for women at risk of deep vein thrombosis and cardiovascular disease. Note that all women with PCOS are at risk of deep vein thrombosis and cardiovascular disease and most of us already have high triglyceride levels. If you do take synthetic hormonal contraceptives, please take them for the shortest time possible.[41,42,43,44,45]

Planned Parenthood has a great overview of all of the most common forms of birth control available today (www.plannedparenthood.org/learn/birth-control). Here are some options to consider.

Do-it-yourself options

There aren't that many non-medical contraceptive options. I don't love spermicide alone or as part of a sponge or cervical cap. Even with perfect use, these methods aren't effective enough, and because spermicide can irritate the vagina, it actually increases your risk of contracting HIV and other sexually transmitted infections.

Here are a couple of do-it-yourself options that I recommend.

Condoms

Condoms are an affordable and effective form of birth control and are one of the absolute best contraceptive options for female health. When used properly every single time, male condoms are 98% effective and female condoms are 95% effective at preventing pregnancy. And condoms are the most reliable way to protect yourself against sexually transmitted infections.

For male condoms, you can now find all natural latex condoms that come with all natural lubricant. But even if you get regular old drug store condoms, at least for most people, you're just not exposed to these chemicals for all that long.

Female condoms are slightly more expensive and complicated to use than male condoms, but they are latex free and female controlled. Also, many couples really like how they feel.

Condoms are hormone-free and protect against sexually transmitted infections. Even when combined with spermicides and lubricants, you don't use that much and you don't have to leave these chemicals in place for hours before and after sex. Hands down, condoms are the healthiest form of highly effective birth control for women, but they are also a form of birth control that women don't have total control over.

Fertility-awareness methods

For some couples, fertility awareness methods provide enough protection while being 100% natural. Also called "natural family planning" or the "rhythm method," fertility-awareness contraceptive methods involve tracking your cycles and your physical signs of fertility, such as cervical mucus and temperature, and abstaining from sex on your fertile days.

These methods are fairly complicated and they are more effective for women with predictable menstrual cycles. However, with a lot of work, they can be reasonably effective. They are completely natural, and they are suitable for couples who have religious concerns with other birth control methods.

Cedar Rivers Medical Clinics offers a nice, medically accurate overview of several fertility-awareness methods: www.birth-control-comparison. info/fertility-awareness.

With-your-doctor options

There are a few other forms of contraception to consider. The copper IUD and the diaphragm are hormone-free, completely under your control, and virtually invisible to your partner. But neither protects you from sexually transmitted infections. Talk to your doctor about the pros and cons of each method.

If you do ultimately choose a hormonal option such as birth control pills, implantations, injections, patches, rings, or a hormonal IUD, remember that the "hormones" are actually hormone-mimicking endocrine disruptors. Use this method for the shortest amount of time possible.

Copper IUD (ParaGard)

The copper IUD is the least bad medical form of birth control. It is hormone-free, which is great. Once it's inserted, you don't have to think about it for up to 10 years. It's basically invisible to your partner. And it's completely reversible. That's the good.

Here's the bad: The copper IUD is inherently inflammatory. That's actually how it works. It creates an inflammatory reaction in the uterus that is toxic to sperm. So, it's not ideal for someone trying to reduce inflammation in her body. But at least it doesn't have endocrine disruptors.[46]

Another newly discovered problem with the copper IUD is that it alters the microbiomes of the cervix, uterus, and vagina. Women with a copper IUD have much higher rates of vaginal infections, particularly bacterial vaginosis (BV), and BV can more than double your risk of contracting sexually transmitted infections.[47,48]

Because both BV and STIs can cause pregnancy complications, I recommend that women who have their copper IUD removed wait six months before attempting to get pregnant. This gives you a chance to get tested for these infections and get all of your microbiomes back in order.

Diaphragm

Another barrier option similar to the condom is the diaphragm. This is a latex cap that you insert over your cervix along with a good dose of spermicide. The diaphragm can be inserted with the spermicide up to two hours before intercourse and then must be left in place for at least six hours after sex. If you have sex again during the six hour time frame, insert more spermicide into your vagina.

A diaphragm is 94% effective at preventing pregnancy. So it's almost as good as a condom, and it is hormone-free, completely under your control, and often can't be detected by your partner. Your partner can still wear a condom and then you've got some super effective barrier birth control!

If you want a diaphragm, you'll need to get fitted by your doctor. It's not the kind of thing you can pick up at the local pharmacy.

Permanent sterilization

If you are 100% sure that you don't want any future children, you or your partner may consider surgical sterilization. The male procedure, a vasectomy, is simpler and safer than the female procedure, a tubal ligation.

A vasectomy cuts or blocks a man's vas deferens, the tubes that carry sperm from the testes to the penis. It's a quick, simple, outpatient procedure that requires very little down-time afterwards. Vasectomies do not alter sexual experience. After a vasectomy, a man will ejaculate exactly the same as he did before, but his semen will be sperm-free. No sperm, no pregnancy.

In a tubal ligation, a woman's fallopian tubes are closed or blocked to prevent eggs from traveling from the ovaries to the uterus. There are a couple of different ways to do this. You should discuss with your doctor what makes the most sense for you. They are all generally safe procedures, but because your fallopian tubes are inside your body, tubal ligation is not as fast and simple as a vasectomy. After a tubal ligation, you will still menstruate normally, but no egg, no pregnancy.

Vasectomies and tubal ligations are completely permanent. You should only get a sterilization procedure if you are positive that you will never want more children. But, once you do them, you'll never have to think about birth control again. Just note that they do not protect against sexually transmitted infections.

Diabetes, type 2

When you have type 2 diabetes, your body loses the ability to control your blood sugar levels. Your pancreas cannot make enough insulin and your body is simultaneously resistant to the insulin you do make. If you've been diagnosed with diabetes or prediabetes, and especially if you are taking medication for your diabetes, you need to do everything, including "do-it-yourself" lifestyle changes, under the care of a physician.

It is beyond the scope of this book to tell you everything you can do and take to improve and reverse your diabetes.

If you are on glucose-lowering medications, you need to be very careful about triggering a hypoglycemic event. This is especially true as you get your blood sugar levels under control.

Do-it-yourself options

Diabetes is a lifetime of disease management. But it is easier and less burdensome if you lose weight, adopt a healthy diet (like the one in this book!), and exercise. There are also several supplements that can help.

If you are a younger woman and/or if you were diagnosed with diabetes within the last ten years, consider going all-in with changing your lifestyle and getting healthy because type 2 diabetes is reversible if you act quickly. With a very healthy lifestyle, you may be able to get off medication and restore normal (or near normal) blood glucose levels. You can do this![49]

Berberine

Berberine (BER-ber-een) is a supplement that comes from traditional Chinese medicine and is extremely effective at controlling blood sugar levels in diabetic patients. In several studies, berberine is as effective at controlling blood glucose levels and insulin resistance as other oral glucose-lowering drugs, including metformin.[50]

In one study, diabetic patients took berberine for 3 months, with no other interventions or lifestyle changes. Over the course of the study, participants' average blood sugar level dropped from 7.0 to 5.6 mmol/L, going from diabetic to normal.[51]

You should take 500 mg three times per day, before meals, for a total of 1500 mg per day. I recommend Thorne Berberine-500 and Berberine Balance by Douglas Laboratories. Note that you should not take berberine if you are pregnant.

Caloric timing

Eat with your circadian rhythm by eating a big breakfast and then smaller meals later in the day. Your body is most insulin sensitive in the morning so take advantage of that. When diabetics shift their calories to earlier in the day, they lose weight. Compared to diabetics eating the exact same foods and calories but later in the day, big breakfast eaters have lower fasting glucose levels, and they use less insulin.[52]

Diet

A healthy diet is one of the best things you can do to mitigate and reverse type 2 diabetes.

You already know that added sugars aren't good for you. If you have diabetes, they really, really aren't good for you. Added sugars spike your blood sugar levels and unnecessarily stress your already struggling pancreas. So you should completely avoid all added sugars.

Highly-processed foods, especially those containing white flour, rice, and potato starch, can also cause significant blood sugar spikes.[53]

For more information on how to reverse type 2 diabetes with diet, I recommend Dr. Fuhrman's book, *The End of Diabetes: The Eat to Live Plan to Prevent and Reverse Diabetes.*

Melatonin

Because most chronic diseases involve circadian rhythm dysfunction, it's not really surprising that melatonin can reduce symptom severity.

In a recent study, a group of 17 obese patients with diabetes were given 3 mg of melatonin at bedtime every night for 12 weeks. That was the only intervention. At the end of 12 weeks, participants' insulin resistance and fasting insulin levels both decreased by about 14%. Participants also lost weight and had visibly reduced acanthosis nigricans, darkened skin caused by insulin resistance. Just from taking melatonin.[54]

So if you have diabetes, take 3 mg of melatonin at bedtime for 12 weeks and monitor your blood sugar. After 12 weeks, you can try to reduce your melatonin to just 1 or 2 mg per night, but if your blood sugar creeps back up, then it's safer to stay at 3 mg per night longterm.

Myo-inositol

Myo-inositol is an insulin mimetic that reduces insulin resistance, and it's a key part of my core supplements for PCOS. All indications are that it is safe to take with glucose-lowering medications that you may already be on, and it improves fasting blood glucose. I give my patients the Pure Encapsulations Inositol (powder) and recommend 4 g (2 scoops) per day.[55]

No mouthwash and antibacterial toothpaste

Protect your oral microbiome. This is covered in detail in the cardiovascular disease section on page 250. Long story short, you need good bacteria in your mouth to help convert nitrates in food to nitric oxide, which is critical for metabolic health. It may sound crazy, but frequent use of mouthwash is an independent risk factor for developing diabetes.[56]

Don't kill your oral microbiome. Check out the gingivitis section (page 262) for mouthwash alternatives if you need them.

With-your-doctor options

To avoid hypoglycemic events, all lifestyle modifications should be done under the supervision of your doctor. Here are a few more intensive treatments you may want to explore.

Fasting

Fasting has been shown to be an effective way to reset metabolism and reduce the severity of type 2 diabetes. However, it also raises the risk of hypoglycemia. If you are interested in fasting, please work with your doctor so she can monitor your blood sugar and suggest possible modifications to your medications. Diabetics who fast under the supervision of their doctor are significantly less likely to experience a hypoglycemic event.[57,58]

Glucagon-like peptide-1 (GLP-1) receptor agonists

This is a whole class of injectable drugs that can help diabetics manage their blood sugar and possibly lose weight. These drugs improve blood sugar control in a variety of ways. They improve insulin production and they slow down the rate that the liver releases glucose. Additionally, these drugs slow down gastric emptying. This means that food stays in your stomach longer, which keeps you full longer and prevents post-eating blood sugar spikes. All of these effects lead to significant weight-loss for many diabetic patients, which further improves glucose control and other metabolic markers.[59]

There are several brands and formulations. Liraglutide (leer-ah-GLOO-tide), sold under the brand names Victoza and Saxenda, seems to work well for PCOS women.

Metformin

Metformin is an insulin-sensitizing pharmaceutical. It has long been used to treat diabetes, and now, more recently it has become a first line pharmaceutical for treating PCOS, even for women without diabetes, which is an off-label use.

If you are taking metformin, you should closely monitor your blood sugar, thyroid function, and vitamin B12 levels. As you improve your diet and lifestyle, watch your blood sugar levels to avoid hypoglycemic events. If you have Hashimoto's thyroiditis, be aware that your thyroid medications may reduce metformin's potency and metformin may change your thyroid function. Check in with your endocrinologist and be sure to get your TSH levels checked frequently. Metformin depletes your body of vitamin B12, so you should annually screen for B12 deficiency.[60,61]

Metformin is not my favorite insulin-sensitizer because I am concerned about its endocrine disrupting properties, particularly during pregnancy. See more about metformin on page 278.

Fatty Liver (NAFLD)

If you've been diagnosed with fatty liver, you have a dysregulated circadian rhythm and a dysbiotic gut. The protocol in this book is the best treatment. Fix your clock and your gut so that your liver is getting the right signals and stops storing fats. Make sure you are doing time-restricted eating and that you are getting a good overnight fast so your body has a chance to switch into fat-burning mode and you can start losing weight. To make a fatty liver less fatty, by definition, you need to lose fat.

Take the core supplements I recommend in the beginning of this book. Several of them, such as NAC and curcumin, protect against fatty liver disease.

And cut out alcohol. Women with PCOS already don't process alcohol well. Once you have fatty liver, even small amounts of alcohol dramatically increase your risk of liver failure.

Gingivitis and periodontal disease

Women with PCOS have an altered oral microbiome, and that puts us at risk for gum and dental diseases. Good oral hygiene is extra important to protect your mouth. Floss, brush twice per day, use a natural non-toxic toothpaste, avoid commercial mouthwash, and visit the dentist twice a year.[62]

Do-it-yourself options

The oral microbiome is a brand new frontier, and scientists are just starting to map the hundreds of microbes living in your mouth. We are beginning to learn who does what, and one bacteria stands out as being particularly problematic — *Streptococcus mutans*. This guy lives on the surface of your teeth and is the instigator of tooth decay, cavities, and gum disease.

Here are some natural ways to reduce *Streptococcus mutans* populations while nurturing a healthy oral microbiome.

Natural mouthwash

Commercial mouthwash is toxic to you and your oral microbiome. Both adults and children have poisoned themselves with mouthwash, so it definitely fails my rule: Don't put toxic chemicals in your mouth.[63]

Fortunately, most people who poison themselves with mouthwash don't die. The same cannot be said of your oral microbiome. Mouthwash kills vast quantities of your oral microbes, including beneficial bacteria essential to producing nitric oxide and lowering your risk of cardiovascular disease and diabetes (see page 251 and page 259 for more info on nitric oxide).

If you are fighting swollen gums, struggling with flossing, or if you really like mouthwash, there are some great alternatives. Try a xylitol mouthwash. There are tons of all-natural ones in a wide variety of flavors. Another option is to use tulsi (also known as holy basil) tea as a mouthwash. Tulsi inhibits *Streptococcus mutans*, and in a head-to-head competition, tulsi mouthwash performed as well as Listerine.[64,65]

Xylitol

Xylitol is an alcohol sugar that completely disables *Streptococcus mutans*. People who use xylitol at least three times per day have significantly less plaque, fewer cavities, and less gum disease. And xylitol seems to do all of this without destroying the oral microbiome. Additionally, it improves the gut microbiome by increasing gram-positive bacteria populations and butyrate production.[66,67]

So use a xylitol toothpaste twice per day and chew xylitol gum or eat xylitol mints sometime in the middle of the day.

However, a note of warning: Too much xylitol works as a laxative. You ideally want 6 g per day for maximum cavity-fighting, but don't go above 8 g per day, or you may regret it.

Hirsutism

Along with acne and alopecia, hirsutism is a sign of elevated testosterone. Hirsutism is when you grow dark body hair in places that women don't usually have dark hair — your face, chest, back, and hands.

The best treatment plan is to permanently remove any unwanted hairs that you already have and stop new hairs from growing by lowering testosterone levels. The plan laid out in this book is a great place to start. Here are a few more tips.

Do-it-yourself options

If you only have a few hairs, you can tweeze, wax, or bleach them. And then try to reduce your testosterone levels naturally to prevent more hairs from growing.

Spearmint Tea and Zinc

The best do-it-yourself options for lowering testosterone are spearmint tea and zinc (page 238). This is the same advice I give for acne and alopecia.

With-your-doctor options

For more extensive hair growth, I recommend cosmetic treatments to permanently zap those dark hairs out of your life forever.

Electrolysis

This is the safest and most permanent form of hair removal, and it is hands down my top recommendation for removing the unwanted hair you already have on your face and other reasonably small parts of your body.

With electrolysis, a licensed and board-certified dermatologist or electrologist inserts a teeny tiny needle into each hair follicle and destroys it by zapping it with a tiny bit of electricity. As you can imagine, it's time consuming, and it takes several sessions to get complete hair removal. But the results are permanent.

Additionally, electrolysis can be done on women with any skin tone, and the risks and side effects are minimal.

Electrolysis is a bit of a dying art form so don't wait too long. It's being replaced by laser hair removal, which is okay but not nearly as good.

Laser Hair Removal

On the plus side, laser hair removal is available everywhere. It's fast and great for large sections of your body like your legs.

Hairy legs, by the way, are not part of hirsutism. They are part of being a normal woman, but if you want to get your face and legs done together, laser hair removal is the way to go. Honestly, I have the Lumenis Diode Laser laser at my office, and because it's so convenient, I've pretty much done my whole body except for my head. Perpetually silky legs are one of the perks of my job.

The laser works by using a laser (surprise!) to zap dark hairs. It really only works on light skinned people with dark hairs because the laser needs to be able to see the hair follicles. On top of that, the results aren't completely permanent.

Get this done by a licensed dermatologist or esthetician. After a few rounds of treatment a few weeks apart, you'll see dramatically reduced hair growth. Maybe even no hairs at all. But you'll probably need a follow-up treatment once a year to maintain the effects.

Spironolactone

This antiandrogen pharmaceutical blocks testosterone receptors. It is useful for acne, alopecia, and hirsutism. See page 243 for more information.

Vaniqa

Vaniqa (VAN-i-kah) is a prescription cream that slows hair growth and may make hairs thinner and lighter. You will still need to pluck, wax, or bleach the hairs that grow in, but much less often. It also may prevent new hairs from growing so your hirsutism doesn't get worse. As with many hair treatments, if you stop using the cream, you will stop seeing results. The hairs will go back to the way they were before.

Irritable Bowel Syndrome (IBS)

IBS is a catch-all diagnosis for people who frequently experience uncomfortable gastrointestinal symptoms without any more serious causes. A good 40% of PCOS women have it. People with IBS may experience cramping, bloating, gas, diarrhea, and constipation.

IBS is different from inflammatory bowel disease (IBD), even though their acronyms are annoyingly similar. IBD is exactly what it sounds like, inflammation of the intestines, and it includes Crohn's disease and ulcerative colitis. If you experience gastrointestinal distress, you need to get a diagnosis from a doctor because IBS can share a lot of the same symptoms with much more serious diseases, including IBD.

Do-it-yourself options

Once you have an IBS diagnosis, there are several things worth trying on your own. One of the best things you can do is eat a healthy, high-fiber diet like the one I recommend. There are strong circadian rhythm components to IBS, so get on the beat. And exercise because nothing keeps your gut moving properly like moving your whole body. Here are a few more tips.

Berberine

Berberine is an ancient Chinese remedy for diarrhea. It slows down gastrointestinal motility and has analgesic properties, so it reduces pain. 500 mg daily is a very effective treatment for diarrhea-dominant IBS. I often give my patients Berberine Balance by Douglas Laboratories or Thorne Berberine-500. Note that you should not take berberine if you are pregnant.[68]

Fiber

Not all fibers behave the same way as they journey through your gut. So although a high fiber diet generally helps normalize digestion, it doesn't do so consistently.

Psyllium fiber is particularly useful for ameliorating both constipation and diarrhea because it is what we call a gelling fiber.

Psyllium absorbs significant water and it does not release this water back to the large intestine. For women with constipation, this fiber softens your stool, increases transit time, and increases bowel movement frequency. It gives you comfortably soft, more frequent poops.

Psyllium holds water in a highly structured gel matrix. Consequently, it minimizes diarrhea as well. Women with diarrhea who take psyllium experience better formed stools, slower transit time, and less frequent bowel movements. You also get comfortably soft (but not too soft) and frequent (but not too frequent) poops.

And because your gut bacteria cannot ferment psyllium, you get these benefits without any increase in gas or bloating.[69]

I recommend Pure Encapsulations G.I. Fortify. It comes in both capsule and powder form. The powder is more effective but it doesn't dissolve well and some people struggle with the taste. I also like Organic India Whole Husk Psyllium. It's an affordable and effective psyllium powder that tastes like bread crumbs. If you take any of these supplements, be sure to drink an extra 8 to 16 ounces of water every day.

Food sensitivities

Many patients with IBS report that their symptoms are triggered by specific foods. Common culprits are lactose, gluten, coffee, and specific fruits and vegetables. You can conduct an elimination challenge on your own or with a knowledgeable nutritionist, integrative or functional medicine doctor, or a naturopathic doctor to figure out what triggers your IBS.[70]

Low-FODMAP diet

FODMAPs are highly fermentable foods that often trigger IBS symptoms. Your gut bacteria eat these fibers and release gas. In some IBS patients, particularly those with small intestinal bacterial overgrowth (SIBO, see page 270), FODMAPs produce lots of bloating and gas, which can be extremely uncomfortable and embarrassing.

Many people with IBS feel better if they reduce or eliminate FODMAPs from their diet for a few weeks. You can get a list of high- and low-FODMAP foods at www.ibsdiets.org. The list is pretty detailed and restrictive, but if you have painful gas, going on a low-FODMAP diet can be life-changing.

One challenge is that most high-FODMAP foods are healthy, high-fiber foods that you need to build a healthy gut microbiome. You shouldn't eat a low-FODMAP diet for longer than necessary. I recommend only six weeks. And then you need to slowly reintroduce foods and see which ones are okay and which ones bring back your symptoms.

Melatonin

Most of the melatonin in your body is produced in your gut so it is critical to normal intestinal function. When constipation-dominant IBS patients take 3 mg of melatonin at bedtime, they report less constipation and significantly less abdominal pain. And they sleep better. This is a safe treatment to try for three months, and then try to taper back to 1 mg to 2 mg per night.[71]

Triphala

This Ayurvedic herbal supplement is made from the dried fruits of three native Indian plants: Amla, Bibhitaki, and Haritaki. These three plants are powerful anti-inflammatories, and combined, they offer extremely effective and gentle constipation relief. I recommend one capsule per day of Douglas Laboratories Ayur-Triphala for anyone suffering from constipation-dominant IBS.[72]

With-your-doctor options

If you have been dealing with IBS for a long time or if it is impacting the way you live your life, I highly recommend that you work with a functional medicine doctor or functional gastroenterologist to develop an individualized treatment plan. Digestive problems like IBS are complicated conditions, and it's easy to haphazardly chase every new remedy that comes your way. You really need a plan.

Remove, Repair, Replace, Repopulate, and Restore the Spirit

The functional medicine principles to heal the gut consist of the five R's — Remove, Repair, Replace, Repopulate, and Restore the Spirit.

- **Remove:** Take all foods out of your diet that are toxic, processed, and allergy provoking. This includes gluten, dairy, and sugar.

- **Repair:** Reestablish a healthy gut mucosal lining by providing intestinal cells with nutrients like L-glutamine, butyrate, and zinc carnosine, and supplementing with coating agents (demulcents) such as slippery elm, aloe vera, marshmallow root, and licorice (DGL).

- **Replace:** Use supplements to bring digestive enzymes, stomach acid, and bile up to their proper levels so the gut can function optimally.

- **Repopulate:** Introduce healthy bacteria to the gut using probiotics.

- **Restore the Spirit:** There is a critical bidirectional relationship between the gut and the brain that is mediated by hormones and neurotransmitters. A sick, unhappy gut leads to an unhealthy, sad brain. A stressed and depressed brain leads to a dysbiotic, leaky gut. To get true and lasting healing, both physical and emotional health must be simultaneously addressed.[73]

I have helped many patients on their journey to heal IBS using this methodology. It's a journey that is hard to take on your own, so if you can find a functional medical doctor to guide you, I cannot recommend that enough.

Small Intestinal Bacterial Overgrowth (SIBO) testing

SIBO occurs when bacteria from the large intestine colonize the small intestine, which is supposed to be nearly bacteria free. These rogue bacteria cause gas, bloating, and sometimes diarrhea and can induce serious nutrient deficiencies.

Current estimates are that almost 80% of patients with IBS may have SIBO, and in these patients, killing the bacteria in the small intestine nearly always leads to complete resolution of IBS symptoms.

You should definitely get tested for SIBO if you start to increase the fiber in your diet and you get painfully bloated and gassy.

Everyone should be a little gassy. That's normal. Bacteria in your large intestines produce gas as they digest fiber, and that's what leads to flatulence. You may not like it, but it shouldn't hurt and it shouldn't change your daily activities.

If you have SIBO, gassiness can impact the way you live your life. Bacteria invade your small intestine, where they ferment fiber in your food and produce gas, often a lot of gas. Not only can this be embarrassing, but because your small intestine is not designed to stretch too much, all of that gas hurts!

The most common test for SIBO is a breath test. It's reasonably but not 100% accurate. If you get a positive SIBO test or if you suspect SIBO, find a functional gastroenterologist who can do more than just run you through antibiotics. SIBO can be hard to treat so get a good team.

Infertility and trying to conceive

The primary cause of infertility for PCOS women is lack of ovulation. For a woman to ovulate, she needs a symphony of well-timed hormonal signals to trigger one of her eggs to grow to maturity and release into her fallopian tubes where it can be fertilized by sperm. When hormones are off, the entire process shuts down.

The absolute best way to restore fertility is to restore health throughout your body. Follow this protocol. Take the core supplements. During the day, get light, eat lots of healthy and high-fiber foods, and exercise. At night, sleep in a dark, dark room. Avoid endocrine disruptors and other toxic chemicals.

It's not the sexiest advice out there. It certainly isn't a one-stop-shopping magic pill. But for the vast majority of women with PCOS, this is the best and healthiest way to restore fertility.

Even more than that, this is the best way to increase your odds of having a healthy, full-term pregnancy. Women with PCOS are at a higher risk of miscarriage, pregnancy complications, and preterm birth. It is impossible to overstate how important it is to get as healthy as you can before you get pregnant.

And by the way, your partner needs to get healthy, too. Healthy sperm are a critical part of the fertility equation.

Bloodwork

Before you even start trying to get pregnant, meet with your doctor and get your bloodwork done. These are the same tests I recommend in the beginning of the book on page 17.

This is also a great time to review any medications and supplements you are taking with your doctor to be sure they are safe during pregnancy. And make sure your vaccinations are up-to-date. Check the CDC for updated vaccination information at www.cdc.gov/vaccines/pregnancy.

Do-it-yourself options

In addition to getting as healthy as possible, there are several things you can do to increase your chances of getting pregnant.

Berberine

Berberine is useful for infertility because it helps control blood sugar and normalizes metabolism. It facilitates losing weight, in particular visceral fat, and it helps normalize triglyceride and cholesterol levels.[74]

Consequently, it improves pregnancy rates for PCOS women.

In a double blind, placebo-controlled study, women with PCOS who had been infertile for at least one year took berberine for six months. 22% of these women got pregnant and delivered a healthy baby.[75]

In another study, women undergoing in vitro fertilization (IVF) were given berberine, metformin, or a placebo. The live birth rate for the berberine group was 48.6%, which was significantly better than the metformin live birth rate (36.8%) and the placebo rate (20.6%).[76]

If you are trying to get pregnant, I recommend that you take 500 mg of berberine three times per day, before meals, for a total of 1500 mg per day. I like Thorne Berberine-500. If you end up needing IVF, keep taking the berberine because it will more than double your chances of getting pregnant and successfully carrying your baby to term.

As soon as you get pregnant, *stop taking the berberine*. Berberine is not safe to take during pregnancy because it may cause a rare birth form of brain damage called kernicterus.[77]

Myo-inositol, plus melatonin

Myo-inositol is one of the core supplements in my protocol for a reason. Myo-inositol is a naturally occurring sugar alcohol. We make it throughout our bodies, particularly in our kidneys and in our brains, and it occurs in fruits, vegetables, and legumes.

It's got a fabulous safety profile, so much so that we give it to preterm infants with breathing problems.[78]

For PCOS women, myo-inositol is an extremely effective insulin-sensitizer. It induces ovulation in 80% of the PCOS women who take it, and 70% of PCOS women taking 4 g of myo-inositol daily will go on to have regular menstrual cycles. On top of that, it also protects your eggs and improves their quality.[79,80]

When compared head-to-head with metformin, myo-inositol induces equal to superior pregnancy outcomes, but with a much stronger safety profile. You can continue taking myo-inositol throughout your pregnancy and it will reduce your risk of developing gestational diabetes by over 50%.[81,82]

I give my patients the Pure Encapsulations Inositol (powder) and recommend 4 g (2 scoops) per day.

Melatonin, which has receptors on the ovaries, further improves the effects of myo-inositol and increases pregnancy success rates. Women with PCOS often have lower quality eggs, which can make getting pregnant and staying pregnant much harder. Melatonin, and especially melatonin plus myo-inositol, improves your egg quality and consequently improves your chances of getting pregnant and having a safe pregnancy. This combination can also be used to improve the success of IVF.[83]

Try taking 3 mg of melatonin per night for three months. Then, cut back to 1 to 2 mg per night.

N-acetyl cysteine (NAC)

NAC is part of my PCOS core supplements because it improves a variety of metabolic markers, including insulin resistance, triglyceride levels, cholesterol levels, and testosterone levels.[84,85]

For women taking Clomid or undergoing assisted reproductive techniques, NAC can improve egg quality, ovulation, pregnancy, and live birth rates. And for women with a history of preterm labor (note that all

PCOS women are at increased risk of preterm labor), NAC helps you stay pregnant longer.[86]

In a study of women with a previous preterm delivery or who had bacterial vaginosis, which increases preterm birth rates, the women were divided into two groups. One group took 17-hydroxyprogesterone caproate (17-OHPC), a form of progesterone that reduces the risk of preterm delivery, with NAC. The other group received 17-OHPC plus a placebo. The women who took NAC delivered on average at 37.4 weeks, versus an average delivery at 34.1 weeks for the placebo group. That extra three weeks makes a *huge* difference in the short term and long term health risks that a baby faces.[87]

I recommend that all PCOS women, and especially those who are pregnant or trying to conceive, take 1800 mg of NAC per day. I like Pure Encapsulations NAC 600 mg. Take 3 capsules per day. There's also a 900 mg version, and then you take 2 capsules per day.

Ovulation trackers

Non-PCOS women can figure out when they are ovulating, more or less, by looking at the calendar. For PCOS women with irregular menstrual cycles, timing sex to your window of peak fertility is much more challenging.

To have the best chance of getting pregnant, you should have sex about every other day, starting a few days before ovulation and continuing through a few days past ovulation. To do this, you need to know when you ovulate.

Fortunately, there are a variety of techniques and products that can help predict when you will next ovulate.

- **Cervical mucus:** If you want to have a baby, you need to become familiar with your cervical mucus because it is one of the best indicators of fertility. A few days before ovulation, your cervical mucus changes dramatically and becomes clear and very stretchy. Some people compare its appearance and consistency to egg whites. You can test your mucus by putting a clean finger in your vagina to pull some out and then seeing how far it will stretch between two fingers. You are looking for clear mucus that can stretch an inch or more. As soon as you see this, you should start having sex every other day.

- **Ovulation predictor kit:** This is a kit that comes with several test strips that can detect the luteinizing hormone (LH) surge that precedes ovulation. You should monitor your cervical mucus and start testing when your mucus becomes stretchy. Otherwise, if you just test all the time, you'll spend a fortune on test strips. Peak LH is about two days before ovulation. This is a great day to have sex.

- **Period tracker apps:** I like the Life app, but there are many that can predict your peak fertility window based on the length of your past menstrual cycles.

- **Thermometer:** Your basal body temperature is your lowest body temperature of the day and you can use it to better understand your fertility cycle. With a very accurate basal body thermometer, take and record your temperature immediately upon waking up at the same time every morning, before you get out of bed. The day after you ovulate, your temperature should go up 0.5 to 1.0 degrees Fahrenheit. This is a great, inexpensive way to confirm ovulation. Combine this data with cervical mucus observations and possibly an ovulation predictor kit to create a detailed picture of your fertility window.

Soy

Add four servings per week of organic soy to your diet to help protect you and your baby from the toxic effects of BPA.

Most women with PCOS have high levels of BPA in their bodies, and high BPA causes elevated testosterone levels and metabolic disease. All of this is bad for fertility. Eating a full serving of soy products like tofu, tempeh, and edamame three to four times per week protects against some of the negative effects of BPA.

This is especially important for women undergoing in vitro fertilization (IVF) where higher BPA levels correspond to lower pregnancy rates and poorer pregnancy outcomes. Women with high levels of BPA who eat soy generally have better IVF success rates.[88]

Supplements

For women who are ovulating, nutritional deficiencies decrease fertility. While you are trying to conceive, you need to eat the healthiest diet you can — the diet in this book is excellent for fertility. Focus on eating mostly plant-based, minimally-processed foods.[89]

Use supplements to reliably fill in any nutritional gaps. Follow the core supplements recommendation on page 19. But swap the regular multivitamin for a good prenatal vitamin that has 800 to 1000 mcg (1 mg) of folate. I suggest that my patients take the Thorne Basic Prenatal.

Also add 400 to 600 mg of magnesium citrate or glycinate. I recommend Pure Encapsulations Magnesium Glycinate. Take 3 to 4 capsules daily with food. This is fine to combine with the Thorne Prenatal.

Weight management

Your body is your baby's first home so before you start trying to get pregnant, you need to get as healthy as possible. In particular, do everything you can to get to a healthy weight.

At the very least, try to get your BMI under 30, and ideally under 25. Find an online BMI calculator to see where you are. This is for you and for your baby. Women with BMIs above 25 have higher rates of gestational diabetes, cesarean section deliveries, and post-delivery complications. And babies born to obese women are up to five times as likely as babies born to healthy-weight mothers to spend time in the neonatal intensive care unit. Oh, and in case you are one of the underweight PCOS outliers, being underweight also makes pregnancy much more dangerous. Do everything you can to get to a healthy weight.[90]

And get on an exercise program. Aerobic exercise, the kind that gets your heartrate up and makes you sweat, is strongly correlated with improved insulin resistance and more regular menstruation. Ideally, aim for one hour of aerobic exercise 3 to 5 days per week.[91]

With-your-doctor options

My patients with persistent infertility usually have failed conception in spite of successful ovulation. I generally refer these women to a fertility center that specializes in the needs of PCOS women. Often, there is a male factor adding to the mix, and sometimes autoimmunity is an issue.

If you are not menstruating, if you are menstruating but you can't get pregnant, or if you've had more than one miscarriage, it may be time to contact a fertility center. Make sure that you choose a clinic that understands the unique needs of PCOS women. We respond differently to many common treatments. For example, women with PCOS ...

- Have double the risk of ovarian hyperstimulation syndrome.[92]
- Respond better to letrozole (LEH-troh-zole) than Clomid.[93]
- Experience higher rates of recurrent pregnancy loss.[94]
- Need to address insulin resistance.

With a fertility clinic, you will have access to a wide range of treatment options — pharmaceuticals like letrozole, Clomid, and metformin, injectable gonadotropins, intrauterine insemination (IUI), and in vitro fertilization (IVF). Make sure you understand the costs and the risks of any procedure.

And remember that lifestyle and the right supplements can increase the success of fertility treatments. Berberine, myo-inositol, melatonin, NAC, soy, and simply losing weight will improve your egg quality, your hormonal profile, and your chances of getting pregnant and successfully delivering a healthy baby.

Here are some things you should know about.

Clomiphene Citrate (Clomid)

Clomid is a pharmaceutical that induces ovulation, and it is considered a first line treatment for anovulatory infertility. I don't love it for PCOS women because as many as 40% of us are Clomid-resistant, and it simply doesn't work. Although more than 40% of non-PCOS women taking Clomid will succeed in having a live birth, the live birth rate for PCOS women with Clomid is just 20%-30%, depending on BMI.[95,96,97,98]

Additionally, PCOS women have a higher than normal risk for developing ovarian hyperstimulation, a painful and potentially dangerous complication of fertility treatments.

> All that being said, my first baby was a Clomid baby. It took several rounds of higher and higher doses, but I did get pregnant and deliver a healthy baby girl.

Letrozole

An alternative to Clomid, letrozole also induces ovulation. This drug is an aromatase inhibitor, which means it blocks the enzyme aromatase and reduces the conversion of testosterone and DHEA-S, another androgen, to estrogen. The drop in estrogen causes the brain to release more ovarian stimulating hormones, which trigger ovulation.

For women with PCOS, letrozole is more effective than Clomid. In a recent study that compared the effectiveness of Clomid to letrozole among women with PCOS, women taking letrozole were 50% more likely to ovulate and had 50% more live births than PCOS women taking Clomid. They also had half the risk of a multiples pregnancy.

Metformin

Metformin is a pharmaceutical competitor to myo-inositol and berberine that sensitizes your body to insulin. Insulin resistance is such a cornerstone of PCOS that for many women, and particularly for lean PCOS women, metformin will regulate hormones and encourage ovulation. In fact, for lean PCOS women, metformin outperforms Clomid for helping PCOS women get pregnant.[99]

It sounds like a dream come true. However, I do not love metformin, and I certainly don't love it as a first line fertility treatment.

Metformin is a powerful endocrine disruptor. It is very widely prescribed for diabetes so it is ending up in all of our waterways. Fish who ingest metformin have a frightening tendency to have intersex babies, that is, babies who have both male and female reproductive systems.[100]

For many years, pregnant women with diabetes and PCOS have been encouraged to stay on metformin to regulate their blood sugar. Their babies appeared healthy so doctors hypothesized that if metformin had any effect on these babies, it would be to improve their metabolic functioning.

We are just now starting to see the effects of metformin on babies, and this hypothesis is wrong. In a study that was published in 2018, children born to PCOS mothers who took metformin during pregnancy had almost double the rate of childhood obesity compared to children whose PCOS mothers did not take metformin. By age four, 32% of the metformin children were overweight or obese.[101]

Metformin simply isn't safe for pregnancy, but this information is so new that your doctor may not know it. If you use metformin to get pregnant, you need to stop taking metformin as soon as you get pregnant. Unfortunately, when you go off this insulin-sensitizing pharmaceutical, your insulin resistance will go back up and this greatly increases your risk of miscarrying and developing gestational diabetes.

I always recommend myo-inositol for insulin-sensitizing before and during pregnancy. While you are trying to conceive, berberine can improve your chances, but stop taking it once you get pregnant.

Liraglutide

Liraglutide is a glucagon-like peptide-1 receptor agonist sold under the brand names Victoza and Saxenda. It is an injectable drug that induces rapid, significant weight-loss.

Overweight and obese PCOS women who take liraglutide for six to seven months will lose, on average, 20 pounds.[102]

Consequently, many fertility centers will recommend that overweight and obese PCOS women take liraglutide for several months before starting fertility treatments. This will increase your chances of becoming pregnant, having a healthy pregnancy, and delivering a healthy baby.

I think this is a reasonable treatment, but obviously, it is a quick-fix that doesn't permanently fix anything. To keep the weight off, you will need to adopt a healthy lifestyle like the one described in this book.

Also, be prepared that many women experience gastrointestinal side effects from liraglutide, including nausea, vomiting, diarrhea, and constipation. These side effects are the worst during the first four weeks of treatment, but most women push through because they are so happy with their weight loss.[103]

Menstrual irregularity

As with infertility and hyperandrogenism, menstrual irregularity is caused by elevated testosterone levels and insulin resistance. The best way to fix these are by following the protocol in this book. Get healthy. Take the core supplements. Get on a fitness routine that includes aerobic exercise, ideally for one hour, three times per week.

Your menstrual cycle, which is essentially a sign of female health, will likely fix itself.

Do-it-yourself options

All of my patients who follow this protocol have begun ovulating and menstruating, and their cycles have become more regular. Even so, they often do not achieve perfectly predictable regularity. So long as you are menstruating once every 21-35 days, you are healthy. But an unpredictable cycle can be annoying, so here are some tips for dealing with the inconveniences of an irregular cycle.

Period tracker app

Use an app to track your period and predict when your next period will come. You can also track symptoms of ovulation like cervical mucus to make your prediction more accurate. My favorite app for PCOS women is Life because it uses your last six cycles to predict your next cycle and it has a nice bar graph that shows you how long each previous cycle was.

Reusable sanitary products

For women with irregular menstrual cycles, you may have a window of time, instead of a day or two, when your period might arrive. You can better relax on these days if you use a just-in-case sanitary product.

You could wear single-use sanitary pads, but it's expensive and wasteful to wear disposable pads day-after-day, waiting for your period to arrive.

In general, I recommend reusable products. For those days when maybe you'll get your period but maybe not, reusable sanitary pads, menstrual cups, and period panties work great. Because they are chemical free, you can use them as often as needed. Just wash them regularly. Reusable products cost more than disposable pads up front, but they last for months or even years and end up being cheaper over the long run.

With-your-doctor options

Unfortunately, there is no miracle medical solution to restore natural menstrual cycles.

Birth control pills

The number one prescribed treatment for irregular or absent menstruation is synthetic hormonal birth control pills. I don't like this solution because essentially what the doctor is saying is, "Your hormones are dysregulated. Let's cover that up with synthetic hormones." This is a treatment that increases your risk for depression, suicide, high blood pressure, cardiovascular disease, and blood clotting. It does not treat your insulin resistance. It does not treat your infertility. If you do decide you want to have a baby, you will be no closer to having healthy hormones than you were the day you started birth control pills.[104,105,106]

Bioidentical progesterone

If it's been several months since you've last menstruated, you need to see your doctor. Women with PCOS have 2.7 times the risk of endometrial cancer, and it's likely linked to long stretches of amenorrhea and prolonged uterine exposure to unshed uterine lining cells, which are hormonally and metabolically active.[107]

Progesterone will cause your uterus to shed its lining through a process called withdrawal bleeding.

When I am working with a patient to restore natural menstruation, I will prescribe her 200 mg of bioidentical progesterone for 14 days of each month for three months to make sure her uterus is cleaned out and healthy. Then I will reduce the prescription to every other month to protect uterine health while making sure we aren't masking natural menstruation.

Your doctor can order bioidentical progesterone through a conventional or compounding pharmacy. A quick note that conventional pharmacies will often deliver progesterone in a peanut oil, so heads up if you have a peanut allergy. I prefer natural bioidentical progesterone over synthetic progestins.

Mood Disorders

If you might harm or hurt yourself, call the National Suicide Prevention Lifeline:

1-800-273-8255

It is free and confidential, and volunteers are available around the clock to help you.

Women with PCOS are seven times more likely to commit suicide than women without PCOS, so please seek help if you need it. Many of your PCOS sisters are in the same boat. You are not alone.[108,109]

Women with PCOS have about 2.5 times the rate of anxiety and 3.5 times as much depression as women without PCOS. And we are five times more likely to have eating disorders, especially binge eating and bulimia (binge eating with purging).[110,111,112,113]

Yes, some of this mental distress is tied to weight, infertility, and the masculinizing effects of hyperandrogenism. But it's more than that. Chronic mood disorders are caused by physical and chemical differences in the brain and the rest of the body. It's not "in your head."

Both PCOS and mood disorders are strongly linked to abnormally high levels of cortisol, elevated testosterone levels, and low estrogen levels. Both PCOS and mood disorders are characterized by neurotransmitter imbalances — low serotonin and dopamine, which are your feel-good neurotransmitters, and high levels of glutamate, a neurotransmitter that damages neurons in high quantities.[114,115,116,117]

Mood disorders themselves change the actual structure of the brain. Both people with depression and obese women with PCOS have less gray matter in their brains than healthy control populations. Gray matter is the tissue in the brain responsible for, among other things, memory, decision making, and emotional control. More is definitely better.[118,119]

Your amygdala is a tiny part of your brain responsible for feelings of fear, worry, and anxiety. In PCOS women, the amygdala is hypersensitized to testosterone, so it is excessively triggered by testosterone, which you have an overabundance of. This can leave you feeling on edge much of the time and can make you overreact in stressful situations.[120]

Feelings are physical things in your body and we have to treat them as such.

Do-it-yourself options

PCOS is an endocrine disorder that disrupts your hormones and neurotransmitters. This literally changes your brain and sets you up for mood disorders. The protocol in this book will help immensely by bringing down testosterone and cortisol, increasing serotonin and estrogen, and supporting brain health.

Here are a few extra, easy things you can try to lower anxiety, raise your mood, and overall increase your mental health.

Ashwagandha

From the whole category of adaptogens, herbs that help the body react to stress, my favorite is ashwagandha. It is both easy to find and well-studied. Women with PCOS tend to have high levels of cortisol, and on top of that, we often have a cortisol peak around bedtime. This leaves us feeling generally anxious and makes it hard to fall asleep.

Ashwagandha lowers cortisol levels and improves mood and sleep. I like to drink it as a tea in the evening a few hours before bed. You can find ashwagandha tea online or in any store that sells medicinal teas. It tastes lovely, especially with a squeeze of lemon. You can also take it as a supplement, either alone or in a combination with other adaptogens.[121]

I recommend Pure Encapsulations Ashwagandha. Take one capsule per day, a few hours before bedtime. I also like Cortisol Manager by Integrative Therapeutics and Adapten-All by Ortho Molecular Products, both of which contain ashwagandha and a blend of additional mood stabilizing nutraceuticals.

Light therapy lamp

Women with depression and anxiety respond as well to morning light therapy as they do to antidepressants, without the side effects. Chronically high cortisol, which is a sign of both stress and circadian rhythm dysregulation, causes anxiety and depression. Bright light in the morning, by setting your master clock and jumpstarting your circadian rhythm, dramatically reduces cortisol levels.

If you are struggling with depression or anxiety, I highly recommend that you invest in a good light therapy lamp, one that emits 10,000 lux, and use it for 30 minutes every single morning. Build it into your schedule so you consistently get your morning light, even on cloudy days.

If you are currently taking antidepressants and can't get off of them, pairing antidepressants with light therapy gives you stronger results.[122]

Low-dose lithium

Another treatment option for depression and especially anxiety is low-dose lithium.

Hear me out on this one. Lithium at very high doses, 600 to 1800 mg, is a powerful antipsychotic used to treat bipolar disorder. But at extremely low doses, 3 mg or less, it's actually a nutritional supplement. It's a naturally occurring trace mineral that humans need for brain health.

Many people are already getting lithium in their water. Depending on your particular water source, you could be getting 1 to 3 mg out of the tap every day. I hope you are because cities with higher levels of lithium in their water have lower suicide rates.[123,124]

At low, nutritional doses, lithium is neuroprotective. It increases serotonin and dopamine, which improves and stabilizes mood. It decreases glutamate and thereby protects neurons. And it is neuroregenerative, increasing overall gray matter in the brain.

It addresses the exact physical and chemical irregularities that we see in PCOS women with depression and anxiety.

And at low doses, it is extremely safe and you can buy it as a supplement without a prescription. Lithium citrate and lithium orotate are both fine. I recommend Lithium Liquid by Pure Encapsulations because it's easy to fine tune your dosage. You can start with as little as 250 micrograms (mcg) per day. A microgram is one thousandth of a milligram (mg), so we are talking about tiny amounts. And you can work your way up to 2 mg a day.

Anything above that and you should work with your doctor to adjust your dosage.

Mediation plus yoga

The amygdala is a part of your brain that initiates stress and anxiety, and in PCOS women, this part of the brain is extra sensitive to testosterone. Bringing down testosterone through the protocol in this book solves half the problem. Calming down your amygdala solves the other half.

Mindfulness meditation actually desensitizes your amygdala so during stressful experiences, there is less activity in that region of your brain.[125,126]

People who suffer from anxiety often have a bigger amygdala that is better connected to the rest of their brain with more synapses. When people combine mindfulness meditation with yoga, their amygdala physically shrinks and they experience better coping skills, particularly in high stress situations.[127,128]

On top of all that, mindfulness meditation also stimulates the growth of brain gray matter, particularly in areas of the brain associated with learning, memory, empathy, and emotional regulation. This is a great, no meds strategy to counteract the gray matter atrophy seen in both PCOS and depression.[129]

Most people start to experience a benefit from mindfulness meditation with as little as five minutes per day on most days of the week. I recommend that people work up to 20 minutes per day, most days of the week. And if you can add 1 or 2 one-hour yoga sessions to your week as well, even better. Of course, the yoga counts towards your exercise plan, so that makes it doubly good for you.

There are all sorts of guided mediation programs that can help you get started. You can listen to podcasts, use an app like Headspace, or check out the mindfulness skills on your Alexa.

With-your-doctor options

If you need help, you should work with a licensed therapist or psychiatrist to develop a treatment plan. I am not a psychiatrist so I never prescribe antidepressants. Most of my patients experience significant improvement in their mood disorders when they sync their circadian rhythm, stabilize their hormones, fix their gut microbiome, and begin exercising. This protocol works wonders for your run-of-the-mill anxiety and depression. But I want to be clear that I am not helping patients through severe psychiatric illnesses.

If you are concerned that you are suffering from a mental illness, discuss your symptoms with your doctor. You need to be to be under the care of a mental health professional.

Depending on your needs, here are some treatments that you might find helpful.

Cognitive Behavioral Therapy (CBT)

CBT is one of the most effective, evidence-based therapy strategies for handling depression and anxiety. It trains your mind to choose helpful, positive thought patterns and behaviors when faced with negative emotions. It's been around since the 1960s and it is backed by literally thousands of studies.

Anyone with mental illness can benefit from CBT and the skills you gain. It reduces anxiety, depression, and stress, and consequently, it improves your stress hormone levels. I highly recommend it.[130]

Estrogen for eating disorders

PCOS in general, and more specifically high testosterone plus low estrogen, causes eating disorders. A promising treatment for eating disorders is estrogen replacement. Some doctors prescribe oral contraceptives, which are pretty effective at reducing or even eliminating bulimic and binge eating behaviors.[131,132]

You already know I don't love birth control pills because they are endocrine disruptors. Instead, I prescribe an estrogen patch, which contains 0.05 mg of bioidentical estradiol, or a compounded 1 mg estradiol cream, to be taken two times per day. For someone who isn't having regular cycles, I pair this with progesterone.

Pregnancy and complications

Once you get pregnant, you need to take extremely good care of yourself and your growing baby. All of the hormonal and metabolic dysfunctions of PCOS make pregnancy more dangerous, and they put your child at risk of developing metabolic dysfunctions, mood disorders, and PCOS itself later in life.

When women with PCOS get pregnant, compared to non-PCOS women, they have much higher rates of early pregnancy loss, gestational diabetes, preeclampsia, and preterm birth. Their babies are much more likely to be large for their gestational age (macrosomia) and have a low Apgar score. As they grow up, these babies are at risk for everything you are dealing with right now. Even boys are affected by their PCOS mothers.[133,134,135]

It's trite but true: Risks are not destiny and knowledge is power.

Pregnancy tracker app

Because your pregnancy is high risk, I recommend that you use a pregnancy tracker app to track all of your stats. There are tons of fun apps out there that will tell you all about your baby's development, but you really need one that lets you track your vitals like weight and blood pressure. Glow Nurture and My Pregnancy A to Z Journal are both pretty good.

Do-it-yourself options

The core protocol in this book — the light therapy, the sleep, the timed eating, the exercise, the gut healthy diet, the clean living — will improve your hormones, lower your insulin resistance, improve your metabolic health, and reduce your exposure to toxic chemicals. You can have a safe pregnancy and a healthy baby.

Blood pressure monitoring

PCOS increases your risk of preeclampsia, dangerously high blood pressure. So I recommend that you buy a home digital blood pressure monitor. Measure your blood pressure every few days and track it in your pregnancy tracker app.[136]

Take this measurement around 8PM after sitting and resting for ten minutes.

If you notice a significant increase from your pre-pregnancy blood pressure (+30 on the top number or +15 on the bottom number) or if your blood pressure ever exceeds 140/90, you should contact your doctor.

BPA and endocrine disruptors

You need to get as close to zero-exposure as possible. Remember that you are predisposed to storing BPA and other toxins in your body, and BPA, specifically, can cause PCOS in your unborn baby. Avoid food + plastic. Eat organic food and use organic products. If you wouldn't give it to your baby, don't expose yourself to it.

Diet

Your diet feeds both you and your baby, so be sure to eat healthy foods.

Focus on eating significant quantities of vegetables. Green leafy veggies, in particular, have lots of calcium and improve your nitric oxide levels. Eat soy three to four times per week to protect your baby from BPA. Drink two cups of spearmint tea every day to lower your testosterone level. Additionally, make sure you eat two servings of protein per day.

Strictly limit sugars and processed foods to reduce your risk of gestational diabetes, macrosomia, and other pregnancy complications. Be sure to follow the government guidelines on what additional foods to avoid during pregnancy: www.foodsafety.gov/risk/pregnant/chklist_pregnancy.html.

Supplements

Pregnant women have much higher nutritional needs than non-pregnant women. My recommendations for pregnancy supplements are the same as they are for pre-pregnancy supplements (page 276).

Take the core supplements (page 19). Swap the regular multivitamin for a good prenatal vitamin, such as Thorne Basic Prenatal, that has 800 to 1000 mcg (1 mg) of folate. Add an additional 400 to 600 mg of magnesium citrate or glycinate. I recommend Pure Encapsulations

Magnesium Glycinate. Take 3 to 4 capsules daily with food. And, check with your doctor to see if you need extra iron, especially in your third trimester.

These supplements are all tested and have shown to be safe and beneficial during pregnancy. I wouldn't add anything else except ginger for nausea.

Be aware that most supplements haven't been tested for safety in pregnancy. Definitely avoid all herbs like berberine.

With-your-doctor options

Find a doctor who is knowledgeable about PCOS and its accompanying risks, one who won't just stick you on metformin and call it a day.

Having PCOS means you have a high-risk pregnancy, so I would strongly recommend getting your prenatal care from a medical doctor and not a midwife. I would also recommend that you deliver in a hospital and not a birth center. Not only are you at risk of a preterm delivery, you are more likely to need a c-section. And if you carry your baby full-term, your baby is at greater risk of meconium aspiration.[137]

All of these conditions, and any pre-existing conditions you might have such as diabetes and hypertension, can be managed much more safely in a hospital setting by a knowledgeable medical doctor.

Glucose tests
Because you are at high risk of gestational diabetes, you need to monitor your blood glucose like a hawk. Most women have their glucose tolerance test done between 24 and 28 weeks. You should have an extra one done earlier, around 12 to 14 weeks.

Metformin vs myo-inositol

I want to repeat this because I feel so strongly about it: I don't like metformin for use during pregnancy unless it's medically necessary to control diabetic blood sugar. The studies on its effectiveness when used as a PCOS treatment for improving pregnancy and live birth outcomes are inconclusive at best. It doesn't protect against miscarriage or gestational diabetes. We do know it's an endocrine disruptor that increases the risk of metabolic dysfunction in children born to mothers who take it.[138]

I greatly prefer myo-inositol as an insulin sensitizer. It is at least as effective as metformin for improving insulin sensitivity in PCOS, but it's not an endocrine disruptor. In pregnancy, it reduces your risk of developing gestational diabetes. I give my patients Pure Encapsulations Inositol (powder) and recommend 4 g (2 scoops) per day.[139,140]

Skin tags

These small skin growths look like tiny balloons, a globby mole connected to the rest of your skin by a small stalk. They are an annoying medical mystery that seem to be connected to abnormal testosterone and estrogen levels. Women with PCOS are prone to get them. They are also more common among obese people.[141]

There are no do-it-yourself creams to remove them. Your best bet is to have a dermatologist snip off the ones that bother you.

Since we don't know exactly what causes them, it's impossible to say for sure how to prevent more from forming. But it's likely that controlling your PCOS and losing weight if you are overweight is the best strategy.

Sleep Disorders

Chapter 6 on page 91 already covers this so I don't want to summarize it here. But sleep disorders are a major problem for women with PCOS, and because they are inextricably linked to circadian rhythm disorder, they are definitely worth the time and energy to fix.

It's so natural to think that we treat sleep disorders at bedtime, but great sleep actually starts with a strong morning routine. Make sure you are getting bright morning light so you get your circadian rhythm synced properly. And then have a calm, dark, consistent evening routine that sets you up for resting slumber.

Use melatonin when you need it, at the lowest levels that work for you. Drink ashwagandha tea a few hours before bedtime. Oh, and if you have sleep apnea, treat that, too.

Stress

As a whole, we PCOS women are a stressed out group. We are predisposed to mental illness. On top of that, we also have these constantly in-your-face symptoms that become a low-grade, always-there source of stress.

PCOS symptoms that affect appearance — acne, hirsutism, alopecia, and obesity — are particularly trying. If you're like me, you may feel like you shouldn't care so much about how you look. But I care. It's normal to care. These symptoms are miserable and for most women, they triple your stress level.[142]

Then there's infertility. If people know that you're trying, there are the cute jokes about how much sex you must be having. If you've kept your dreams of children secret, then there's the loneliness of pretending that everything is fine and normal. Either way, you find that the world is practically full of happy pregnant women. Infertility is immensely stressful.[143]

And there's life itself. Sometimes, we go through inherently stressful experiences like divorce, death of a loved one, financial insecurity, and life transitions. Even when you have a very good reason for being stressed, you should treat your stress because it can make you sick.

In all cases, stress makes the symptoms of PCOS worse. It causes cortisol to go up, which increases insulin resistance, which increases testosterone and metabolic dysfunction. It's all a huge, vicious cycle, and reducing stress is critical to restoring health.

Do-it-yourself options

All of the tips suggested for mood disorders (page 283) earlier in this chapter apply to stress as well. Here are a few more things to try on your own or with a licensed practitioner.

Acupuncture

No one really knows why acupuncture works. Maybe it's meridians, maybe not. It's hard to tell and there's a lot of passion, history, and culture tied up in it. But acupuncture creates physically observable changes in the human body and in people's overall feelings of well-being. It improves your immune system, eases pain, and reduces psychological distress. I've been offering acupuncture in my office for 20 years. If you get your treatments done by a licensed acupuncturist, they are very safe and effective.[144]

Guided imagery

Guided imagery is a simple, passive form of guided meditation that is completely foolproof. All you need is a quiet comfortable space and a recorded imagery to listen to. Then press play.

Several studies show that daily guided imagery can significantly reduce stress and fatigue in as little as four weeks.[145,146,147]

It also serves as an excellent stepping stone to more advanced forms of mindfulness like meditation.

I personally love and use www.HealthJourneys.com as a trusted, excellent, affordable source of guided imageries.

Massage and other relaxation therapies

There are now hundreds of different types of massage and they all claim to be good for you. In general the risks to massage therapy are low; just don't get anything too aggressive. Massage immediately alleviates stress and anxiety. Although a single session doesn't have a significant impact on long-term mental health, an hour-long session once per week for two to three months does reduce chronic stress levels.[148,149]

And if massage isn't your thing, other relaxation therapies work equally well. It shouldn't be surprising, but we humans respond really well to things that feel good. Get a spa treatment. Hang out in a sauna or jacuzzi. Do something once a week that nurtures your body and makes you feel totally pampered and relaxed.[150]

Weight loss

If you are overweight, losing weight will improve your PCOS symptoms. Find a BMI calculator online. Overweight is generally defined as a BMI over 25. It's an imperfect tool and it doesn't account for muscle weight and visceral versus subcutaneous fat. But it's a reasonable guideline for most people.

I'm sure you are beyond tired of hearing this, but if you are overweight or even at the upper end of normal weight, every 5% of your body weight that you lose will dramatically improve your hormonal and metabolic health.

That being said, I am still not a fan of dieting. Calorie restriction works in the short term, but it puts you at risk of weight yo-yoing, and it's just so unpleasant. Getting healthy shouldn't feel bad.

I truly believe the tips and strategies in this book are the way to go. Weight gain is a sign of circadian, metabolic, and hormonal dysregulation. Fix those and eat reasonable, healthy foods, and your weight will go down.

Do-it-yourself options

Everything in this book will contribute to weight loss, but these are the most effective tips for fixing your metabolism and shedding pounds.

Fasting, time-restricted eating, and caloric timing
Not to repeat myself, but these are my best when-to-eat tips for losing weight.

- Eat a big breakfast, a moderate lunch, and a tiny dinner.
- Fast for at least 12 hours overnight, every night.
- Explore longer fasts.

If you eat all the time, your body stays in storage mode. You need to take extended breaks from eating so your body can transition through all of the stages of metabolism and get into fat burning mode. If you don't do this, you cannot lose weight.

Fiber
Fiber rich foods are good for your health, the health of your microbiome, and the size of your waistline. The more fiber people eat, the less they weigh.[151]

There are numerous reasons for this. High-fiber foods are nutrient dense and calorically sparse. High-fiber foods control blood sugar levels and regulate insulin. High-fiber foods fill you up for longer. High-fiber foods support a healthy microbiome, protect against leaky gut, and lower systemic inflammation.[152]

So eat fiber-rich, plant-based foods. They are good for you in a thousand ways, and they'll help you lose weight.

Morning sun

People who get bright morning light every day have lower BMIs than people who don't, even when all of their other risk factors are taken into account. Morning light sets your circadian rhythm, which normalizes your hormones and metabolism, which improves weight loss. So get sunshine every morning, and if you live someplace where that isn't feasible, get your morning light through a light therapy lamp.

With-your-doctor options

If your weight has created urgent health problems and you simply cannot lose weight, you may want to consider medical interventions. These are last option treatments, but in some cases, the risk of a treatment is less than the risk of doing nothing.

Bariatric surgery

This is a catch-all term for a variety of weight loss surgical procedures, including gastric bypass and gastric banding. Bariatric surgery may be considered for women with a BMI over 40 or for women with a BMI greater than 35 and additional, serious, weight-related illnesses. It should be a last resort procedure because, as with all surgeries, it carries risk, and many of these procedures are permanent.

If you are extremely obese and nothing else works, the risks of surgery may be less than the risks associated with remaining at your current weight. The short term safety of these procedures has improved greatly over the last 20 years, but we still don't know what the long-term prognosis and potential complications are for these patients.[153]

Liraglutide

Liraglutide, sold under the brand names Victoza and Saxenda, is an injectable drug that induces rapid, significant weight loss. See page 260 and page 280. It's a short-term solution for initiating weight loss. You will still need to make all of the changes in this book to keep the weight off.

A quick summary

PCOS is a complex syndrome that affects every system and organ in your body.

With PCOS, you absolutely have to be a powerful advocate for your own health. You need to understand the treatments available and the potential risks of traditional versus integrative options because many doctors don't. I hope this chapter and the ones before it give you a natural plan to reclaim your health.

- Follow my protocol.
- For any bothersome symptoms that have not resolved, pick additional therapies to add to your plan.
- Work with a trusted team of doctors to develop the safest, most effective treatment plan that meets your particular needs.
- Be your own best advocate.

Don't be afraid to question your doctor. No doctor knows everything, not even me! New studies and treatments are coming out all the time. Just because something was a standard treatment a few years ago doesn't mean that it still is today. If a doctor doesn't make you feel empowered to understand and contribute to your treatment plan, then you need a new doctor.

No one will ever know your body better than you, and no one will ever look out for your best interests better than you and your loved ones.

I hope this chapter and this book help you feel informed and empowered to make decisions about your healthcare. If some of the advice in these pages doesn't work for you, don't do it. If something works great for you but isn't in this book, I'm so happy you learned about it. Please contact me through my webpage at www.felicelgershmd.com and tell me about it. Maybe I'll include it in an updated edition!

You control your health. I am honored to be a part of your healthcare journey.

CHAPTER 12

PCOS – Today and into the future

So, now you've read a whole book (or maybe skimmed part of it because, hey, we are all busy!). Now what? Will you set it down with a, "Hmm, that's interesting. Someday, I really should do those things?" Or are you going to grab onto this lifeline and make these changes, starting today?

I so hope that you will make these changes. Do it for yourself because you are worth the time, energy, and money that it takes to live a healthy, happy life. You and every other woman with PCOS deserve it.

Healthy habits

The easiest way to change your behavior is to swap an unhealthy habit for a healthy habit. We don't break habits. We replace them.

A habit is a behavior that you mindlessly do as a response to an external cue. More simply put, every time Event A happens, you automatically do Action B. For example, every time you use the toilet (Event A), you habitually wash your hands (Action B). You'll know it's a habit when it feels weird to not do it.[1]

So if you want to change your behaviors, you need to tie them to everyday cues and make the new behaviors automatic and easy.

Now that you've read through this book, go back and look through the healthy habits at the end of each step in this protocol. Hopefully, you've already knocked off a few, but whether you have or haven't started yet, I'm sure there are a bunch left to work on.

Try these techniques to make them easier to adopt.

- **Physical proximity:** Put two things close together so you start doing them together. For example, if you want to take a bedtime melatonin after dinner, put the melatonin bottle next to the kitchen sink so you take your pill while you clean up the dishes.

- **Path of least resistance:** Make the healthiest choice the easiest choice. For example, keep a bowl of fruit on your kitchen table so it's easier to grab a banana than a bag of chips. Also, don't even buy the chips so they are extra inconvenient.

- **One, and done:** Replace an unhealthy item with a healthy item. For example, replace your plastic water bottle with a stainless steel water bottle. Change is done. Check it off your to-do list!

- **One, then two:** Always follow one action with another one. For example, always take a short walk after dinner.

The "one, and done" actions are the fastest changes to make. Do them and you're done.

Forming new behavioral habits takes longer. A recent research study into building habits shows that, on average, new behaviors take about 10 weeks to become automatic, at which point study participants describe behaviors as "second nature" and say that they feel "quite strange" if they don't do them. When you feel this way, congratulations, your new behavior has become a habit. And it's time to start working on some new healthy habits.[2]

How many habits can you work on at once? Conventional wisdom says people can only make one change at a time. But new research suggests that with structure, support, and determination, people can make dramatic, sweeping improvements to their lifestyle routines.[3]

You know yourself best. What will work for you? Make a plan that sets you up for success.

Long-term prognosis

A woman with PCOS has PCOS for her whole life. She is born with it. It is most severe during her reproductive years. And it follows her into menopause and old age.

For the longest time, PCOS has been treated as an infertility problem. It's only recently that the medical community has looked beyond reproduction to study what PCOS means for a woman's health over a much broader timescale. And so there's been very little research into how PCOS manifests in a woman's later years.

In fact, a woman can't even be diagnosed with PCOS after menopause because ovulation and menstruation are part of the definition. You can have it but you can't be diagnosed with it. Wrap your head around that one!

But we do know a bit about how PCOS impacts women leading into and beyond their menopause years, and what we know is mostly positive.

Fertility

As your hormones normalize with age, your menstrual cycle may also normalize. For most women with PCOS, menstruation and ovulatory regularity increase with age, up to menopause.[4]

Most women with PCOS menstruate less regularly and less frequently than non-PCOS women, so they maintain a larger reserve of healthy eggs as they age, and PCOS women go through menopause, on average, two years later than their non-PCOS peers.[5]

This means that women with PCOS have a longer fertility window. There's never a point at which we become more fertile than non-PCOS women, but after age 35, we are much more similar. So much so that after 35, PCOS and non-PCOS women have the same IVF success rates.[6,7]

By no means does this mean that you should wait to get pregnant. Your chances are still better when you are younger, and advanced maternal age brings additional risks. But, the window is there.

Another interesting thing to note: If you have children, then parenting, weirdly enough, seems to be a good treatment for PCOS. Pregnancy may actually reset your hormones. And whether you have biological children or adopt, parenting forces most people to lead healthier, more circadian-rhythmic lives.

Women with children eat more fruits and vegetables and they sleep more regular hours than women without children. Consequently, they have lower testosterone levels and more regular menstrual cycles.[8]

Hyperandrogenism

If you have acne today, one silver lining is that all of the oil in your skin protects it from aging. Your skin will stay younger longer; your wrinkles will develop later. And simultaneously, as you age, your acne may begin to go away all on its own.[9]

All women, as they age, produce less testosterone. So all of your signs of hyperandrogenism should become less pronounced as you get older.[10]

Long-term chronic conditions

For conditions such as type 2 diabetes, heart disease, autoimmune disease, and cancer, the story is mixed. On the one hand, the risk for PCOS women stays pretty stable. It doesn't go up much as you age. But it certainly doesn't go down either.

In fact, we say that your risk "normalizes." This is because for non-PCOS women, menopause induces many of the hormonal and metabolic changes that you have already gone through. Post-menopausal women become insulin resistant. They acquire visceral fat around their bellies. Their blood pressure and risk of heart disease go up. Their risk of cancer and autoimmune diseases go up. Basically, they catch up so that, going into old age, we are all in the same crappy, old boat.

That is, unless you actively counteract those natural trends. You can be healthy into menopause doing the same things that help you live a healthy life with PCOS. So, if you follow my advice, you'll actually be ahead of the game and perfectly set up to vibrantly enter your silver years.

Caring for our daughters

If you have a daughter, you are likely wondering how you can protect her from PCOS. I think about this all of the time. I have young granddaughters and I want nothing more than for these little girls to be happy and healthy throughout their hopefully very long lives.

Can we prevent PCOS? Maybe. If a mother does everything possible to treat her own PCOS before and during pregnancy, if she is able to keep her testosterone level down to a normal female non-PCOS level and avoid all BPA and other endocrine disruptors, then her daughter has a good chance of avoiding PCOS altogether.

But if that perfect situation doesn't happen, there is still a ton that we can do to mold a young girl's PCOS into the ancient, non-disease phenotype. This requires a lot of healthy food and healthy living.

Antibiotics

Carefully weigh the risks and benefits before using antibiotics. These are powerful, lifesaving drugs that are commonly overprescribed. Avoid them if you can, especially during the first two years of life. We used to give antibiotics to every kid with an ear infection. Now, the new guidelines for most mild infections are to just watch them. The majority will go away on their own.

When you do use these drugs, pair them with probiotics and then, after the course of treatment, focus on feeding your child lots of high-fiber fruits and vegetables to encourage healthy microbes to grow back. This is time-critical because if you allow dysbiotic bacteria to populate her gut microbiome, it's very hard to get rid of them later.

Clean living

Keep your daughter away from toxins and toxic chemicals.

If you have PCOS, then your daughter is at risk of developing PCOS.

Women with PCOS are what we call "poor detoxers." We do not metabolize BPA as well as non-PCOS women. We tend to store a wide range of endocrine disruptors and other toxic chemicals in our bodies.

Your daughter may be a poor detoxer, too. She likely cannot metabolize BPA well and if she is exposed to BPA and other endocrine disruptors, these toxic chemicals will likely accumulate in her body.

Remember, BPA can cause PCOS. For children and adolescent girls, elevated BPA blood levels are strongly correlated with an eventual PCOS diagnosis.[11]

So protect your daughter from plastics and pesticides. Do not let those chemicals poison her and reprogram her genes. Live the cleanest life you can.

Diet

Feed your daughter a healthy, high-fiber, low-sugar diet full of fruits and vegetables. Eat gluten free and dairy free to reduce inflammation and the risk of autoimmune disease. Nurture a healthy gut microbiome.

Additionally, the foods you feed your daughter now will shape her food preferences later in life. If you teach her to love healthy foods, she will never have to diet as an adult.[12]

Hygiene

Although you need to avoid toxic chemicals, you don't want to keep your daughter too clean. Dirt is actually critical to the development of a healthy immune system. Children need to be exposed to natural microbes on their skin, in their mouths, and in their guts to develop a healthy immune response to environmental compounds.[13]

Let her play outside, especially in places where the grass isn't covered in weedkiller. Take her to natural places. Get a pet, especially a dog. And don't over-bathe your daughter. Bathing is linked to eczema and immune disorders, so unless she smells or has visible dirt on her, I promise you, she's fine.[14,15]

Sleep

Make sure your daughter gets plenty of sleep in a very dark room. Children's large pupils make them more sensitive than adults to light and the circadian rhythm disruption it causes.[16]

Poor sleep is linked to every behavior disorder under the sun. Anyone who has ever observed a tired toddler will agree that tired children display a bizarre range of maladaptive behaviors. Chronically tired children get misdiagnosed with all sorts of disorders, especially attention-deficit/hyperactivity disorder (ADHD), and existing mood and behavior disorders are magnified when children are tired.[17,18]

Good sleep is extra important for little girls because it helps prevent early puberty. Children exposed to a lot of evening light have lower levels of melatonin, and chronically low melatonin can trigger the onset of puberty.[19]

Early puberty exacerbates many of the risks of PCOS. It increases girls' risks of obesity, metabolic disease, and breast cancer, and early puberty is linked to mental health problems.[20,21]

So get that girl to bed early. Ditch the nightlight, or swap it for a dim, red bulb that won't affect melatonin production. Get her a sleep mask.

Melatonin supplements are safe to use with children. Give them to your child an hour or two before bedtime. My grandchildren take Tired Teddies chewable 0.3 mg melatonin. For middle-of-the-night awakenings, my grandchildren take 1 mg melatonin dissolvable tablets from Douglas Laboratories. They say they taste like marshmallows.

Supplements

For better or worse, until they can swallow pills, you can only give your kids vitamins that are chewable and decent-tasting. Ortho Molecular makes a kids supplements line called Springboard. Metagenics also makes a great kids line. If your child can swallow pills, Thorne makes an excellent children's multivitamin.

Several of my grandchildren take:

- Ortho Molecular Products Springboard SuperNutes Chewable Multivitamins
- Pure Encapsulations Inositol (powder): 2 g (1 scoop) per day

- Metagenics UltraFlora Children's Daily Probiotic
- Metagenics OmegaGenics
- Natures Plus Animal Parade MagKidz Children's Magnesium

One of my granddaughters with allergies also takes Ortho Molecular Products D-Hist JR Tablets.

After puberty, your daughter can take the same supplements that you do.

Time-restricted eating

Children need to eat with the clock. Yes, they eat more frequently than adults. Young children, in particular, need to eat several times per day. But as with adults, breakfast is still the most important meal of the day. Kids and teens who eat breakfast perform better academically and behaviorally. And again, as with adults, kids who eat breakfast have a lower risk of becoming overweight.[22,23]

Once kids are in elementary school, they should be fasting overnight. Feed older children and teens a moderate dinner and avoid late-night snacks.

Please note that fasts longer than 12 hours are appropriate for adults only.

Weight

Little girls and teenagers need to maintain a healthy weight. Extra fat causes insulin resistance and higher testosterone. It causes early puberty and acne. Overweight children are at risk for fatty liver disease and diabetes. And overweight girls will likely go on to develop a more severe form of PCOS later in life.[24,25]

Talk to your child's doctor to figure out what a healthy weight for your child is because it changes dramatically as kids age.

Caring for our sons

All of the recommendations for your daughter apply to your son as well. Men don't develop PCOS, per se, but the sons of women with PCOS generally weigh more and are at increased risk of developing insulin resistance and metabolic disorder.[26]

So you'll need to be extra careful with your son's health as well.

Final Thoughts

PCOS is a natural female genetic variant. It's not a disease by default. It is an endocrine difference and it is a vulnerability. In today's culture, PCOS puts you at high risk of developing serious endocrine dysfunctions, metabolic disorders, and infertility.

Your ancestors were strong, powerful women. They didn't have all of the "comforts" and "conveniences" of the modern day. They couldn't stay up late and eat food wrapped in cellophane, filled with pesticides and plasticizers. They spent their days out in the world, not holed up in a dark office on a computer. They didn't have Netflix and Instacart and cellphones. And so they didn't get sick from PCOS.

Today, PCOS has exploded into a disease that doctors manage with ever more pharmaceuticals, but this approach never gets at the underlying problems of circadian and metabolic dysfunction.

Young women are parked on birth control pills to give them regular menstrual cycles. Not only does this not treat insulin resistance, metabolic disease, and the broader hormonal irregularities that characterize PCOS, it actually makes some of the problems worse! It increases depression and raises triglycerides and blood pressure. It elevates the risk of fatty liver and thrombosis. At the same time, birth control does nothing to reduce a woman's risk of diabetes and her propensity to gain weight. And, it simply pushes her infertility problems off to the future, assuming that whenever that time comes, she can take metformin or Clomid or try her hand at IVF.

This treatment plan doesn't make you healthy. It gives you drugs to treat your current biggest problems, and it assumes you will get more drugs over time as your health gets worse.

I do not agree with this treatment plan. I know we can do better.

If we look beyond pills and invasive medical procedures, if we acknowledge the body's capacity to heal, if we embrace the power of diet, lifestyle, and the earth's rhythms that we are all a part of, then we can do more than treat PCOS. We can stop its progression and undo the downward health spiral.

By living the way our bodies were designed to live and by supporting our bodies with nutrients, supplements, and healthy habits, we can reverse the course of our PCOS. We can heal.

This isn't a popular philosophy. It's easier for everyone involved to rely on pills.

Pills are simple. Pills are transactional. I get sick; I go to the doctor; I leave with pills.

Lifestyle changes are hard. They take time. They are not something that a doctor can simply give you. Supplements are expensive. They aren't covered by insurance, and when you take a bunch of them, you can feel like a pill-popper. Eating healthy means trading convenient, tasty, comfort food for homemade fare that may sometimes miss the mark. It can be boring to be the person who always goes to bed at a reasonable time.

But for all of this effort, you will be rewarded with something that a pill cannot give you: health.

You can feel good. You can look good. You can finally match your vibrant mind with an equally vibrant body. And if you want children someday, you will have a body that is capable of creating new life.

We will always have PCOS. And that's okay. Our grandmothers had it. Our grandmothers' grandmothers had it. We come from a long line of ancestors who were strong women and strong mothers because they had PCOS.

I live the protocol that I've laid out in this book. I've shared it with my patients and my daughters. And I am sharing it with you because it works.

I hope that you find within these pages the keys to restoring your health and living the life that you choose. I hope that you make peace with the unique characteristics of your PCOS body, accepting its limitations and finding its limitless potential. I hope that you tap into its strength and resilience. I hope that you find beauty in your own skin.

Most of all, I hope that you are healthy and happy and whole.

APPENDIX A

———

Additional testing and bloodwork

*W*hen I am treating a patient, I always want to deeply understand what is going on in her body. Diagnostic tests are one of a doctor's best tools for creating a comprehensive picture of a patient's health and then monitoring the effectiveness of a treatment plan.

Often, doctors simply treat patients until they stop complaining and stop returning. But I don't want my patients to simply go away! I want them to be healthy.

Yes, health is a feeling, an ability to move comfortably through the world with joy and resilience. But at the same time, we know know that long-term, sustainable health corresponds to specific results on medical tests.

Tests can tell you about your current health, and they can also predict your risk of developing illnesses down the road. I want you to be healthy today and tomorrow. And tomorrow's health depends on making well-informed, meaningful, healthy choices today.

Here are many of the tests that I use to assess and monitor my patients' health. You should discuss these with your doctor to decide which ones would be useful for guiding your personal treatment plan.

Many of these tests are cutting edge and not offered through your average medical laboratory. I've included the laboratories that I use and trust for the harder-to-find tests.

Autoimmunity and allergy testing
Cyrex Laboratories (www.cyrexlabs.com/CyrexTestsArrays) offers a wide range of tests that can help pinpoint autoimmune diseases, allergies, and sensitivities. Array 11, Chemical Immune Reactivity Screen, and Array 12, Pathogen-Associated Immune Reactivity Screen, often reveal surprising immune responses to environmental toxins and chemicals.

Celiac testing
Symptoms for celiac disease can be very subtle and diverse, so I recommend celiac testing for any patients with chronic health conditions or signs of autoimmunity. Any lab can order a basic celiac panel.

I will often order celiac testing from Vibrant America because they test for advanced markers of gluten autoimmunity and leaky gut (www.vibrant-america.com/celiac-disease).

Zonulin is a valuable marker of gluten sensitivity and intestinal permeability. You can order a zonulin test from Doctor's Data (www.doctorsdata.com/zonulin).

Cortisol four point test
Cortisol plays a critical role in the circadian rhythm dysfunction, sleep disorders, and mood disorders that many PCOS women experience. You can map your daily cortisol rhythm with a simple salivary test.

ZRT Laboratory offers a Cortisol Saliva Test Kit that you can order online. I order them directly from ZRT, but they are also available on Amazon.

Environmental toxic chemical exposures testing

I use Genova Diagnostics to test my patients for exposure to toxic chemicals such as BPA, phthalates, and solvents. You can order the tests individually, but I usually order the Toxic Effects Core panel (www.gdx.net/tests/by-product-line#environmental).

Glucose and insulin testing

Because all PCOS women are likely insulin resistant, I recommend that all of my PCOS patients do periodic glucose and insulin testing. If you have additional diabetes risk factors or if you are pregnant, you should definitely get these tests. There is no reason to wait until you are prediabetic or diabetic to start treating insulin resistance.

Hopefully, you get your fasting blood sugar done as part of your Comprehensive Metabolic Panel (see page 18). I also recommend:

- **Fasting insulin:** Many doctors just test glucose, but insulin is more sensitive and allows for earlier detection of blood sugar control problems. You could have a borderline glucose result with a very high insulin result.

- **Hemoglobin A1c (HgbA1C):** This tests the stability of your blood sugar over three months and measures the toxic effect of persistently high blood sugar on hemoglobin. HgbA1C is useful for diagnosing diabetes and for determining how well a diabetes treatment plan is working.

Hormones and neurotransmitters testing

To better understand and track a patient's hormones and neurotransmitters, I will order panels from ZRT Laboratory (www.zrtlab.com/test-specialties). For PCOS patients, the fertility panel is often useful. Depending on a patient's symptoms, I will sometimes also order a neurotransmitters panel, a thyroid panel, or a sleep panel.

I also often order an anti-müllerian hormone (AMH) test to get a more detailed PCOS profile and insight into a patient's fertility. I order this test from Quest Diagnostics.

Imaging studies

Sometimes, you need to look at an organ to understand what's going on. Here are a few totally pain-free imaging tests that can help diagnose medical conditions and risks.

- **Abdominal ultrasound:** This is a great test that I recommend for all PCOS women. It allows your doctor to take a look at all of your abdominal organs. I'll look at the ovaries and uterus, the pancreas, and especially the liver. An abdominal ultrasound is one of the best way to assess whether someone has fatty liver, and if they do, this test provides insight into the severity.

- **Carotid intima-media thickness test (CIMT):** I recommend this test for all PCOS patients over age 40 or with risk factors for cardiovascular disease. A CIMT is an ultrasound of the main artery in your neck and allows your doctor to detect early signs of atherosclerosis, thickening of your arteries, which is a significant risk factor for a heart attack or stroke. If your test shows signs of arterial thickening, you should consider taking a nitric oxide supplement (page 251) to help soften your artery walls.

- **Echocardiogram:** This is an ultrasound of your heart. I recommend this test for all PCOS women over age 40 and all women with cardiovascular risk factors or symptoms. PCOS causes estrogen deficiency, and estrogen deficiency can cause heart muscle deficiency. An echocardiogram can show that a woman has a stiffer heart that doesn't relax normally. The official name for this condition is left ventricular diastolic dysfunction (LVDD). It's a symptom that is often ignored so you may need to ask about it, but it is a significant risk for heart failure and arrhythmias. If your test result is abnormal, estrogen therapy can help reverse LVDD.[1,2]

- **Transvaginal ultrasound:** In this test, a small ultrasound wand is inserted two to three inches inside your vagina to get detailed pictures of your uterus and ovaries. It is useful for identifying polycystic ovaries and other reproductive organ abnormalities.

Inflammation markers testing

Inflammation is a foundational component of PCOS. Understanding how inflammation is affecting various systems and organs in your body can help you address critical health risks before you get critically ill. I order the Inflammation Panel through Cleveland Heart Lab (www.clevelandheartlab.com/test-menu). These tests are particularly valuable for identifying early risk factors for cardiovascular disease and kidney damage.

Nutrients testing

Women with PCOS tend to have several nutrient deficiencies that can impede healing. Once identified, they can usually be corrected through diet and supplements.

I often order the Vitamins Panel from Cleveland Heart Lab (www.clevelandheartlab.com), which includes COQ10, folate, vitamin B12, and vitamin D. I order the OmegaCheck panel, which shows omega-3 and omega-6 levels and ratios. On top of that, I'll add copper, zinc, and magnesium.

For more extensive nutrient testing, I'll order the NutrEval panel from Genova Diagnostics (www.gdx.net/product/nutreval-fmv-nutritional-test-blood-urine). This is a highly sensitive and extensive test that can diagnose a wide range of nutritional deficiencies. It also tests for heavy metals, signs of oxidative stress, and toxin markers.

APPENDIX B

PCOS science, advocacy, and community

$\mathcal{T}$he future of medicine is constantly shaped by the science happening today. This science relies on curiosity, ingenuity, passion, dedication, attention to detail, and careful analysis. It also relies on funding.

By virtue of having PCOS, you are a de facto member of a vibrant community. Here's how you can get involved and advance the treatment of PCOS. Do it for yourself, for your PCOS sisters, and for all the little girls out there who will someday join our PCOS family.

Join an organization

I am involved in several organizations that advocate for research into PCOS. You should consider following the work of these organizations. They are great sources of information and I recommend that you sign up for their newsletters. If you'd like to give back to the PCOS community, these organizations are always looking for donations and volunteers, and they sometimes need people to contact their representatives to promote PCOS funding and awareness on a national level.

The Androgen Excess and Polycystic Ovary Syndrome Society

www.ae-society.org

I am a member of the AE-PCOS Society because I support their mission to "promote knowledge and original clinical and basic research" in PCOS and other androgen excess conditions. They have been instrumental in defining PCOS as a whole-body endocrine disorder and not just a fertility disorder. In 2009, they published the modern diagnosis criteria for PCOS that established androgen excess as a required feature of PCOS.

They fund research into PCOS and host an annual conference where doctors from around the world gather to learn about the latest studies on PCOS and other androgen conditions. Periodically, they release position statements on the proper screening and treatment of women with PCOS. It is primarily a professional organization of doctors and researchers, but it is also a great source of scientific information. Anyone can donate to them and contribute to the advancement of quality PCOS care.

PCOS Awareness Association

www.pcosaa.org

This non-profit raises awareness about PCOS. Today, at least half of all women with PCOS don't know they have it. PCOS Awareness Association hosts events and provides informational resources to women around the world to teach them about PCOS symptoms and connect them to the treatment they need.

If you volunteer or donate money to this organization, you will be helping to improve access to healthcare for women with PCOS around the world.

PCOS Challenge

www.pcoschallenge.org

PCOS Challenge is a global non-profit organization dedicated to raising awareness about PCOS and closing the gap between the widespread impact of this common condition and the relatively tiny amount of funding dedicated to understanding and treating it.

I volunteer on their Medical/Scientific Advisory Board. In 2017, PCOS Challenge sponsored Senate Resolution 336, which passed unanimously, officially recognizing PCOS as a serious condition in need of further research and designating September as PCOS Awareness Month. On May 18, 2018, I spoke at the very first PCOS Advocacy Day on Capitol Hill in Washington, D.C.

In addition to national advocacy work, PCOS Challenge supports patient care. If you are struggling to pay for skin and hair treatments related to your PCOS, you should look into their Confidence Grant. PCOS Challenge and my friend, Amy Medling of PCOS Diva, are helping women obtain needed hair and skin treatments that insurance otherwise doesn't cover (www.pcoschallenge.org/confidence-grant).

This is an extremely active organization that I recommend every PCOS woman join. At the very least, you should subscribe to their bi-monthly online magazine.

Keep your eye on these amazing areas of research

Innovative new research is coming out all of the time. Here are some of the studies and topics that may impact healthcare for PCOS women.

Anti-müllerian hormone (AMH)

AMH is a hormone that plays a critical role in female ovulation. A recent study showed that elevated AMH may play a role in how PCOS is passed from one generation to the next. Pregnant PCOS women have higher levels of AMH than pregnant non-PCOS women do. In rodents, treating pregnant mice with AMH caused PCOS symptoms to develop in female offspring.[3]

Some people hope that this study may lead to a cure for PCOS or a way of stopping its mother-to-daughter transmission. I think this study offers fascinating new insights into PCOS, but I am less optimistic than some of my peers that AMH will be the PCOS panacea. AMH is part of the unique hormonal profile of PCOS but it operates downstream of the true cause of PCOS — poor aromatization that leads to high testosterone and low estrogen.

That being said, I am keenly watching research into this field with the hope that these researchers develop new therapies that improve PCOS symptoms. And in fact, I am hoping that I am wrong and they do develop a way to protect babies from PCOS. That would be game-changing, indeed!

Chronotyping blood test

A team of researchers at Northwestern University have developed a blood test that can identify your body's circadian rhythm and determine how much it varies from Earth's 24-hour day. The test, TimeSignature, requires two blood draws and is currently accurate to 1.5 hours.[4]

This opens a whole world of scientific study and personalized medical treatment. Researchers will be able to study in detail the effects of misaligned circadian rhythm on a wide range of diseases. We already know that circadian rhythm dysfunction plays a role in Alzheimer's disease, diabetes, and cardiovascular disease. Hopefully, this test will help us better understand the mechanisms at play, identify patients at higher risk, and lead to more treatment options. I'm sure we will discover circadian features in a wide range of other diseases as well.

I am also very excited about the potential for chronotherapy, incorporating a patient's unique circadian rhythm into her medical care. Many treatments such as chemotherapy, vaccinations, pharmaceuticals, and surgery, are more or less effective with more or less severe side effects, depending on the time of day they are administered. Many recent studies have shown conflicting results. A specific treatment at a specific time of day may improve survival rates by as much as 500% for some groups of patients but the exact same chronotherapy will have zero impact for other patients. Age and gender seem to be important factors.[5,6,7]

I am optimistic that the TimeSignature test will help researchers identify differences between these groups so that all patients can time their therapies to the time of day that will lead to the best results.

Continuous glucose monitoring

Continuous glucose monitoring devices are powerful new tools that will likely improve the care of PCOS women.

A continuous glucose monitoring device is exactly what it sounds like — a small device that you attach to your upper arm or abdomen that monitors your blood sugar level around the clock. The device has a tiny needle that you insert with an applicator into your skin and the whole thing is held in place with adhesive. The device takes a blood glucose reading every five minutes around the clock.

There are currently a handful of FDA approved devices and they need to be replaced every seven to ten days.

For people with type 1 or type 2 diabetes, and for women with PCOS and insulin resistance, continuous monitoring means that you can understand how certain foods, such as fruits and grains, and certain activities, such as exercise and fasting, affect your blood sugar level. With this detailed information, you will be able to make better lifestyle decisions, and if you are diabetic, you can fine-tune your treatment plan to avoid hypoglycemic events.

I'm particularly optimistic that continuous glucose monitoring will make pregnancy safer for PCOS women and their babies. PCOS increases your risk of gestational diabetes and macrosomia, having a baby large for its gestational age. Controlling your blood sugar and identifying blood sugar regulation problems early could significantly improve pregnancy outcomes.

DOGMA theory of PCOS

DOGMA, which stands for "Dysbiosis of Gut Microbiota," came to the forefront of PCOS research in 2012 when Dr. Tremellen and Dr. Pearce released their groundbreaking paper, *Dysbiosis of Gut Microbiota (DOGMA) – A novel theory for the development of Polycystic Ovarian Syndrome*[8].

By identifying many pathways through which an unhealthy gut microbiome exacerbates all of the symptoms of PCOS, this theory has spawned numerous avenues of research into diet, probiotics, hormones, exercise, fecal transplants, immunotherapies, and other means of healing the gut microbiome.

My own PCOS protocol is highly influenced by this research, and I am very optimistic that future research into the unique PCOS gut microbiome will lead to many new and novel therapies for PCOS.

Fasting mimicking diet

The ProLon fasting mimicking diet is particularly effective at normalizing metabolic functions. I have prescribed this treatment to many of my PCOS patients with great results. Observationally, the fasting mimicking diet leads to significant weight loss, improved insulin sensitivity, and normalized hormone levels. Many of my patients begin to menstruate.

I am collaborating with USC Professor Dr. Valter Longo, who developed ProLon, to research the effects of ProLon on the clinical markers and symptoms of PCOS, and I am optimistic that our study will show that a fasting mimicking diet is a safe and effective part of a PCOS treatment plan.

Fecal transplants

In a fecal transplant, stool from a healthy donor is transplanted into a patient's colon to restore a healthy gut microbiome. It is a low-risk, fairly easy procedure.

Today, fecal transplants are only approved to treat recurrent C. difficile colitis infections, for which they are extremely effective. But there are indications that they may be useful in treating a wide range of additional conditions, including PCOS.

The unique, dysbiotic gut microbiome of PCOS women plays a critical role in maintaining high testosterone levels and low estrogen levels. In rat models, fecal transplants from non-PCOS rats to PCOS rats improve estrogen levels, lower testosterone, and normalize ovarian function and appearance.[9]

Future studies will show if fecal transplants improve PCOS hormones and fertility in humans and whether probiotics are an effective alternative.

Hormonal testing

There are all sorts of new tests coming out that help doctors identify medical conditions and monitor the progress of treatments. For PCOS, I recommend hormonal testing to better understand a patient's specific version of PCOS.

This already allows for personalized medical care. A menstrual cycle map can help pinpoint subtle hormonal problems in ovulation and a fertility profile can identify hormonal irregularities that contribute to infertility. With this knowledge, I can formulate treatment plans that best address a woman's particular PCOS symptoms, and I can monitor the impact of those treatments in real time so we can make adjustments quickly if something doesn't seem to be working the way we expected.

In the future, as more studies come out on the use of bioidentical hormones and rhythmic hormonal treatments, I believe that hormonal testing will facilitate highly individualized hormone replacement therapies.

LuCI, a new weight loss pill

Diet pills have a frightening history that includes fraud, poisoning, addiction, and the deaths of countless people. Please don't rely on diet pills because many of them are dangerous.[10]

However, I am watching a new pharmaceutical, LuCI," short for "luminal coating of the intestine." It's a treatment being developed at Harvard that relies on sucralfate, a drug that doctors have been using for decades to treat ulcers. It has a long, strong safety profile and it causes minimal side effects.

LuCI works by temporarily coating the digestive tract with a pasty substance that prevents the body from absorbing calories. After six to eight hours, the lining dissolves and passes harmlessly through the digestive tract.[11,12,13]

If you used it long term, you'd develop nutritional deficiencies. But short-term, it could be used to mimic fasts or to limit calorie absorption in the evenings. And for obese women with serious weight-related health problems, it could be a safer and reversible alternative to gastric bypass surgery.

Male contraception

If you are in a long-term, monogamous relationship, keep an eye on male contraceptive options. I'm not too excited about the male birth control pill currently being tested because instead of giving synthetic hormones to women, we are giving them to men. But I am intrigued by Vasalgel (www.parsemus.org/projects/vasalgel). In this treatment, a polymer is injected into a man's vas deferens and blocks the tube that carries sperm to the penis. The idea is that the polymer can later be flushed out. So this is essentially a reversible vasectomy that is hormone-free and surgery-free. Testing is still under way and until I truly know it is safe and reversible, I can't recommend it. But it's an innovative, totally hormone-free contraception possibility.

Microbiome testing

Incredible and rapid advancements are happening in the world of microbiome mapping, and we are in the early stages of using these tests as diagnostic tools. Ubiome (ubiome.com) is one industry leader and offers several different microbiome tests. There is a basic microbiome profile that they sell directly to consumers that lets you compare your gut microbiome to microbiomes from around the world and, if you are embarking on a lifestyle change, you can track the health of your microbiome over time. Ubiome also offers clinical tests that link microbiome abnormalities to specific medical conditions; these tests must be ordered by a physician.

Today, a test of your microbiome can help diagnose and inform the treatment of gastrointestinal conditions, cardiovascular disease, diabetes, non-alcoholic fatty liver disease, and chronic kidney disease. Women can also sequence their vaginal microbiome to assess vaginal health and identify vaginal infections and sexually transmitted infections.

At this point, these tests can diagnose dysbiotic microbiomes and link them to microbiome patterns commonly associated with specific disease conditions, but there aren't clear protocols on how to use this information to improve patient health. That will come with more time, more data, and more research.[14]

For many conditions, studies have shown that improving the health of the gut microbiome leads to decreased disease symptoms. I am confident that in the future, we will have a wide array of microbiome-targeted therapies that will be part of the standard treatment for a wide array of health conditions, including PCOS.

Rhythmic estrogen

There are very few research studies on the use of rhythmic bioidentical estrogen to treat PCOS but I am extremely optimistic about its potential use as a powerful therapy.[15]

In bioidentical rhythmic estrogen, doctors prescribe bioidentical estrogen, which you can get through a compounding pharmacy. The estrogen dose varies over the course of 28 days to mirror the naturally cycling estrogen levels of a non-PCOS woman.

Doctors are currently prescribing this treatment, and observationally, the results are promising. But we need rigorous scientific studies to back up this protocol before it can be widely recommended.

Consequently, I am working with a group of doctors and pharmacies who have set up a nonprofit, Women's Hormone Network (www.womenshormonenetwork.org), to fund these studies. As the Director of Clinical Affairs, I promote research and education into bioidentical hormone therapies.

Sirtuins

Recently, several research teams have identified sirtuins, a class of proteins, as critical players in human metabolism. As one of their many functions, sirtuins maintain mitochondrial function in our cells. Your mitochondria are cell organelles that literally create the energy that your cells use to stay alive.

As part of the aging process, our sirtuins become less active. PCOS women, even young PCOS women, have less active sirtuins than similarly aged non-PCOS women. Increased sirtuin activity is associated with weight loss, healthy circadian rhythm regulation, reduced incidence of chronic disease, and overall increased life span.[16,17,18,19]

There are a number of ways to upregulate your sirtuins. Fasting is a powerful sirtuin activator, and this may be one of the reasons that the fasting mimicking diet has such a profound impact on metabolic diseases. A vast array of supplements improve sirtuin function, including melatonin, resveratrol, quercetin, and curcumin.[20,21,22]

Another interesting compound is nicotinamide adenine dinucleotide (NAD⁺), a coenzyme that regulates sirtuin activity. As people age, NAD⁺ availability decreases and in tandem, sirtuin activity declines. So, the hope is that if we can boost NAD⁺, we can upregulate sirtuins. That should improve metabolic health and consequently, improve PCOS symptoms and reduce the symptoms of aging.

Scientists are studying a related compound called nicotinamide riboside (NR), a NAD⁺ precursor that people can take as a supplement and convert to NAD⁺. Early research is promising that NR leads to increased sirtuin activity. Although NR is on the market today, I'd like to see more robust studies confirming its long term efficacy and safety before I recommend it. For now, I am watching with hopeful anticipation.[23]

Participate in research

There are many important studies going on right now that you can participate in. These projects need the involvement of large groups of people to produce meaningful data. When you join, you help research move faster.

All of Us Research Program
allofus.nih.gov

Run by the National Institutes of Health, the program has a goal "to gather data from one million or more people living in the United States to accelerate research and improve health." This information will be part of a national research platform that will accelerate the rate of medical research.

American Gut

humanfoodproject.com/americangut

Hosted by the Human Food Project, an organization founded by microbiome expert, Jeff Leach, The American Gut is a data collection research project based on open-source, open-access principles. You pay for the kit and shipping and they'll send you back information on your gut microbiome. Then, your gut data will be anonymously available to researchers advancing the science of the gut microbiome.

If you live in the United Kingdom, you can participate in the sister project, the British Gut (britishgut.org). If you're in Asia, check out the Asian Gut (www.asiangut.com).

Northwestern PCOS Research Study

www.pcos.northwestern.edu

The PCOS team at Northwestern University is creating a registry of PCOS women and their daughters to explore the causes of PCOS and the symptoms related to it. The more people who join the study, the better the data they collect will be.

Ubiome

ubiome.com

If you get your microbiome sequenced with Ubiome, you can opt to anonymously include your information in their microbiome database, which is the largest microbiome database in the world, combining data from hundreds of thousands of people. Ubiome works with thousands of scientists, including many from top universities, to further research into the microbiome and how it relates to human health. This is an active scientific community that has produced hundreds of papers, dozens of patents, and is constantly pushing for new scientific breakthroughs.

APPENDIX C

Professional relationship disclosures

I actively contribute to the PCOS and nutraceutical communities in a variety of ways. As part of this, I have professional relationships with several companies.

I am a salaried consultant for Pure Encapsulations, which is a brand under the umbrella company, Atrium Innovations, and for L-Nutra, the company that developed the ProLon fasting mimicking diet.

Part of what I do for these companies is speak at professional conferences, develop webinars, and present research in order to educate my fellow doctors about integrative medical approaches to diseases and how supplements and fasting can aid in treatment. Equally exciting, I get to advise on new products, develop treatment protocols, and participate in research studies. Consequently, I've been able to direct significant energy and attention toward PCOS issues.

With Pure Encapsulations, I've developed an entire set of nutraceutical protocols called PureWoman: www.pureencapsulations.com /purewoman. These are protocols targeted at integrative physicians and naturopathic doctors to inform their treatment of women with cardiovascular disease, metabolic disease, detoxification needs, PMS, and, of course, PCOS.

With L-Nutra, I've piloted informal observational studies on the impact of the fasting mimicking diet on women with PCOS. And based on early, favorable results, we are now designing a formal study on fasting and the metabolic and hormonal markers in women with PCOS.

There are a few other companies that I frequently collaborate with. I am an educator and speaker for the Cleveland Heart Lab, a clinical laboratory that develops cutting edge biomarker tests with the goal to change the landscape for cardiovascular and inflammatory diseases. I am an educational speaker and webinar instructor for ZRT Laboratory. And I volunteer on the medical advisory board of Ubiome.

References

*H*ere are all of the scientific studies and articles that this book is based on. Most of these resources are freely available online. Where available, I have included articles' digital object identifier (DOI) numbers. A DOI is a unique, searchable ID number associated with a specific online article. Googling a DOI will bring up the exact article I referenced.

Some of the articles are pretty technical and can be hard to read. Another option is to Google the title of an article along with the lead researcher's name. You'll often find a wide array of synopses and response articles that will explain the study and its implications. If you go this route, make sure you read several different study interpretations to get a balanced understanding of the topic.

Forwords

1. Melanie Gibson-Helm, Helena Teede, Andrea Dunaif, Anuja Dokras; Delayed Diagnosis and a Lack of Information Associated With Dissatisfaction in Women With Polycystic Ovary Syndrome, *The Journal of Clinical Endocrinology & Metabolism*, Volume 102, Issue 2, 1 February 2017, Pages 604–612, https://doi.org/10.1210/jc.2016-2963
2. Annie W Lin, Elena J Bergomi, Jamie S Dollahite, Jeffery Sobal, Kathleen M Hoeger, Marla E Lujan; Trust in Physicians and Medical Experience Beliefs Differ Between Women With and Without Polycystic Ovary Syndrome, *Journal of the Endocrine Society*, Volume 2, Issue 9, 1 September 2018, Pages 1001–1009, https://doi.org/10.1210/js.2018-00181

Introduction

1. Bulent O. Yildiz, Eric S. Knochenhauer, Ricardo Azziz; Impact of Obesity on the Risk for Polycystic Ovary Syndrome, *The Journal of Clinical Endocrinology & Metabolism*, Volume 93, Issue 1, 1 January 2008, Pages 162–168, https://doi.org/10.1210/jc.2007-1834
2. Wing, R. R., Lang, W., Wadden, T. A., Safford, M., Knowler, W. C., Bertoni, A. G., Hill, J. O., Brancati, F. L., Peters, A., Wagenknecht, L., Look AHEAD Research Group (2011). Benefits of modest weight loss in improving cardiovascular risk factors in overweight and obese individuals with type 2 diabetes. *Diabetes care*, 34(7), 1481-6, https://doi.org/10.2337/dc10-2415

Chapter 1

1. Carly R. Pacanowski and David A. Levitsky, "Frequent Self-Weighing and Visual Feedback for Weight Loss in Overweight Adults," *Journal of Obesity*, vol. 2015, Article ID 763680, 9 pages, 2015. https://doi.org/10.1155/2015/763680.
2. Reading the new blood pressure guidelines. [Accessed November 6, 2018]; *Harvard's Men's Health Watch*. Available from: https://www.health.harvard.edu/heart-health/reading-the-new-blood-pressure-guidelines
3. Pedro-Antonio Regidor and Adolf Eduard Schindler, "Myoinositol as a Safe and Alternative Approach in the Treatment of Infertile PCOS Women: A German Observational Study," *International Journal of Endocrinology*, vol. 2016, Article ID 9537632, 5 pages, 2016. https://doi.org/10.1155/2016/9537632.
4. Unfer, V., Facchinetti, F., Orrù, B., Giordani, B., & Nestler, J. (2017). Myo-inositol effects in women with PCOS: a meta-analysis of randomized controlled trials. *Endocrine connections*, 6(8), 647-658. https://doi.org/10.1530/EC-17-0243.
5. R. D'Anna, V. Di Benedetto, P. Rizzo, E. Raffone, M. L. Interdonato, F. Corrado & A. Di Benedetto(2012) Myo-inositol may prevent gestational diabetes in PCOS women, *Gynecological Endocrinology*, 28:6, 440-442, https://doi.org/10.3109/09513590.2011.633665.
6. Wang, Z., Zhai, D., Zhang, D., Bai, L., Yao, R., Yu, J., ... Yu, C. (2017). Quercetin Decreases Insulin Resistance in a Polycystic Ovary Syndrome Rat Model by Improving Inflammatory Microenvironment. *Reproductive Sciences*, 24(5), 682–690. https://doi.org/10.1177/1933719116667218
7. Rezvan, N., Moini, A., Gorgani-Firuzjaee, S., & Hosseinzadeh-Attar, M. J. (2017). Oral Quercetin Supplementation Enhances Adiponectin Receptor Transcript Expression in Polycystic Ovary Syndrome Patients: A Randomized Placebo-Controlled Double-Blind Clinical Trial. *Cell journal*, 19(4), 627-633. doi: [10.22074/cellj.2018.4577]
8. Jahan, S., Abid, A., Khalid, S., Afsar, T., Qurat-Ul-Ain, Shaheen, G., Almajwal, A., Razak, S. (2018) Therapeutic potentials of Quercetin in management of polycystic ovarian syndrome using Letrozole induced rat model: a histological and a biochemical study, *Journal of Ovarian Research*, 11:26, https://doi.org/10.1186/s13048-018-0400-5.
9. Cheraghi, E., Soleimani Mehranjani, M., Shariatzadeh, S., Nasr Esfahani, M. H., & Alani, B. (2017). N-Acetylcysteine Compared to Metformin, Improves The Expression Profile of Growth Differentiation Factor-9 and Receptor Tyrosine Kinase c-Kit in The Oocytes of Patients with Polycystic Ovarian Syndrome. *International journal of fertility & sterility*, 11(1), 270-278. doi: [10.22074/ijfs.2018.5142].
10. Thakker, D., Raval, A., Patel, I., & Walia, R. (2015). N-acetylcysteine for polycystic ovary syndrome: a systematic review and meta-analysis of randomized controlled clinical trials. *Obstetrics and gynecology international*, 2015, 817849. doi: [10.1155/2015/817849].
11. Khoshbaten, M., Aliasgarzadeh, A., Masnadi, K., Tarzamani, M. K., Farhang, S., Babaei, H., Kiani, J., Zaare, M., ... Najafipoor, F. (2010). N-acetylcysteine improves liver function in patients with non-alcoholic Fatty liver disease. *Hepatitis monthly*, 10(1), 12-6.
12. Rahmani, A. H., Alsahli, M. A., Aly, S. M., Khan, M. A., & Aldebasi, Y. H. (2018). Role of Curcumin in Disease Prevention and Treatment. *Advanced biomedical research*, 7, 38. doi:10.4103/abr.abr_147_16. doi: [10.4103/abr.abr_147_16]

13. Fleet, J. C., DeSmet, M., Johnson, R., & Li, Y. (2012). Vitamin D and cancer: a review of molecular mechanisms. *The Biochemical journal*, 441(1), 61-76. doi: [10.1042/BJ20110744]
14. Gominak, Stasha & E Stumpf, W. (2012). The world epidemic of sleep disorders is linked to vitamin D deficiency. *Medical hypotheses*. 79. 132-5. 10.1016/j.mehy.2012.03.031.
15. Lin, M. W., & Wu, M. H. (2015). The role of vitamin D in polycystic ovary syndrome. *The Indian journal of medical research*, 142(3), 238-40. doi: [10.4103/0971-5916.166527]
16. Charan, J., Goyal, J. P., Saxena, D., & Yadav, P. (2012). Vitamin D for prevention of respiratory tract infections: A systematic review and meta-analysis. *Journal of pharmacology & pharmacotherapeutics*, 3(4), 300-3. doi: [10.4103/0976-500X.103685]
17. Aragon, G., Graham, D. B., Borum, M., & Doman, D. B. (2010). Probiotic therapy for irritable bowel syndrome. *Gastroenterology & hepatology*, 6(1), 39-44.
18. Karamali, M., Eghbalpour, S., Rajabi, S., Jamilian, M., Bahmani, F., Tajabadi-Ebrahimi, M., Keneshlou, F., Mirhashemi, SM., Chamani, M., Hashem Gelougerdi, S., Asemi, Z. (2018). Effects of Probiotic Supplementation on Hormonal Profiles, Biomarkers of Inflammation and Oxidative Stress in Women With Polycystic Ovary Syndrome: A Randomized, Double-Blind, Placebo-Controlled Trial. *Arch Iran Med*. 2018 Jan 1;21(1):1-7.
19. Wallace, C., & Milev, R. (2017). The effects of probiotics on depressive symptoms in humans: a systematic review. *Annals of general psychiatry*, 16, 14. doi:10.1186/s12991-017-0138-2
20. Nordqvist M, Jacobsson B, Brantsæter A, et al. Timing of probiotic milk consumption during pregnancy and effects on the incidence of preeclampsia and preterm delivery: a prospective observational cohort study in Norway. *BMJ Open* 2018;8:e018021. doi: 10.1136/bmjopen-2017-018021
21. Shoda, H., Yanai, R., Yoshimura, T., Nagai, T., Kimura, K., Sobrin, L., Connor, K. M., Sakoda, Y., Tamada, K., Ikeda, T., ... Sonoda, K. H. (2015). Dietary Omega-3 Fatty Acids Suppress Experimental Autoimmune Uveitis in Association with Inhibition of Th1 and Th17 Cell Function. *PloS one*, 10(9), e0138241. doi:10.1371/journal.pone.0138241
22. Mohebi-Nejad, A., & Bikdeli, B. (2014). Omega-3 supplements and cardiovascular diseases. *Tanaffos*, 13(1), 6-14.
23. (2015). Long-chain omega-3 fatty acids and the brain: a review of the independent and shared effects of EPA, DPA and DHA. *Frontiers in aging neuroscience*, 7, 52. doi:10.3389/fnagi.2015.00052

Chapter 2

1. Androgen Excess and PCOS Society: http://www.ae-society.org/sub/education.php
2. Giudice, Linda C., Endometrium in PCOS: Implantation and predisposition to endocrine CA. *Best Practice & Research Clinical Endocrinology & Metabolism*, Volume 20 , Issue 2 , 235 - 244. https://doi.org/10.1016/j.beem.2006.03.005
3. Alessandro Pacchiarotti, Gianfranco Carlomagno, Gabriele Antonini & Arianna Pacchiarotti (2016)Effect of myo-inositol and melatonin versus myo-inositol, in a randomized controlled trial, for improving in vitro fertilization of patients with polycystic ovarian syndrome, *Gynecological Endocrinology*, 32:1, 69-73, DOI: 10.3109/09513590.2015.1101444
4. Kamalanathan, S., Sahoo, J. P., & Sathyapalan, T. (2013). Pregnancy in polycystic ovary syndrome. *Indian journal of endocrinology and metabolism*, 17(1), 37-43. doi: [10.4103/2230-8210.107830]
5. Defining Adult Overweight and Obesity. [Accessed November 6, 2018] Centers for Disease Control and Prevention. Available from: https://www.cdc.gov/obesity/adult/defining.html.
6. Enrico Carmina, Salvo Bucchieri, Antonella Esposito, Antonio Del Puente, Pasquale Mansueto, Francesco Orio, Gaetana Di Fede, GiovamBattista Rini; Abdominal Fat Quantity and Distribution in Women with Polycystic Ovary Syndrome and Extent of Its Relation to Insulin Resistance, *The Journal of Clinical Endocrinology & Metabolism*, Volume 92, Issue 7, 1 July 2007, Pages 2500–2505, https://doi.org/10.1210/jc.2006-2725
7. Lindheim, L., Bashir, M., Münzker, J., Trummer, C., Zachhuber, V., Pieber, T., Gorkiewicz, G, Obermayer-Pietsch, B. (2016) The Salivary Microbiome in Polycystic Ovary Syndrome (PCOS) and Its Association with Disease-Related Parameters: A Pilot Study. *Frontiers in Microbiology*. Volume 7. DOI=10.3389/fmicb.2016.01270
8. Akcalı, A., Bostanci, N., Özçaka, Ö., Öztürk-Ceyhan, B., Gümüş, P., Buduneli, N., & Belibasakis, G. N. (2014). Association between polycystic ovary syndrome, oral microbiota and systemic antibody responses. *PloS one*, 9(9), e108074. doi:10.1371/journal.pone.0108074
9. Varela Kellesarian, Sergio & Ros Malignaggi, Vanessa & Varela Kellesarian, Tammy & Alkhuraif, Abdulaziz & M Alwageet, M & Malmström, Hans & Romanos, Georg & Javed, Fawad. (2017). Association between periodontal disease and polycystic ovary syndrome: a systematic review. *International Journal of Impotence Research*. 29. 10.1038/ijir.2017.7.
10. Nordqvist, Christian. All you need to know about skin tags. [Accessed November 6, 2018]; *Medical News Today*. Available from: https://www.medicalnewstoday.com/articles/67317.php.

11. Fernandez, R. C., Moore, V. M., Van Ryswyk, E. M., Varcoe, T. J., Rodgers, R. J., March, W. A., Moran, L. J., Avery, J. C., McEvoy, R. D., ... Davies, M. J. (2018). Sleep disturbances in women with polycystic ovary syndrome: prevalence, pathophysiology, impact and management strategies. *Nature and science of sleep*, 10, 45-64. doi:10.2147/NSS.S127475

12. N. Shreeve, F. Cagampang, K. Sadek, M. Tolhurst, A. Houldey, C.M. Hill, N. Brook, N. Macklon, Y. Cheong; Poor sleep in PCOS; is melatonin the culprit?, *Human Reproduction*, Volume 28, Issue 5, 1 May 2013, Pages 1348–1353, https://doi.org/10.1093/humrep/det013

13. Tasoula Tsilchorozidou, John W. Honour, Gerard S. Conway; Altered Cortisol Metabolism in Polycystic Ovary Syndrome: Insulin Enhances 5α-Reduction But Not the Elevated Adrenal Steroid Production Rates, *The Journal of Clinical Endocrinology & Metabolism*, Volume 88, Issue 12, 1 December 2003, Pages 5907–5913, https://doi.org/10.1210/jc.2003-030240

14. Alexandros N. Vgontzas, Richard S. Legro, Edward O. Bixler, Allison Grayev, Anthony Kales, George P. Chrousos; Polycystic Ovary Syndrome Is Associated with Obstructive Sleep Apnea and Daytime Sleepiness: Role of Insulin Resistance, *The Journal of Clinical Endocrinology & Metabolism*, Volume 86, Issue 2, 1 February 2001, Pages 517–520, https://doi.org/10.1210/jcem.86.2.7185

15. Institute of Medicine (US) Committee on Sleep Medicine and Research; Colten HR, Altevogt BM, editors. *Sleep Disorders and Sleep Deprivation: An Unmet Public Health Problem*. Washington (DC): National Academies Press (US); 2006. 3, Extent and Health Consequences of Chronic Sleep Loss and Sleep Disorders. Available from: https://www.ncbi.nlm.nih.gov/books/NBK19961/

16. Mobeen, H., Afzal, N., & Kashif, M. (2016). Polycystic Ovary Syndrome May Be an Autoimmune Disorder. *Scientifica*, 2016, 4071735. doi: [10.1155/2016/4071735]

17. Du, D., & Li, X. (2013). The relationship between thyroiditis and polycystic ovary syndrome: a meta-analysis. *International journal of clinical and experimental medicine*, 6(10), 880-9.

18. Janssen OE, Mehlmauer N, Hahn S, Offner AH, Gartner R. High prevalence of autoimmune thyroiditis in patients with polycystic ovary syndrome. *Eur J Endocrinol* (2004) 150(3):363–9. doi:10.1530/eje.0.1500363

19. Dumesic, D.A., & Lobo, R.S. (2013). Cancer risk and PCOS. *Steroids*, 78 8, 782-5. DOI: 10.1016/j.steroids.2013.04.004

20. John A. Barry, Mallika M. Azizia, Paul J. Hardiman; Risk of endometrial, ovarian and breast cancer in women with polycystic ovary syndrome: a systematic review and meta-analysis, *Human Reproduction Update*, Volume 20, Issue 5, 1 September 2014, Pages 748–758, https://doi.org/10.1093/humupd/dmu012

21. Aus Tariq Ali*, "Fertility Drugs and Ovarian Cancer", Current Cancer Drug Targets (2018) 18: 567. https://doi.org/10.2174/1568009617666170620102049

22. Katrine Hass Rubin, Dorte Glintborg, Mads Nybo, Bo Abrahamsen, Marianne Andersen; Development and Risk Factors of Type 2 Diabetes in a Nationwide Population of Women With Polycystic Ovary Syndrome, *The Journal of Clinical Endocrinology & Metabolism*, Volume 102, Issue 10, 1 October 2017, Pages 3848–3857, https://doi.org/10.1210/jc.2017-01354

23. Busiah K, Colmenares A, Bidet M, Tubiana-Rufi N, Levy-Marchal C, Delcroix C, Jacquin P, Martin D, Benadjaoud L, Jacqz-Aigrain E, Laborde K, Robert J, -J, Samara-Boustani D, Polak M: High Prevalence of Polycystic Ovary Syndrome in Type 1 Diabetes Mellitus Adolescents: Is There a Difference Depending on the NIH and Rotterdam Criteria? *Hormone Research in Paediatrics* 2017;87:333-341. doi: 10.1159/000471805

24. (2014). Nonalcoholic fatty liver disease and polycystic ovary syndrome. *World journal of gastroenterology*, 20(26), 8351-63.

25. Noreen Hossain, Maria Stepanova, Arian Afendy, Fatema Nader, Youssef Younossi, Nila Rafiq, Zachary Goodman & Zobair M. Younossi (2011) Non-alcoholic steatohepatitis (NASH) in patients with polycystic ovarian syndrome (PCOS), *Scandinavian Journal of Gastroenterology*, 46:4, 479-484, DOI: 10.3109/00365521.2010.539251

26. Kumarendran, B., O'Reilly, M. W., Manolopoulos, K. N., Toulis, K. A., Gokhale, K. M., Sitch, A. J., Wijeyaratne, C. N., Coomarasamy, A., Arlt, W., ... Nirantharakumar, K. (2018). Polycystic ovary syndrome, androgen excess, and the risk of nonalcoholic fatty liver disease in women: A longitudinal study based on a United Kingdom primary care database. *PLoS medicine*, 15(3), e1002542. doi:10.1371/journal.pmed.1002542

27. Tan, J., Wang, Q. Y., Feng, G. M., Li, X. Y., & Huang, W. (2017). Increased Risk of Psychiatric Disorders in Women with Polycystic Ovary Syndrome in Southwest China. *Chinese medical journal*, 130(3), 262-266. doi: [10.4103/0366-6999.198916]

28. Suzette Bishop, Samuel Basch, and Walter Futterweit (2009) Polycystic Ovary Syndrome, Depression, and Affective Disorders. *Endocrine Practice*: July 2009, Vol. 15, No. 5, pp. 475-482. https://doi.org/10.4158/EP09083.RAR

29. Bernadett, M., Szemán-N, A. (2016) Prevalence of eating disorders among women with polycystic ovary syndrome [Article in Hungarian] *Psychiatria Hungarica*. 31(2):136-45.

30. Stefano Palomba, Marlieke A. de Wilde, Angela Falbo, Maria P.H. Koster, Giovanni Battista La Sala, Bart C.J.M. Fauser; Pregnancy complications in women with polycystic ovary syndrome, *Human Reproduction Update*, Volume 21, Issue 5, 1 September 2015, Pages 575–592, https://doi.org/10.1093/humupd/dmv029

31. Roos, N., Kieler, H., Sahlin, L., Ekman-Ordeberg, G., Falconer, H., & Stephansson, O. (2011). Risk of adverse pregnancy outcomes in women with polycystic ovary syndrome: population based cohort study. BMJ (Clinical research ed.), 343, d6309. doi:10.1136/bmj.d6309

Chapter 3

1. Das, M., Djahanbakhch, O., Hacihanefioglu, B., Saridogan, E., Ikram, M., Ghali, L., Raveendran, M., ... Storey, A. (2007). Granulosa cell survival and proliferation are altered in polycystic ovary syndrome. The Journal of clinical endocrinology and metabolism, 93(3), 881-7. doi: [10.1210/jc.2007-1650]
2. Yang, F., Ruan, Y., Yang, Y., Wang, K., Liang, S., Han, Y., Teng, X., & Yang, J. (2015). Follicular hyperandrogenism downregulates aromatase in luteinized granulosa cells in polycystic ovary syndrome women, REPRODUCTION, 150(4), 289-296. Retrieved Nov 6, 2018, from https://rep.bioscientifica.com/view/journals/rep/150/4/289.xml
3. Mickey S. Coffler, Ketan Patel, Michael H. Dahan, Pamela J. Malcom, Toana Kawashima, Reena Deutsch, R. Jeffrey Chang; Evidence for Abnormal Granulosa Cell Responsiveness to Follicle-Stimulating Hormone in Women with Polycystic Ovary Syndrome, The Journal of Clinical Endocrinology & Metabolism, Volume 88, Issue 4, 1 April 2003, Pages 1742-1747, https://doi.org/10.1210/jc.2002-021280
4. Mariana Hulchiy, Åsa Nybacka, Lena Sahlin, Angelica Lindén Hirschberg; Endometrial Expression of Estrogen Receptors and the Androgen Receptor in Women With Polycystic Ovary Syndrome: A Lifestyle Intervention Study, The Journal of Clinical Endocrinology & Metabolism, Volume 101, Issue 2, 1 February 2016, Pages 561-571, https://doi.org/10.1210/jc.2015-3803
5. Tayebeh Artimani, Massoud Saidijam, Reza Aflatoonian, Iraj Amiri, Mahnaz Ashrafi, Nooshin Shabab, Nooshin Mohammadpour & Mehdi Mehdizadeh (2015) Estrogen and progesterone receptor subtype expression in granulosa cells from women with polycystic ovary syndrome, Gynecological Endocrinology, 31:5, 379-383, DOI: 10.3109/09513590.2014.1001733
6. Drummond, A., & Fuller, P. (2010). The importance of ERα signalling in the ovary, Journal of Endocrinology, 205(1), 15-23. Retrieved Nov 6, 2018, from https://joe.bioscientifica.com/view/journals/joe/205/1/15.xml
7. Alonso-Magdalena, P., Ropero, A. B., Carrera, M. P., Cederroth, C. R., Baquié, M., Gauthier, B. R., Nef, S., Stefani, E., ... Nadal, A. (2008). Pancreatic insulin content regulation by the estrogen receptor ER alpha. PloS one, 3(4), e2069. doi:10.1371/journal.pone.0002069
8. Qiu, S., Vazquez, J.T., Boulger, E., Liu, H., Xue, P., Hussain, M.A., & Wolfe, A. (2017). Hepatic estrogen receptor α is critical for regulation of gluconeogenesis and lipid metabolism in males. Scientific Reports. DOI:10.1038/s41598-017-01937-4
9. Osamu Wada-Hiraike, Otabek Imamov, Haruko Hiraike, Kjell Hultenby, Thomas Schwend, Yoko Omoto, Margaret Warner, Jan-Åke Gustafsson. Role of estrogen receptor β in colonic epithelium. Proceedings of the National Academy of Sciences. Feb 2006, 103 (8) 2959-2964; DOI:10.1073/pnas.0511271103
10. Kovats, S. Estrogen receptors regulate innate immune cells and signaling pathways. Cellular Immunology. 2015 Apr;294(2):63-9. doi: 10.1016/j.cellimm.2015.01.018.
11. Mollerup, Steen et al. Expression of estrogen receptors α and β in human lung tissue and cell lines. Lung Cancer, Volume 37 , Issue 2 , 153 - 159. DOI: https://doi.org/10.1016/S0169-5002(02)00039-9
12. (2013). Estrogens and aging skin. Dermato-endocrinology, 5(2), 264-70. doi: [10.4161/derm.23872]

Chapter 4

1. Skovlund CW, Mørch LS, Kessing LV, Lidegaard Ø. Association of Hormonal Contraception With Depression. JAMA Psychiatry. 2016;73(11):1154-1162. doi:10.1001/jamapsychiatry.2016.2387
2. Chasan-Taber, Lisa & Willett, Walter & E. Manson, JoAnn & Spiegelman, Donna & J. Hunter, David & Curhan, Gary & Colditz, Graham & J. Stampfer, Meir. (1996). Prospective Study of Oral Contraceptives and Hypertension Among Women in the United States. Circulation. 94. 483-9. 10.1161/01.CIR.94.3.483.
3. Kaminski, Pawel & Szpotanska-Sikorska, Monika & Wielgos, Miroslaw. (2013). Cardiovascular risk and the use of oral contraceptives. Neuro endocrinology letters. 34. 587-9.
4. Jick H, Jick SS, Gurewich V, Myers MW, Vasilakis C. Risk of idiopathic cardiovascular death and nonfatal venous thromboembolism in women using oral contraceptives with differing progestagen components. Lancet [1995]
5. McIntosh, James. The impact of shift work on health. [Accessed November 6, 2018] Medical News Today. Available from: https://www.medicalnewstoday.com/articles/288310.php
6. Magrini, A & Pietroiusti, Antonio & Coppeta, Luca & Babbucci, A & Barnaba, E & Papadia, C & Iannaccone, U & Boscolo, Paolo & Bergamaschi, Enrico & Bergamaschi, A. (2006). Shift work and autoimmune thyroid disorders. International journal of immunopathology and pharmacology. 19. 31-6.

7.   Mínguez-Alarcón, L., Souter, I., Williams, P. L., Ford, J. B., Hauser, R., Chavarro, J. E., Gaskins, A. J., Earth Study Team (2017). Occupational factors and markers of ovarian reserve and response among women at a fertility centre. *Occupational and environmental medicine*, 74(6), 426-431. doi: [10.1136/oemed-2016-103953]

8.   Yu, Xiaofei, Rollins, Darcy, Ruhn, Kelly A., Stubblefield, Jeremy J., Green, Carla B., Kashiwada, Masaki, Rothman, Paul B., Takahashi, Joseph S., Hooper, Lora V. TH17 Cell Differentiation Is Regulated by the Circadian Clock. *Science.* 08 Nov 2013 : 727-730 DOI: 10.1126/science.1243884

9.   Sutton, Caroline & Finlay, Conor & Raverdeau, Mathilde & Early, James & Decourcey, Joseph & Zaslona, Zbigniew & A. J. O'Neill, Luke & Mills, Kingston & Curtis, Anne. (2017). Loss of the molecular clock in myeloid cells exacerbates T cell-mediated CNS autoimmune disease. *Nature Communications.* 8. 10.1038/s41467-017-02111-0.

10.   Roberto Salgado-Delgado, Araceli Tapia Osorio, Nadia Saderi, and Carolina Escobar, "Disruption of Circadian Rhythms: A Crucial Factor in the Etiology of Depression," *Depression Research and Treatment*, vol. 2011, Article ID 839743, 9 pages, 2011. https://doi.org/10.1155/2011/839743.

Chapter 5

1.   Wright, K. P., McHill, A. W., Birks, B. R., Griffin, B. R., Rusterholz, T., & Chinoy, E. D. (2013). Entrainment of the human circadian clock to the natural light-dark cycle. *Current biology: CB*, 23(16), 1554-8. doi: [10.1016/j.cub.2013.06.039]

2.   American Academy of Sleep Medicine. (2008, June 13). Delayed Sleep Phase Syndrome Linked To Irregular Menstrual Cycles, Premenstrual Symptoms In Women. *ScienceDaily*. Retrieved November 7, 2018 from www.sciencedaily.com/releases/2008/06/080610072156.htm

3.   Burgess, H. J., & Eastman, C. I. (2008). Human tau in an ultradian light-dark cycle. *Journal of biological rhythms*, 23(4), 374-6. doi: [10.1177/0748730408318592]

4.   Konturek, P.C. & Brzozowski, Thomas & Konturek, S.J.. (2011). Gut clock: Implication of circadian rhythms in the gastrointestinal tract. *Journal of physiology and pharmacology : an official journal of the Polish Physiological Society*. 62. 139-50.

5.   Terman, M. and Terman, J.S., Controlled Trial of Naturalistic Dawn Simulation and Negative Air Ionization for Seasonal Affective Disorder. *American Journal of Psychiatry* 2006 163:12, 2126-2133 DOI: 10.1176/ajp.2006.163.12.2126

6.   Danilenko, Konstantin & Ivanova, I.A.. (2015). Dawn simulation vs. bright light in seasonal affective disorder: Treatment effects and subjective preference. *Journal of affective disorders*. 180. 87-89. DOI: 10.1016/j.jad.2015.03.055.

7.   Thorn, L. et al. The effect of dawn simulation on the cortisol response to awakening in healthy participants. *Psychoneuroendocrinology*, Volume 29 , Issue 7 , 925 - 930. DOI: 10.1016/j.psyneuen.2003.08.005

8.   Leppamaki S, Meesters Y, Haukka J, et al. Effect of simulated dawn on quality of sleep—a community-based trial. BMC *Psychiatry.* 2003;3:14.

9.   Avery, David H et al. Dawn simulation and bright light in the treatment of SAD: a controlled study *Biological Psychiatry*, Volume 50 , Issue 3 , 205 - 216 DOI: https://doi.org/10.1016/S0006-3223(01)01200-8

10.   Viola, A., Gabel, V., Chellappa, S., Schmidt, C., Hommes, V., Tobaldini, E., Montano, N., Cajochen, C. Dawn simulation light: a potential cardiac events protector. *Sleep Medicine*, Volume 16 , Issue 4 , 457 - 461

11.   Boyles, Salynn. (2011) Heart Attacks in the Morning Are More Severe. WebMD. Available from: https://www.webmd.com/heart-disease/news/20110427/heart-attacks-in-the-morning-are-more-severe

12.   Rachel Leproult, Egidio F. Colecchia, Mireille L'Hermite-Balériaux, Eve Van Cauter; Transition from Dim to Bright Light in the Morning Induces an Immediate Elevation of Cortisol Levels, *The Journal of Clinical Endocrinology & Metabolism*, Volume 86, Issue 1, 1 January 2001, Pages 151–157, https://doi.org/10.1210/jcem.86.1.7102

13.   Ivy N. Cheung, Phyllis C. Zee, Dov Shalman, Roneil G. Malkani, Joseph Kang, Kathryn J. Reid. Morning and Evening Blue-Enriched Light Exposure Alters Metabolic Function in Normal Weight Adults. PLoS ONE, 2016; 11 (5): e0155601 DOI: 10.1371/journal.pone.0155601

14.   Reid KJ, Santostasi G, Baron KG, Wilson J, Kang J, Zee PC (2014) Timing and Intensity of Light Correlate with Body Weight in Adults. PLoS ONE 9(4): e92251. https://doi.org/10.1371/journal.pone.0092251

15.   Lam RW, Levitt AJ, Levitan RD, et al. Efficacy of Bright Light Treatment, Fluoxetine, and the Combination in Patients With Nonseasonal Major Depressive DisorderA Randomized Clinical Trial. JAMA *Psychiatry.* 2016;73(1):56–63. doi:10.1001/jamapsychiatry.2015.2235

16.   Whiteman, Honor. (2015) Study sheds light on link between PCOS and mental health. *Medical News Today*. Available from: https://www.medicalnewstoday.com/articles/301822.php

17. E. Jedel, M. Waern, D. Gustafson et al. Anxiety and depression symptoms in women with polycystic ovary syndrome compared with controls matched for body mass index. *Hum. Reprod.* 25(2), 450–456 (2010).

18. J Burgess, Helen & F Fogg, Louis & Young, Michael & Eastman, Charmane. (2004). Bright Light Therapy for Winter Depression—Is Phase Advancing Beneficial?. *Chronobiology International.* 21. 759-75. 10.1081/CBI-200025979.

19. Figueiro, Mariana G. et al., The impact of daytime light exposures on sleep and mood in office workers. *Sleep Health: Journal of the National Sleep Foundation,* Volume 3 , Issue 3 , 204 - 215. DOI: https://doi.org/10.1016/j.sleh.2017.03.005

20. Shin-Jung Park & Hiromi Tokura (1999) Bright Light Exposure During the Daytime Affects Circadian Rhythms of Urinary Melatonin and Salivary Immunoglobulin A, *Chronobiology International,* 16:3,359-371, DOI: 10.3109/07420529909116864

21. Nair, R., & Maseeh, A. (2012). Vitamin D: The "sunshine" vitamin. *Journal of pharmacology & pharmacotherapeutics,* 3(2), 118-26. doi: [10.4103/0976-500X.95506]

22. Lin, M. W., & Wu, M. H. (2015). The role of vitamin D in polycystic ovary syndrome. *The Indian journal of medical research,* 142(3), 238-40. doi: [10.4103/0971-5916.166527]

23. University of Southampton. (2014, January 17). Here comes the sun to lower your blood pressure. *ScienceDaily.* Retrieved November 7, 2018 from www.sciencedaily.com/releases/2014/01/140117090139.htm

24. Matsui, M. S., Pelle, E., Dong, K., & Pernodet, N. (2016). Biological Rhythms in the Skin. *International journal of molecular sciences,* 17(6), 801. doi:10.3390/ijms17060801

25. Krishna, Meera & Joseph, Annu & Litto Thomas, Philip & Dsilva, Belinda & M Pillai, Sathy & Laloraya, Malini. (2017). Impaired Arginine Metabolism Coupled to a Defective Redox Conduit Contributes to Low Plasma Nitric Oxide in Polycystic Ovary Syndrome. *Cellular physiology and biochemistry : international journal of experimental cellular physiology, biochemistry, and pharmacology.* 43. 1880-1892. 10.1159/000484107.

26. Plataforma SINC. (2017, March 8). How much sun is good for our health?. *ScienceDaily.* Retrieved November 7, 2018 from www.sciencedaily.com/releases/2017/03/170308083938.htm

27. Maria-Antonia Serrano, Javier Cañada, Juan Carlos Moreno, Gonzalo Gurrea. Solar ultraviolet doses and vitamin D in a northern mid-latitude. *Science of The Total Environment,* 2017; 574: 744 DOI: 10.1016/j.scitotenv.2016.09.102

28. Gringras, P., Middleton, B., Skene, D. J., & Revell, V. L. (2015). Bigger, Brighter, Bluer-Better? Current Light-Emitting Devices - Adverse Sleep Properties and Preventative Strategies. *Frontiers in public health,* 3, 233. doi:10.3389/fpubh.2015.00233

29. Carter, B., Rees, P., Hale, L., Bhattacharjee, D., & Paradkar, M. S. (2016). Association Between Portable Screen-Based Media Device Access or Use and Sleep Outcomes: A Systematic Review and Meta-analysis. *JAMA pediatrics,* 170(12), 1202-1208. doi: [10.1001/jamapediatrics.2016.2341]

30. Suttie, Jill. (2015, December 7) How Smartphones Are Killing Conversation. *Greater Good Science Center at UC Berkeley.* Retrieved November 7, 2018 from https://greatergood.berkeley.edu/article/item/how_smartphones_are_killing_conversation

31. Yuichi Esaki, Tsuyoshi Kitajima, Yasuhiro Ito, Shigefumi Koike, Yasumi Nakao, Akiko Tsuchiya, Marina Hirose & Nakao Iwata (2016) Wearing blue light-blocking glasses in the evening advances circadian rhythms in the patients with delayed sleep phase disorder: An open-label trial, *Chronobiology International,* 33:8, 1037-1044, DOI: 10.1080/07420528.2016.1194289

32. Leung, T. W., Li, R. W., & Kee, C. S. (2017). Blue-Light Filtering Spectacle Lenses: Optical and Clinical Performances. *PloS one,* 12(1), e0169114. doi:10.1371/journal.pone.0169114

33. Figueiro, M. G., & Rea, M. S. (2012). Preliminary evidence that light through the eyelids can suppress melatonin and phase shift dim light melatonin onset. *BMC research notes,* 5, 221. doi:10.1186/1756-0500-5-221

34. I Mason, D Grimaldi, R G Malkani, K J Reid, P C Zee; 0117 Impact of Light Exposure during Sleep on Cardiometabolic Function, *Sleep,* Volume 41, Issue suppl_1, 27 April 2018, Pages A46, https://doi.org/10.1093/sleep/zsy061.116

35. Mariana G. Figueiro and Mark S. Rea, "The Effects of Red and Blue Lights on Circadian Variations in Cortisol, Alpha Amylase, and Melatonin," *International Journal of Endocrinology,* vol. 2010, Article ID 829351, 9 pages, 2010. https://doi.org/10.1155/2010/829351.

36. Kopcso, Krisztina and Lang, Andras. Nighttime Fears of Adolescents and Young Adults. November 03, 2017. Available from: http://www.smgebooks.com/anxiety-disorders/chapters/ANXD-17-03.pdf

37. E.R. Stothard, A.W. McHill, C.M. Depner, B.R. Birks, et al.Circadian entrainment to the natural light-dark cycle across seasons and the weekend. *Current Biology,* 27 (2017), pp. 508-513 DOI: https://doi.org/10.1016/j.cub.2016.12.041

38. Wright KP, McHill AW, Birks BR, Griffin BR, Rusterholz T, Chinoy ED. Entrainment of the Human Circadian Clock to the Natural Light-Dark Cycle. *Current biology: CB.* 2013;23(16):1554-1558. doi:10.1016/j.cub.2013.06.039.

39.   Aan Het Rot, M., Miloserdov, K., Buijze, ALF, Meesters,Y., Gordijn, MCM. Premenstrual mood and empathy after a single light therapy session. *Psychiatry Research.* 2017 Oct;256():212-218. doi: 10.1016/j.psychres.2017.06.052.

Chapter 6

1.   Romm, Cari. (2017, January 26) What It Actually Means to Get a Good Night's Sleep, by the Numbers. *The Cut.* Retrieved November 7, 2018 from https://www.thecut.com/2017/01/what-a-good-nights-sleep-looks-like-by-the-numbers.html

2.   L.J. Moran, W.A. March, M.J. Whitrow, L.C. Giles, M.J. Davies, V.M. Moore; Sleep disturbances in a community-based sample of women with polycystic ovary syndrome, *Human Reproduction*, Volume 30, Issue 2, 1 February 2015, Pages 466–472, https://doi.org/10.1093/humrep/deu318

3.   Fernandez, R. C., Moore, V. M., Van Ryswyk, E. M., Varcoe, T. J., Rodgers, R. J., March, W. A., Moran, L. J., Avery, J. C., McEvoy, R. D., … Davies, M. J. (2018). Sleep disturbances in women with polycystic ovary syndrome: prevalence, pathophysiology, impact and management strategies. *Nature and science of sleep*, 10, 45-64. doi:10.2147/NSS.S127475

4.   Pizzino, G., Irrera, N., Cucinotta, M., Pallio, G., Mannino, F., Arcoraci, V., Squadrito, F., Altavilla, D., … Bitto, A. (2017). Oxidative Stress: Harms and Benefits for Human Health. *Oxidative medicine and cellular longevity*, 2017, doi: [10.1155/2017/8416763]

5.   Mora Murri, Manuel Luque-Ramírez, María Insenser, Miriam Ojeda-Ojeda, Hector F. Escobar-Morreale; Circulating markers of oxidative stress and polycystic ovary syndrome (PCOS): a systematic review and meta-analysis, *Human Reproduction Update*, Volume 19, Issue 3, 1 May 2013, Pages 268-288, https://doi.org/10.1093/humupd/dms059

6.   Jain P, Jain M, Haldar C, Singh TB, Jain S. Melatonin and its correlation with testosterone in polycystic ovarian syndrome. *Journal of Human Reproductive Sciences* 2013;6:253-8. Available from: http://www.jhrsonline.org/text.asp?2013/6/4/253/126295

7.   N. Shreeve, F. Cagampang, K. Sadek, M. Tolhurst, A. Houldey, C.M. Hill, N. Brook, N. Macklon, Y. Cheong; Poor sleep in PCOS; is melatonin the culprit?, *Human Reproduction*, Volume 28, Issue 5, 1 May 2013, Pages 1348-1353, https://doi.org/10.1093/humrep/det013

8.   Song, X. et al., (2015 Dec) Family association study between melatonin receptor gene polymorphisms and polycystic ovary syndrome in Han Chinese. *European Journal of Obstetrics and Gynecology and Reproductive Biology*, Volume 195 , 108 - 112 DOI: 10.1016/j.ejogrb.2015.09.043

9.   Tasoula Tsilchorozidou, John W. Honour, Gerard S. Conway; Altered Cortisol Metabolism in Polycystic Ovary Syndrome: Insulin Enhances 5α-Reduction But Not the Elevated Adrenal Steroid Production Rates, *The Journal of Clinical Endocrinology & Metabolism*, Volume 88, Issue 12, 1 December 2003, Pages 5907-5913, https://doi.org/10.1210/jc.2003-030240

10.   Rupert Lanzenberger, Wolfgang Wadsak, Christoph Spindelegger, Markus Mitterhauser, Elena Akimova, Leonhard-Key Mien, Martin Fink, Ulrike Moser, Markus Savli, Georg S. Kranz, Andreas Hahn, Kurt Kletter, Siegfried Kasper; Cortisol plasma levels in social anxiety disorder patients correlate with serotonin-1A receptor binding in limbic brain regions, *International Journal of Neuropsychopharmacology*, Volume 13, Issue 9, 1 October 2010, Pages 1129-1143, https://doi.org/10.1017/S1461145710000581

11.   Marcos A. López-Patiño, Manuel Gesto, Marta Conde-Sieira, José L. Soengas, Jesús M. Míguez. Stress inhibition of melatonin synthesis in the pineal organ of rainbow trout (Oncorhynchus mykiss) is mediated by cortisol. *Journal of Experimental Biology.* 2014 217: 1407-1416; doi: 10.1242/jeb.087916

12.   (2007). Insomnia: definition, prevalence, etiology, and consequences. *Journal of clinical sleep medicine : JCSM : official publication of the American Academy of Sleep Medicine*, 3(5 Suppl), S7-10.

13.   Fernandez, R. C., Moore, V. M., Van Ryswyk, E. M., Varcoe, T. J., Rodgers, R. J., March, W. A., Moran, L. J., Avery, J. C., McEvoy, R. D., … Davies, M. J. (2018). Sleep disturbances in women with polycystic ovary syndrome: prevalence, pathophysiology, impact and management strategies. *Nature and science of sleep*, 10, 45-64. doi:10.2147/NSS.S127475

14.   Grzegorz Franik, Krzysztof Krysta, Paweł Madej, Beata Gimlewicz-Pięta, Barbara Oślizło, Justina Trukawka & Magdalena Olszanecka-Glinianowicz (2016) Sleep disturbances in women with polycystic ovary syndrome, *Gynecological Endocrinology*, 32:12, 1014-1017, DOI: 10.1080/09513590.2016.1196177

15.   Alexandros N. Vgontzas, Richard S. Legro, Edward O. Bixler, Allison Grayev, Anthony Kales, George P. Chrousos; Polycystic Ovary Syndrome Is Associated with Obstructive Sleep Apnea and Daytime Sleepiness: Role of Insulin Resistance, *The Journal of Clinical Endocrinology & Metabolism*, Volume 86, Issue 2, 1 February 2001, Pages 517-520, https://doi.org/10.1210/jcem.86.2.7185

16.   Monahan, K., & Redline, S. (2011). Role of obstructive sleep apnea in cardiovascular disease. *Current opinion in cardiology*, 26(6), 541-7. doi: [10.1097/HCO.0b013e32834b806a]

17.   Ruchała, M., Bromińska, B., Cyrańska-Chyrek, E., Kuźnar-Kamińska, B., Kostrzewska, M., & Batura-Gabryel, H. (2016). Obstructive sleep apnea and hormones - a novel insight. *Archives of medical science : AMS*, 13(4), 875-884. doi: [10.5114/aoms.2016.61499]

18.	Husse J, Hintze SC, Eichele G, Lehnert H, Oster H (2012) Circadian Clock Genes Per1 and Per2 Regulate the Response of Metabolism-Associated Transcripts to Sleep Disruption. PLoS ONE 7(12): e52983. https://doi.org/10.1371/journal.pone.0052983

19.	Gangwisch, J. E., Heymsfield, S. B., Boden-Albala, B., Buijs, R. M., Kreier, F., Pickering, T. G., Rundle, A. G., Zammit, G. K., … Malaspina, D. (2007). Sleep duration as a risk factor for diabetes incidence in a large U.S. sample. *Sleep*, 30(12), 1667-73.

20.	Obesity Society. "Insulin sensitivity: One night of poor sleep could equal six months on a high-fat diet, study in dogs suggests." *ScienceDaily*. ScienceDaily, 4 November 2015. <www.sciencedaily.com/releases/2015/11/151104134039.htm>.

21.	Covassin, N., & Singh, P. (2016). Sleep Duration and Cardiovascular Disease Risk: Epidemiologic and Experimental Evidence. *Sleep medicine clinics*, 11(1), 81-9. doi: [10.1016/j.jsmc.2015.10.007]

22.	Luca, A., Luca, M., & Calandra, C. (2013). Sleep disorders and depression: brief review of the literature, case report, and nonpharmacologic interventions for depression. *Clinical interventions in aging*, 8, 1033-9. doi: [10.2147/CIA.S47230]

23.	Cooke, Rachel. (2017, 24 Sep) 'Sleep should be prescribed': what those late nights out could be costing you. *The Guardian*. Retrieved November 7, 2018 from https://www.theguardian.com/lifeandstyle/2017/sep/24/why-lack-of-sleep-health-worst-enemy-matthew-walker-why-we-sleep

24.	Yi-Han Hsiao, Yung-Tai Chen, Ching-Min Tseng, Li-An Wu, Wei-Chen Lin, Vincent Yi-Fong Su, Diahn-Warng Perng, Shi-Chuan Chang, Yuh-Min Chen, Tzeng-Ji Chen, Yu-Chin Lee, Kun-Ta Chou; Sleep Disorders and Increased Risk of Autoimmune Diseases in Individuals without Sleep Apnea, *Sleep*, Volume 38, Issue 4, 1 April 2015, Pages 581–586, https://doi.org/10.5665/sleep.4574

25.	Matsui, M. S., Pelle, E., Dong, K., & Pernodet, N. (2016). Biological Rhythms in the Skin. *International journal of molecular sciences*, 17(6), 801. doi:10.3390/ijms17060801

26.	Oyetakin-White, P. , Suggs, A. , Koo, B. , Matsui, M. S., Yarosh, D. , Cooper, K. D. and Baron, E. D. (2015), Does poor sleep quality affect skin ageing?. *Clinical and Experimental Dermatology*, 40: 17-22. doi:10.1111/ced.12455

27.	Matthew P. Pase, Jayandra J. Himali, Natalie A. Grima, Alexa S.Beiser, Claudia L. Satizabal, Hugo J. Aparicio, Robert J. Thomas, Daniel J. Gottlieb, Sandford H. Auerbach, Sudha Seshadri. Sleep architecture and the risk of incident dementia in the community. *Neurology* Sep 2017, 89 (12) 1244-1250; DOI:10.1212/WNL.0000000000004373

28.	Kristen L. Knutson & Malcolm von Schantz (2018) Associations between chronotype, morbidity and mortality in the UK Biobank cohort, *Chronobiology International*, 35:8, 1045-1053, DOI: 10.1080/07420528.2018.1454458

29.	Ohkuma, Toshiaki et al., U-shaped association of sleep duration with metabolic syndrome and insulin resistance in patients with type 2 diabetes: The Fukuoka Diabetes Registry. *Metabolism - Clinical and Experimental*, Volume 63 , Issue 4 , 484 - 491. DOI: https://doi.org/10.1016/j.metabol.2013.12.001

30.	Koopman, A., Rauh, S. P., van 't Riet, E., Groeneveld, L., van der Heijden, A. A., Elders, P. J., Dekker, J. M., Nijpels, G., Beulens, J. W., … Rutters, F. (2017). The Association between Social Jetlag, the Metabolic Syndrome, and Type 2 Diabetes Mellitus in the General Population: The New Hoorn Study. *Journal of biological rhythms*, 32(4), 359-368. doi: [10.1177/0748730417713572]

31.	N. Shreeve, F. Cagampang, K. Sadek, M. Tolhurst, A. Houldey, C.M. Hill, N. Brook, N. Macklon, Y. Cheong; Poor sleep in PCOS; is melatonin the culprit?, *Human Reproduction*, Volume 28, Issue 5, 1 May 2013, Pages 1348–1353, https://doi.org/10.1093/humrep/det013

32.	Jain, P., Jain, M., Haldar, C., Singh, T. B., & Jain, S. (2013). Melatonin and its correlation with testosterone in polycystic ovarian syndrome. *Journal of human reproductive sciences*, 6(4), 253-8. doi: [10.4103/0974-1208.126295]

33.	Ferracioli-Oda E, Qawasmi A, Bloch MH (2013) Meta-Analysis: Melatonin for the Treatment of Primary Sleep Disorders. PLoS ONE 8(5): e63773. https://doi.org/10.1371/journal.pone.0063773

34.	Rai, Seema & Basheer, Muddasir. (2015). Melatonin Attenuates Free Radical Load and Reverses Histologic Architect and Hormone Profile Alteration in Female Rat: An In vivo Study of Pathogenesis of Letrozole Induced Poly Cystic Ovary. *Journal of Clinical & Cellular Immunology*. 06. 10.4172/2155-9899.1000384.

35.	Alessandro Pacchiarotti, Gianfranco Carlomagno, Gabriele Antonini & Arianna Pacchiarotti (2016)Effect of myo-inositol and melatonin versus myo-inositol, in a randomized controlled trial, for improving *in vitro* fertilization of patients with polycystic ovarian syndrome, *Gynecological Endocrinology*, 32:1, 69-73, DOI: 10.3109/09513590.2015.1101444

36.	Tagliaferri, Valeria & Romualdi, Daniela & Scarinci, Elisa & De Cicco, Simona & Di Florio, Christian & Immediata, Valentina & Tropea, Anna & Mariaflavia Santarsiero, Carla & Lanzone, Antonio & Apa, Rosanna. (2017). Melatonin Treatment May Be Able to Restore Menstrual Cyclicity in Women With PCOS: A Pilot Study. *Reproductive Sciences*. 25. 193371911771126. 10.1177/1933719117711262.

37.	Zizhen Xie, Fei Chen, William A. Li, Xiaokun Geng, Changhong Li, Xiaomei Meng, Yan Feng, Wei Liu & Fengchun Yu (2017) A review of sleep disorders and melatonin, *Neurological Research*, 39:6, 559-565, DOI: 10.1080/01616412.2017.1315864

38. Silman, R.E., Melatonin: a contraceptive for the nineties. *European Journal of Obstetrics & Gynecology*, Volume 49 , Issue 1 , 3 - 9

39. (2013). Effects of odor on emotion, with implications. *Frontiers in systems neuroscience*, 7, 66. doi:10.3389/fnsys.2013.00066

40. Kim, I. H., Kim, C., Seong, K., Hur, M. H., Lim, H. M., & Lee, M. S. (2012). Essential oil inhalation on blood pressure and salivary cortisol levels in prehypertensive and hypertensive subjects. *Evidence-based complementary and alternative medicine* : eCAM, 2012, 984203.

41. Kim, I. H., Kim, C., Seong, K., Hur, M. H., Lim, H. M., & Lee, M. S. (2012). Essential oil inhalation on blood pressure and salivary cortisol levels in prehypertensive and hypertensive subjects. *Evidence-based complementary and alternative medicine* : eCAM, 2012, 984203.

42. Knight, L., A. Levin, AND C. Mendenhall. Candles and Incense as Potential Sources of Indoor Air Pollution: Market Analysis And Literature Review (EPA/600/R-01/001). U.S. Environmental Protection Agency, Washington, D.C., 2001.

43. Kim, I. H., Kim, C., Seong, K., Hur, M. H., Lim, H. M., & Lee, M. S. (2012). Essential oil inhalation on blood pressure and salivary cortisol levels in prehypertensive and hypertensive subjects. *Evidence-based complementary and alternative medicine* : eCAM, 2012, 984203.

44. Chandrasekhar, K., Kapoor, J., & Anishetty, S. (2012). A prospective, randomized double-blind, placebo-controlled study of safety and efficacy of a high-concentration full-spectrum extract of ashwagandha root in reducing stress and anxiety in adults. *Indian journal of psychological medicine*, 34(3), 255-62.

45. Gannon, J. M., Forrest, P. E., & Roy Chengappa, K. N. (2014). Subtle changes in thyroid indices during a placebo-controlled study of an extract of Withania somnifera in persons with bipolar disorder. *Journal of Ayurveda and integrative medicine*, 5(4), 241-5.

46. Šrámek, P., Šimečková, M., Janský, L. et al. *European Journal of Applied Physiology and Occupational Physiology* (2000) 81: 436. https://doi.org/10.1007/s004210050065

47. Kanda, K., Tochihara, Y. & Ohnaka, T. *European Journal of Applied Physiology and Occupational Physiology* (1999) 80: 71. https://doi.org/10.1007/s004210050560

48. Pascoe, MC., Thompson, DR., Jenkins, ZM., Ski, CF. Mindfulness mediates the physiological markers of stress: Systematic review and meta-analysis. *Journal of Psychiatric Research*. Volume 95, December 2017, Pages 156-178. DOI: 10.1016/j.jpsychires.2017.08.004

49. Hölzel, B. K., Carmody, J., Vangel, M., Congleton, C., Yerramsetti, S. M., Gard, T., & Lazar, S. W. (2010). Mindfulness practice leads to increases in regional brain gray matter density. *Psychiatry research*, 191(1), 36-43.

50. Nieber K. The Impact of Coffee on Health. *Planta Med.* 2017 Nov;83(16):1256-1263. doi: 10.1055/s-0043-115007.

51. Fernandez, R. C., Moore, V. M., Van Ryswyk, E. M., Varcoe, T. J., Rodgers, R. J., March, W. A., Moran, L. J., Avery, J. C., McEvoy, R. D., … Davies, M. J. (2018). Sleep disturbances in women with polycystic ovary syndrome: prevalence, pathophysiology, impact and management strategies. *Nature and science of sleep*, 10, 45-64. doi:10.2147/NSS.S127475

52. Jara SM, Hopp ML, Weaver EM. Association of Continuous Positive Airway Pressure Treatment With Sexual Quality of Life in Patients With Sleep ApneaFollow-up Study of a Randomized Clinical Trial. *JAMA Otolaryngol Head Neck Surg.* 2018;144(7):587-593. doi:10.1001/jamaoto.2018.0485

53. Sleep Apnea. *Mayo Clinic.* Retrieved November 7, 2018 from https://www.mayoclinic.org/diseases-conditions/sleep-apnea

54. Simou, E., Britton, J., & Leonardi-Bee, J. (2018). Alcohol and the risk of sleep apnoea: a systematic review and meta-analysis. *Sleep medicine*, 42, 38-46.

55. Alexandros N. Vgontzas, Richard S. Legro, Edward O. Bixler, Allison Grayev, Anthony Kales, George P. Chrousos; Polycystic Ovary Syndrome Is Associated with Obstructive Sleep Apnea and Daytime Sleepiness: Role of Insulin Resistance, *The Journal of Clinical Endocrinology & Metabolism*, Volume 86, Issue 2, 1 February 2001, Pages 517-520, https://doi.org/10.1210/jcem.86.2.7185

56. Sivertsen, Børge & Lallukka, Tea & J Petrie, Keith & Steingrímsdóttir, Ólöf & Stubhaug, Audun & Sivert Nielsen, Christopher. (2015). Sleep and Pain Sensitivity in Adults. Pain. 27. 10.1097/j.pain.0000000000000131.

57. (2011). Nocturnal gastroesophageal reflux: assessment and clinical implications. *Journal of neurogastroenterology and motility*, 17(2), 105-7.

58. Tharwat S Kandil; Amany A Mousa; Ahmed A El-Gendy; Amr M Abbas. The Potential Therapeutic Effect of Melatonin in Gastro-esophageal Reflux Disease. BMC *Gastroenterology*. 2010;10:7

59. Sahbaie P, Sun Y, Liang DY, Shi XY, Clark JD. Curcumin treatment attenuates pain and enhances functional recovery after incision. *Anesthesia & Analgesia*. 118(6):1336-1344, JUN 2014. doi: 10.1213/ANE.0000000000000189.

60. June J. Pilcher PhD, Kristin R. Michalowski & Renee D. Carrigan (2001) The Prevalence of Daytime Napping and Its Relationship to Nighttime Sleep, *Behavioral Medicine*, 27:2, 71-76, DOI: 10.1080/08964280109595773

61. Jones, Jeffery. (2013, December 19) In U.S., 40% Get Less Than Recommended Amount of Sleep. *Gallup.* Retrieved November 7, 2018 from https://news.gallup.com/poll/166553/less-recommended-amount-sleep.aspx

62. Herxheimer A, Petrie KJ. Melatonin for the prevention and treatment of jet lag. *Cochrane Database of Systematic Reviews* 2002, Issue 2. Art. No.: CD001520. DOI: 10.1002/14651858.CD001520.
63. (2017). What do hypnotics cost hospitals and healthcare?. *F1000Research*, 6, 542. doi:10.12688/f1000research.11328.2
64. Chelsie B. Heesch (2014) The long-term use of sedative hypnotics in chronic insomnia. *Mental Health Clinician*: March 2014, Vol. 4, No. 2, pp. 78-81. https://doi.org/10.9740/mhc.n190097
65. Ashish Kumar U, Palatty PL (2013) Comparative Action of Sedative Hypnotics on Neurophysiology of Sleep. *J Sleep Disord Ther* 2:150. doi:10.4172/2167-0277.1000150
66. Baker FC, Mitchell D, Driver HS. Oral contraceptives alter sleep and raise body temperature in young women. *Pflügers Arch - Eur J Physiol* (2001) 442: 729. https://doi.org/10.1007/s004240100582

Chapter 7

1. Gill, S., & Panda, S. (2015). A Smartphone App Reveals Erratic Diurnal Eating Patterns in Humans that Can Be Modulated for Health Benefits. *Cell metabolism*, 22(5), 789-98. doi: [10.1016/j.cmet.2015.09.005]
2. Slingerland, A. E., Schwabkey, Z., Wiesnoski, D. H., & Jenq, R. R. (2017). Clinical Evidence for the Microbiome in Inflammatory Diseases. *Frontiers in immunology*, 8, 400. doi:10.3389/fimmu.2017.00400
3. Gill, S., & Panda, S. (2015). A Smartphone App Reveals Erratic Diurnal Eating Patterns in Humans that Can Be Modulated for Health Benefits. *Cell metabolism*, 22(5), 789-98. doi: [10.1016/j.cmet.2015.09.005]
4. Wu, H. J., & Wu, E. (2012). The role of gut microbiota in immune homeostasis and autoimmunity. *Gut microbes*, 3(1), 4-14. doi: [10.4161/gmic.19320]
5. (2014). The gut microbiome and the brain. *Journal of medicinal food*, 17(12), 1261-72. doi: [10.1089/jmf.2014.7000]
6. Yano, J. M., Yu, K., Donaldson, G. P., Shastri, G. G., Ann, P., Ma, L., Nagler, C. R., Ismagilov, R. F., Mazmanian, S. K., … Hsiao, E. Y. (2015). Indigenous bacteria from the gut microbiota regulate host serotonin biosynthesis. *Cell*, 161(2), 264-76. doi: [10.1016/j.cell.2015.02.047]
7. Gerard Clarke, Roman M. Stilling, Paul J. Kennedy, Catherine Stanton, John F. Cryan, Timothy G. Dinan; Minireview: Gut Microbiota: The Neglected Endocrine Organ, *Molecular Endocrinology*, Volume 28, Issue 8, 1 August 2014, Pages 1221–1238, https://doi.org/10.1210/me.2014-1108
8. Sender, R., Fuchs, S., & Milo, R. (2016). Revised Estimates for the Number of Human and Bacteria Cells in the Body. *PLoS biology*, 14(8), e1002533. doi:10.1371/journal.pbio.1002533
9. Gnocchi, D., Pedrelli, M., Hurt-Camejo, E., & Parini, P. (2015). Lipids around the Clock: Focus on Circadian Rhythms and Lipid Metabolism. *Biology*, 4(1), 104-32. doi:10.3390/biology4010104
10. Newman, T. (2018, March 2). "What does the liver do?." *Medical News Today*. Retrieved from https://www.medicalnewstoday.com/articles/305075.php.
11. Scharping, Nathaniel. (2017, May 4) "The Liver Grows by Day, Shrinks by Night." *Discover*. Retrieved from: http://blogs.discovermagazine.com/d-brief/2017/05/04/liver-grow-and-shrink/
12. Berg JM, Tymoczko JL, Stryer L. Biochemistry. 5th edition. New York: W H Freeman; 2002. Section 16.3, *Glucose Can Be Synthesized from Noncarbohydrate Precursors*. Available from: https://www.ncbi.nlm.nih.gov/books/NBK22591
13. Flore Sinturel, Alan Gerber, Daniel Mauvoisin, Jingkui Wang, David Gatfield, Jeremy J. Stubblefield, Carla B. Green, Frédéric Gachon, Ueli Schibler. Diurnal Oscillations in Liver Mass and Cell Size Accompany Ribosome Assembly Cycles. *Cell*, 2017; 169 (4): 651 DOI: 10.1016/j.cell.2017.04.015
14. Paschos, P., & Paletas, K. (2009). Non alcoholic fatty liver disease and metabolic syndrome. *Hippokratia*, 13(1), 9-19.
15. Thaler, J. P., Yi, C. X., Schur, E. A., Guyenet, S. J., Hwang, B. H., Dietrich, M. O., Zhao, X., Sarruf, D. A., Izgur, V., Maravilla, K. R., Nguyen, H. T., Fischer, J. D., Matsen, M. E., Wisse, B. E., Morton, G. J., Horvath, T. L., Baskin, D. G., Tschöp, M. H., … Schwartz, M. W. (2011). Obesity is associated with hypothalamic injury in rodents and humans. *The Journal of clinical investigation*, 122(1), 153-62. doi: [10.1172/JCI59660]
16. WU, Tao & YAO, Cencen & HUANG, Liangfeng & MAO, Youxiang & Wanjing, Zhang & JIANG, Jianguo & Fu, Zhengwei. (2015). Nutrients and Circadian Rhythms in Mammals. *Journal of Nutritional Science and Vitaminology*. 61. S89–S91. doi: 10.3177/jnsv.61.S89.
17. Td Lopes, Md Borba, Rd Lopes, S L Paim, V V Teodoro, R Fisberg, I Z Zimberg, C Crispim; 0471 The Effect of Meal Timing on Sleep Parameters and Apnea Severity in Sleep Apnea Patients, *Sleep*, Volume 41, Issue suppl_1, 27 April 2018, Pages A178, https://doi.org/10.1093/sleep/zsy061.470
18. Haraguchi, Atsushi et al. "Night eating model shows time-specific depression-like behavior in the forced swimming test." *Scientific Reports* (2018). DOI:10.1038/s41598-018-19433-8
19. Daniela Jakubowicz, Maayan Barnea, Julio Wainstein, Oren Froy. Effects of caloric intake timing on insulin resistance and hyperandrogenism in lean women with polycystic ovary syndrome. *Clinical Science*, 2013; 125 (9): 423 DOI: 10.1042/CS20130071

20. Patterson, R. E., Laughlin, G. A., LaCroix, A. Z., Hartman, S. J., Natarajan, L., Senger, C. M., Martínez, M. E., Villaseñor, A., Sears, D. D., Marinac, C. R., … Gallo, L. C. (2015). Intermittent Fasting and Human Metabolic Health. *Journal of the Academy of Nutrition and Dietetics*, 115(8), 1203-12. doi: [10.1016/j.jand.2015.02.018]

21. Marinac CR, Nelson SH, Breen CI, et al. Prolonged Nightly Fasting and Breast Cancer Prognosis. *JAMA Oncol*. 2016;2(8):1049–1055. doi:10.1001/jamaoncol.2016.0164

22. Jakubowicz, D. , Barnea, M. , Wainstein, J. and Froy, O. (2013), High Caloric intake at breakfast vs. dinner differentially influences weight loss of overweight and obese women. *Obesity*, 21: 2504-2512. doi:10.1002/oby.20460

23. Daniela Jakubowicz, Maayan Barnea, Julio Wainstein, Oren Froy. Effects of caloric intake timing on insulin resistance and hyperandrogenism in lean women with polycystic ovary syndrome. *Clinical Science*, 2013; 125 (9): 423 DOI: 10.1042/CS20130071

24. Marinac CR, Sears DD, Natarajan L, Gallo LC, Breen CI, Patterson RE. Frequency and Circadian Timing of Eating May Influence Biomarkers of Inflammation and Insulin Resistance Associated with Breast Cancer Risk. *PLoS One*. 2015 Aug 25;10(8):e0136240. doi: 10.1371/journal.pone.0136240. eCollection 2015.

25. Jakubowicz, Daniela & Froy, Oren & Wainstein, Julio & Boaz, Mona. "Meal timing and composition influence ghrelin levels, appetite scores and weight loss maintenance in overweight and obese adults" *Steroids* 77 (2012) 323–331. 10.1016/j.steroids.2011.12.006.

26. Andrew Scholey, Lauren Owen; Effects of chocolate on cognitive function and mood: a systematic review, *Nutrition Reviews*, Volume 71, Issue 10, 1 October 2013, Pages 665–681, https://doi.org/10.1111/nure.12065

27. Hess, J. M., Jonnalagadda, S. S., & Slavin, J. L. (2016). What Is a Snack, Why Do We Snack, and How Can We Choose Better Snacks? A Review of the Definitions of Snacking, Motivations to Snack, Contributions to Dietary Intake, and Recommendations for Improvement. *Advances in nutrition (Bethesda, Md.)*, 7(3), 466-75. doi:10.3945/an.115.009571

28. D Capaldi, Elizabeth & Quinn Owens, Jacqueline & J Privitera, Gregory. (2006). Isocaloric meal and snack foods differentially affect eating behavior. *Appetite*. 46. 117-23. doi:10.1016/j.appet.2005.10.008.

29. Ikeda, A., Miyamoto, J. J., Usui, N., Taira, M., & Moriyama, K. (2018). Chewing Stimulation Reduces Appetite Ratings and Attentional Bias toward Visual Food Stimuli in Healthy-Weight Individuals. *Frontiers in psychology*, 9, 99. doi:10.3389/fpsyg.2018.00099

30. Söderling, E., ElSalhy, M., Honkala, E. et al. *Clin Oral Invest* (2015) 19: 237. https://doi.org/10.1007/s00784-014-1229-y

31. Xu, J., Xiao, X., Li, Y., Zheng, J., Li, W., Zhang, Q., & Wang, Z. (2015). The effect of gum chewing on blood GLP-1 concentration in fasted, healthy, non-obese men. *Endocrine*, 50(1), 93-8. doi: [10.1007/s12020-015-0566-1]

32. Bian, X., Chi, L., Gao, B., Tu, P., Ru, H., & Lu, K. (2017). The artificial sweetener acesulfame potassium affects the gut microbiome and body weight gain in CD-1 mice. *PloS one*, 12(6), e0178426. doi:10.1371/journal.pone.0178426

33. Jotham Suez, Tal Korem, Gili Zilberman-Schapira, Eran Segal & Eran Elinav (2015) Non-caloric artificial sweeteners and the microbiome: findings and challenges, *Gut Microbes*, 6:2, 149-155, DOI: 10.1080/19490976.2015.1017700

34. Lindsay, Jessica. (2018, 2 Aug) Did you know most chewing gum contains plastic? *Metro*. Retrieved November 7, 2018 from https://metro.co.uk/2018/08/02/know-chewing-gum-contains-plastic-7790722/

35. Nathan Watemberg, Manar Matar, Miki Har-Gil, Muhammad Mahajnah. The Influence of Excessive Chewing Gum Use on Headache Frequency and Severity Among Adolescents. *Pediatric Neurology*, 2013; DOI: 10.1016/j.pediatrneurol.2013.08.015

36. Alirezaei, M., Kemball, C. C., Flynn, C. T., Wood, M. R., Whitton, J. L., & Kiosses, W. B. (2010). Short-term fasting induces profound neuronal autophagy. *Autophagy*, 6(6), 702-10. doi: [10.4161/auto.6.6.12376]

37. Bronwen Martin, Michele Pearson, Lisa Kebejian, Erin Golden, Alex Keselman, Meredith Bender, Olga Carlson, Josephine Egan, Bruce Ladenheim, Jean-Lud Cadet, Kevin G. Becker, William Wood, Kara Duffy, Prabhu Vinayakumar, Stuart Maudsley, Mark P. Mattson; Sex-Dependent Metabolic, Neuroendocrine, and Cognitive Responses to Dietary Energy Restriction and Excess, *Endocrinology*, Volume 148, Issue 9, 1 September 2007, Pages 4318–4333, https://doi.org/10.1210/en.2007-0161

38. Martin B, Pearson M, Brenneman R, Golden E, Wood W III, Prabhu V, et al. (2009) Gonadal Transcriptome Alterations in Response to Dietary Energy Intake: Sensing the Reproductive Environment. *PLoS ONE* 4(1): e4146. https://doi.org/10.1371/journal.pone.0004146

39. Harvie, M., & Howell, A. (2017). Potential Benefits and Harms of Intermittent Energy Restriction and Intermittent Fasting Amongst Obese, Overweight and Normal Weight Subjects-A Narrative Review of Human and Animal Evidence. *Behavioral sciences (Basel, Switzerland)*, 7(1), 4. doi:10.3390/bs7010004

40. Li, Guolin & Xie, Cen & Lu, Siyu & Nichols, Robert & Tian, Yuan & Li, Licen & Patel, Daxesh & Ma, Yinyan & N. Brocker, Chad & Yan, Tingting & W. Krausz, Kristopher & Xiang, Rong & Gavrilova, Oksana & Patterson, Andrew & J. Gonzalez, Frank. (2017). Intermittent Fasting Promotes White Adipose Browning and Decreases Obesity by Shaping the Gut Microbiota. *Cell Metabolism.* doi: 26. 10.1016/j.cmet.2017.08.019.

41. Hoddy, K. K., Kroeger, C. M., Trepanowski, J. F., Barnosky, A. R., Bhutani, S., & Varady, K. A. (2015). Safety of alternate day fasting and effect on disordered eating behaviors. *Nutrition journal*, 14, 44. doi:10.1186/s12937-015-0029-9

42. Khodadadi, S., Sobhani, N., Mirshekar, S., Ghiasvand, R., Pourmasoumi, M., Miraghajani, M., & Dehsoukhteh, S. S. (2017). Tumor Cells Growth and Survival Time with the Ketogenic Diet in Animal Models: A Systematic Review. *International journal of preventive medicine*, 8, 35. doi:10.4103/2008-7802.207035

43. Brandhorst, Sebastian & Choi, In Young & Wei, Min & Cheng, Chia-Wei & Sedrakyan, Sargis & Navarrete, Gerardo & Dubeau, Louis & Peng Yap, Li & Park, Ryan & Vinciguerra, Manlio & Di Biase, Stefano & Mirzaei, Hamed & Mirisola, Mario & Childress, Patra & Ji, Lingyun & Groshen, Susan & Penna, Fabio & Odetti, Patrizio & Perin, Laura & D. Longo, Valter. (2015). A Periodic Diet that Mimics Fasting Promotes Multi-System Regeneration, Enhanced Cognitive Performance, and Healthspan. *Cell Metabolism.* doi: 22. 10.1016/j.cmet.2015.05.012.

44. Cheng, C. W., Adams, G. B., Perin, L., Wei, M., Zhou, X., Lam, B. S., Da Sacco, S., Mirisola, M., Quinn, D. I., Dorff, T. B., Kopchick, J. J., ... Longo, V. D. (2014). Prolonged fasting reduces IGF-1/PKA to promote hematopoietic-stem-cell-based regeneration and reverse immunosuppression. *Cell stem cell*, 14(6), 810-23. doi: [10.1016/j.stem.2014.04.014]

45. Mojto, Viliam & Gvozdjakova, Anna & Kucharska, J & Rausova, Zuzana & Vancova, Olga & Valuch, J. (2018). Effects of complete water fasting and regeneration diet on kidney function, oxidative stress and antioxidants. *Bratislava Medical Journal.* doi: 119. 107-111. 10.4149/BLL_2018_020.

46. Zhang, X. D., Wu, T. X., Cai, L. S., & Zhu, Y. F. (2007). Influence of fasting on muscle composition and antioxidant defenses of market-size Sparus macrocephalus. *Journal of Zhejiang University. Science.* B, 8(12), 906-11. doi: [10.1631/jzus.2007.B0906]

47. (2016 April 26) Fasting for Longevity: 9 Questions for Dr. Valter D. Longo. Retrieved November 7, 2018 from https://www.bluezones.com/2016/04/fasting-for-longevity/

48. Longo, V. D., & Panda, S. (2016). Fasting, Circadian Rhythms, and Time-Restricted Feeding in Healthy Lifespan. *Cell metabolism*, 23(6), 1048-1059. doi: [10.1016/j.cmet.2016.06.001]

49. Choi, I. Y., Piccio, L., Childress, P., Bollman, B., Ghosh, A., Brandhorst, S., Suarez, J., Michalsen, A., Cross, A. H., Morgan, T. E., Wei, M., Paul, F., Bock, M., ... Longo, V. D. (2016). A Diet Mimicking Fasting Promotes Regeneration and Reduces Autoimmunity and Multiple Sclerosis Symptoms. *Cell reports*, 15(10), 2136-2146. doi: [10.1016/j.celrep.2016.05.009]

50. I Berlin, A Grimaldi, C Landault, F Cesselin, A J Puech; Suspected postprandial hypoglycemia is associated with beta-adrenergic hypersensitivity and emotional distress, *The Journal of Clinical Endocrinology & Metabolism*, Volume 79, Issue 5, 1 November 1994, Pages 1428–1433, https://doi.org/10.1210/jcem.79.5.7962339

51. Noon, M. J., Khawaja, H. A., Ishtiaq, O., Khawaja, Q., Minhas, S., Niazi, A. K., Minhas, A., ... Malhi, U. R. (2016). Fasting with diabetes: a prospective observational study. *BMJ global health*, 1(2), e000009. doi:10.1136/bmjgh-2015-000009

52. Arnason, T. G., Bowen, M. W., & Mansell, K. D. (2017). Effects of intermittent fasting on health markers in those with type 2 diabetes: A pilot study. *World journal of diabetes*, 8(4), 154-164.

53. Kahleova, H., Belinova, L., Malinska, H., Oliyarnyk, O., Trnovska, J., Skop, V., Kazdova, L., Dezortova, M., Hajek, M., Tura, A., Hill, M., ... Pelikanova, T. (2014). Eating two larger meals a day (breakfast and lunch) is more effective than six smaller meals in a reduced-energy regimen for patients with type 2 diabetes: a randomised crossover study. *Diabetologia*, 57(8), 1552-60. doi: [10.1007/s00125-014-3253-5]

54. Ganda, Om. (2016). Fasting Until Noon Triggers Increased Postprandial Hyperglycemia and Impaired Insulin Response After Lunch and Dinner in Individuals With Type 2 Diabetes: A Randomized Clinical Trial. Diabetes Care 2015;38:1820-1826. *Diabetes Care.* 39. e28-e28. doi 10.2337/dc15-2362.

55. Li C, Sadraie B, Steckhan N, Kessler C, Stange R, Jeitler M, Michalsen A. Effects of A One-week Fasting Therapy in Patients with Type-2 Diabetes Mellitus and Metabolic Syndrome - A Randomized Controlled Explorative Study. *Exp Clin Endocrinol Diabetes.* 2017 Oct;125(9):618-624. doi: 10.1055/s-0043-101700.

56. Gotthardt, J. D., Verpeut, J. L., Yeomans, B. L., Yang, J. A., Yasrebi, A., Roepke, T. A., & Bello, N. T. (2015). Intermittent Fasting Promotes Fat Loss With Lean Mass Retention, Increased Hypothalamic Norepinephrine Content, and Increased Neuropeptide Y Gene Expression in Diet-Induced Obese Male Mice. *Endocrinology*, 157(2), 679-91. doi: [10.1210/en.2015-1622]

57. (2011). Science behind human saliva. *Journal of natural science, biology, and medicine*, 2(1), 53-8. doi: [10.4103/0976-9668.82322]

58. Leanne M. Redman, Steven R. Smith, Jeffrey H. Burton, Corby K. Martin, Dora Il'yasova, Eric Ravussin. Metabolic Slowing and Reduced Oxidative Damage with Sustained Caloric Restriction Support the Rate of Living and Oxidative Damage Theories of Aging. *Cell Metabolism*, 2018; DOI: 10.1016/j.cmet.2018.02.019

59. Taylor, Kate (2007, April 23) Eating for Fewer Than One. *Slate*. Retrieved November 7, 2018 from http://www.slate.com/articles/health_and_science/medical_examiner/features/2007/eating_for_fewer_than_one/is_calorie_restriction_really_different_from_anorexia.html

Chapter 8

1.   Redman, L. M., Elkind-Hirsch, K., & Ravussin, E. (2011). Aerobic exercise in women with polycystic ovary syndrome improves ovarian morphology independent of changes in body composition. *Fertility and sterility*, 95(8), 2696-9. doi: [10.1016/j.fertnstert.2011.01.137]

2.   Jedel, Elizabeth & Labrie, Fernand & Odén, Anders & Holm, Göran & Nilsson, Lars & Janson, Per & Lind, Anna-Karin & Ohlsson, Claes & Stener-Victorin, Elisabet. (2010). Impact of electro-acupuncture and physical exercise on hyperandrogenism and oligo/amenorrhea in women with polycystic ovary syndrome: A randomized controlled trial. American journal of physiology. *Endocrinology and metabolism*. 300. E37-45. doi: 10.1152/ajpendo.00495.2010.

3.   Giallauria, F. , Palomba, S. , Maresca, L. , Vuolo, L. , Tafuri, D. , Lombardi, G., Colao, A. , Vigorito, C. and , (2008), Exercise training improves autonomic function and inflammatory pattern in women with polycystic ovary syndrome (PCOS). *Clinical Endocrinology*, 69: 792-798. doi:10.1111/j.1365-2265.2008.03305.x

4.   Conte, F., Banting, L., Teede, H. J., & Stepto, N. K. (2014). Mental health and physical activity in women with polycystic ovary syndrome: a brief review. *Sports medicine (Auckland, N.Z.)*, 45(4), 497-504. doi: [10.1007/s40279-014-0291-6]

5.   Mosca, A., Leclerc, M., & Hugot, J. P. (2016). Gut Microbiota Diversity and Human Diseases: Should We Reintroduce Key Predators in Our Ecosystem?. *Frontiers in microbiology*, 7, 455. doi:10.3389/fmicb.2016.00455

6.   Lindheim L, Bashir M, Münzker J, Trummer C, Zachhuber V, Leber B, et al. (2017) Alterations in Gut Microbiome Composition and Barrier Function Are Associated with Reproductive and Metabolic Defects in Women with Polycystic Ovary Syndrome (PCOS): A Pilot Study. PLoS ONE 12(1): e0168390. https://doi.org/10.1371/journal.pone.0168390

7.   Pedro J Torres, Martyna Siakowska, Beata Banaszewska, Leszek Pawelczyk, Antoni J Duleba, Scott T Kelley, Varykina G Thackray; Gut Microbial Diversity in Women With Polycystic Ovary Syndrome Correlates With Hyperandrogenism, *The Journal of Clinical Endocrinology & Metabolism*, Volume 103, Issue 4, 1 April 2018, Pages 1502-1511, https://doi.org/10.1210/jc.2017-02153

8.   (2016). The Gut Microbiome and Its Role in Obesity. *Nutrition today*, 51(4), 167-174. doi: [10.1097/NT.0000000000000167]

9.   Carding, S., Verbeke, K., Vipond, D. T., Corfe, B. M., & Owen, L. J. (2015). Dysbiosis of the gut microbiota in disease. *Microbial ecology in health and disease*, 26, 26191. doi:10.3402/mehd.v26.26191

10. Jacob M. Allen, Lucy J. Mailing, Grace M. Niemiro, Rachel Moore, Mark D. Cook, Bryan A. White, Hannah D. Holscher, Jeffrey A. Woods. Exercise Alters Gut Microbiota Composition and Function in Lean and Obese Humans. *Medicine & Science in Sports & Exercise*, 2017; 1 DOI: 10.1249/MSS.0000000000001495

11. University of Illinois at Urbana-Champaign. (2017, December 4). Exercise changes gut microbial composition independent of diet, team reports. *ScienceDaily*. Retrieved November 8, 2018 from www.sciencedaily.com/releases/2017/12/171204144757.htm

12. Tahara, Yu & Yamazaki, Mayu & Sukigara, Haruna & Motohashi, Hiroaki & Sasaki, Hiroyuki & Miyakawa, Hiroki & Haraguchi, Atsushi & Ikeda, Yuko & Fukuda, Shinji & Shibata, Shigenobu. (2018). Gut Microbiota-Derived Short Chain Fatty Acids Induce Circadian Clock Entrainment in Mouse Peripheral Tissue. *Scientific Reports*. 8. doi: 10.1038/s41598-018-19836-7.

13. S. Manfredo Vieira, M. Hiltensperger, V. Kumar, D. Zegarra-Ruiz, C. Dehner, N. Khan, F. R. C. Costa, E. Tiniakou, T. Greiling, W. Ruff, A. Barbieri, C. Kriegel, S. S. Mehta, J. R. Knight, D. Jain, A. L. Goodman, M. A. Kriegel. Translocation of a gut pathobiont drives autoimmunity in mice and humans. *Science*, 2018; 359 (6380): 1156 DOI: 10.1126/science.aar7201

14. Paddock, Catharine. (2008, April 21) Menstrual Disorder May Help Female Athletes, Thesis. *Medical News Today*. Retrieved November 7, 2018 from https://www.medicalnewstoday.com/articles/104747.php

15. Gislaine Satyko Kogure, Rafael Costa Silva, Fabiene K. Picchi Ramos, Cristiana Libardi Miranda-Furtado, Lucia Alves da Silva Lara, Rui Alberto Ferriani & Rosana Maria dos Reis (2015) Women with polycystic ovary syndrome have greater muscle strength irrespective of body composition, *Gynecological Endocrinology*, 31:3, 237-242, DOI: 10.3109/09513590.2014.982083

16. Seo, D. Y., Lee, S., Kim, N., Ko, K. S., Rhee, B. D., Park, B. J., & Han, J. (2013). Morning and evening exercise. *Integrative medicine research*, 2(4), 139-144. doi: [10.1016/j.imr.2013.10.003]

17. Alizadeh, Z. , Younespour, S. , Rajabian Tabesh, M. and Haghravan, S. (2017), Comparison between the effect of 6 weeks of morning or evening aerobic exercise on appetite and anthropometric indices: a randomized controlled trial. *Clin Obes*, 7: 157-165. doi:10.1111/cob.12187

18. (2015). Sick of sitting. *Diabetologia*, 58(8), 1751-8. doi: [10.1007/s00125-015-3624-6]

19. Chatchawan, U., Jupamatangb, U., Chanchitc, S., Puntumetakul, R., Donpunha, W., & Yamauchi, J. (2015). Immediate effects of dynamic sitting exercise on the lower back mobility of sedentary young adults. *Journal of physical therapy science*, 27(11), 3359-63. doi: [10.1589/jpts.27.3359]

20. Koepp, G. A., Moore, G. K., & Levine, J. A. (2016). Chair-based fidgeting and energy expenditure. *BMJ open sport & exercise medicine*, 2(1), e000152. doi:10.1136/bmjsem-2016-000152

21. Hartman, S. J., Nelson, S. H., & Weiner, L. S. (2018). Patterns of Fitbit Use and Activity Levels Throughout a Physical Activity Intervention: Exploratory Analysis from a Randomized Controlled Trial. *JMIR mHealth and uHealth*, 6(2), e29. doi:10.2196/mhealth.8503

22. Colberg, Sheri R. et al., Exercise Effects on Postprandial Glycemia, Mood, and Sympathovagal Balance in Type 2 Diabetes. *Journal of the American Medical Directors Association*, 2014 Apr; Volume 15 , Issue 4, 261 - 266 doi: 10.1016/j.jamda.2013.11.026

23. Cocotos, Tom. (2012, May 23) What's Your Golf Mileage? *Golf Digest*. Retrieved November 7, 2018 from https://www.golfdigest.com/story/kaspriske-fitness-column-2009-10

24. Buist I, Bredeweg SW. Higher risk of injury in overweight novice runners. *British Journal of Sports Medicine* 2011;45:338.

25. van Marken Lichtenbelt, Wouter & Kingma, Boris & van der Lans, Anouk & Schellen, Lisje. (2014). Cold exposure – an approach to increasing energy expenditure in humans. *Trends in endocrinology and metabolism: TEM*. 25. doi: 10.1016/j.tem.2014.01.001.

26. Choudhary, Nidhi & Padmalatha, Venkatram & Nagarathna, Raghuram & Ram, Amritanshu. (2012). Effects of a Holistic Yoga Program on Endocrine Parameters in Adolescents with Polycystic Ovarian Syndrome: A Randomized Controlled Trial. *Journal of alternative and complementary medicine* (New York, N.Y.). 19. 10.1089/acm.2011.0868.

27. McPhee, J. S., French, D. P., Jackson, D., Nazroo, J., Pendleton, N., & Degens, H. (2016). Physical activity in older age: perspectives for healthy ageing and frailty. *Biogerontology*, 17(3), 567-80. doi: [10.1007/s10522-016-9641-0]

28. Kim, T. W., Lee, S. H., Choi, K. H., Kim, D. H., & Han, T. K. (2015). Comparison of the effects of acute exercise after overnight fasting and breakfast on energy substrate and hormone levels in obese men. *Journal of physical therapy science*, 27(6), 1929-32. doi: [10.1589/jpts.27.1929]

29. Hanlon B, Larson MJ, Bailey BW, LeCheminant JD. Neural response to pictures of food after exercise in normal-weight and obese women. *Med Sci Sports Exerc*. 2012 Oct;44(10):1864-70. doi: 10.1249/MSS.0b013e31825cade5.

30. Schroeder, A. M., Truong, D. , Loh, D. H., Jordan, M. C., Roos, K. P. and Colwell, C. S. (2012), Voluntary scheduled exercise alters diurnal rhythms of behaviour, physiology and gene expression in wild-type and vasoactive intestinal peptide-deficient mice. *The Journal of Physiology*, 590: 6213-6226. doi:10.1113/jphysiol.2012.233676

31. Eirik. (2016, September 5) Obesity: A Cause or Consequence of Physical Inactivity? *Darwinian Medicine*. Retrieved November 7, 2018 from http://darwinian-medicine.com/obesity-a-cause-or-consequence-of-physical-inactivity/

32. (2003). The effectiveness of personal training on changing attitudes towards physical activity. *Journal of sports science & medicine*, 2(1), 10-4.

33. Rogers, T., Milkman, K. L., John, L. K., & Norton, M. I. (2015). Beyond good intentions: Prompting people to make plans improves follow-through on important tasks. *Behavioral Science & Policy*, 1(2).

34. A. Treiber, Frank & Baranowski, Tom & S. Braden, David & B. Strong, William & Levy, Maurice & Knox, Willie. (1991). Social support for exercise: Relationship to physical activity in young adults. *Preventive medicine*. 20. 737-50. 10.1016/0091-7435(91)90068-F.

35. Vatansever-Ozen, S., Tiryaki-Sonmez, G., Bugdayci, G., & Ozen, G. (2011). The effects of exercise on food intake and hunger: relationship with acylated ghrelin and leptin. *Journal of sports science & medicine*, 10(2), 283-91.

36. Mitchell, J. E., Roerig, J., & Steffen, K. (2013). Biological therapies for eating disorders. *The International journal of eating disorders*, 46(5), 470-7. doi: [10.1002/eat.22104]

37. Zhang, H., Tong, T. K., Qiu, W., Zhang, X., Zhou, S., Liu, Y., & He, Y. (2017). Comparable Effects of High-Intensity Interval Training and Prolonged Continuous Exercise Training on Abdominal Visceral Fat Reduction in Obese Young Women. *Journal of diabetes research*, 2017, 5071740. doi: [10.1155/2017/5071740]

Chapter 9

1. Gill, Steven & Pop, Mihai & T Deboy, Robert & Eckburg, Paul & Turnbaugh, Peter & Samuel, Buck & I Gordon, Jeffrey & Relman, David & M Fraser-Liggett, Claire & E Nelson, Karen. (2006). Metagenomic Analysis of the Human Distal Gut Microbiome. *Science* (New York, N.Y.). 312. 1355-9. 10.1126/science.1124234.

2. Rowland, I., Gibson, G., Heinken, A. et al. *Eur J Nutr* (2018) 57: 1. https://doi.org/10.1007/s00394-017-1445-8

3. H. Zeisel, Steven & Warrier, Manya. (2017). Trimethylamine N -Oxide, the Microbiome, and Heart and Kidney Disease. *Annual Review of Nutrition.* 37. 10.1146/annurev-nutr-071816-064732.

4. (2015). TMAO is both a biomarker and a renal toxin. *Circulation research,* 116(3), 396-7. doi: [10.1161/CIRCRESAHA.114.305680]

5. (2011). Microflora modulation of motility. *Journal of neurogastroenterology and motility,* 17(2), 140-7. doi: [10.5056/jnm.2011.17.2.140]

6. Lee BJ, Bak YT. Irritable Bowel Syndrome, Gut Microbiota and Probiotics. *J Neurogastroenterol Motil* 2011;17:252-266. https://doi.org/10.5056/jnm.2011.17.3.252

7. Mathur, R., Ko, A., Hwang, L.J. et al. *Dig Dis Sci* (2010) 55: 1085. https://doi.org/10.1007/s10620-009-0890-5

8. Distrutti, E., Monaldi, L., Ricci, P., & Fiorucci, S. (2016). Gut microbiota role in irritable bowel syndrome: New therapeutic strategies. *World journal of gastroenterology,* 22(7), 2219-41. doi: [10.3748/wjg.v22.i7.2219]

9. Belkaid, Y., & Hand, T. W. (2014). Role of the microbiota in immunity and inflammation. *Cell,* 157(1), 121-41. doi: [10.1016/j.cell.2014.03.011]

10. Vighi, G., Marcucci, F., Sensi, L., Di Cara, G., & Frati, F. (2008). Allergy and the gastrointestinal system. *Clinical and experimental immunology,* 153 Suppl 1(Suppl 1), 3-6. doi: [10.1111/j.1365-2249.2008.03713.x]

11. Yano, J. M., Yu, K., Donaldson, G. P., Shastri, G. G., Ann, P., Ma, L., Nagler, C. R., Ismagilov, R. F., Mazmanian, S. K., ... Hsiao, E. Y. (2015). Indigenous bacteria from the gut microbiota regulate host serotonin biosynthesis. *Cell,* 161(2), 264-76. doi: [10.1016/j.cell.2015.02.047]

12. Frazer A, Hensler JG. Serotonin Involvement in Physiological Function and Behavior. In: Siegel GJ, Agranoff BW, Albers RW, et al., editors. Basic Neurochemistry: Molecular, Cellular and Medical Aspects. 6th edition. Philadelphia: Lippincott-Raven; 1999. Available from: https://www.ncbi.nlm.nih.gov/books/NBK27940/

13. Evrensel, A., & Ceylan, M. E. (2015). The Gut-Brain Axis: The Missing Link in Depression. *Clinical psychopharmacology and neuroscience : the official scientific journal of the Korean College of Neuropsychopharmacology,* 13(3), 239-44. doi: [10.9758/cpn.2015.13.3.239]

14. Jackson, M. L., Butt, H., Ball, M., Lewis, D. P., & Bruck, D. (2015). Sleep quality and the treatment of intestinal microbiota imbalance in Chronic Fatigue Syndrome: A pilot study. *Sleep science* (Sao Paulo, Brazil), 8(3), 124-33. doi: [10.1016/j.slsci.2015.10.001]

15. Krueger, J. M., & Opp, M. R. (2016). Sleep and Microbes. *International review of neurobiology,* 131, 207-225. doi: [10.1016/bs.irn.2016.07.003]

16. Maryann Kwa, Claudia S. Plottel, Martin J. Blaser, Sylvia Adams; The Intestinal Microbiome and Estrogen Receptor–Positive Female Breast Cancer, JNCI: *Journal of the National Cancer Institute,* Volume 108, Issue 8, 1 August 2016, djw029, https://doi.org/10.1093/jnci/djw029

17. Barbara J. Fuhrman, Heather Spencer Feigelson, Roberto Flores, Mitchell H. Gail, Xia Xu, Jacques Ravel, and James J. Goedert. Associations of the Fecal Microbiome With Urinary Estrogens and Estrogen Metabolites in Postmenopausal Women. *The Journal of Clinical Endocrinology & Metabolism,* 2014 DOI: 10.1210/jc.2014-2222

18. Baker, James M. et al. Estrogen–gut microbiome axis: Physiological and clinical implications, *Maturitas.* 2017, Sept. Volume 103, 45 - 53 DOI: 10.1016/j.maturitas.2017.06.025

19. Guo Y, Qi Y, Yang X, Zhao L, Wen S, Liu Y, et al. (2016) Association between Polycystic Ovary Syndrome and Gut Microbiota. PLoS ONE 11(4): e0153196. https://doi.org/10.1371/journal.pone.0153196

20. Qi, J., You, T., Li, J., Pan, T., Xiang, L., Han, Y., & Zhu, L. (2017). Circulating trimethylamine N-oxide and the risk of cardiovascular diseases: a systematic review and meta-analysis of 11 prospective cohort studies. *Journal of cellular and molecular medicine,* 22(1), 185-194. doi: [10.1111/jcmm.13307]

21. Sawicki, C. M., Livingston, K. A., Obin, M., Roberts, S. B., Chung, M., & McKeown, N. M. (2017). Dietary Fiber and the Human Gut Microbiota: Application of Evidence Mapping Methodology. *Nutrients,* 9(2), 125. doi:10.3390/nu9020125

22. Fields, Helen. (2015, November) The Gut: Where Bacteria and Immune System Meet. *John Hopkins Medicine.* Retrieved November 7, 2018 from https://www.hopkinsmedicine.org/research/advancements-in-research/fundamentals/in-depth/the-gut-where-bacteria-and-immune-system-meet

23. Kwon, Diana. (2018, May 8) Does Parkinson's Begin in the Gut? *Scientific American.* Retrieved November 7, 2018 from https://www.scientificamerican.com/article/does-parkinsons-begin-in-the-gut/

24. Maldarelli, Claire. (2017, August 24) The gut microbes of modern hunter-gatherers reveal one big problem with your diet. *Popular Science.* Retrieved November 7, 2018 from https://www.popsci.com/hunter-gatherer-gut-microbiome-diverse-fiber

25. U.S. Department of Health and Human Services and U.S. Department of Agriculture. 2015 – 2020 Dietary Guidelines for Americans. 8th Edition. December 2015. Available at https://health.gov/dietaryguidelines/2015/guidelines/.

26. Leach, Jeff. (2015, July 10) Paleo versus Vegetarian – who eats more fiber? *Human Food Project.* http://humanfoodproject.com/paleo-versus-vegetarian-who-eats-more-fiber/

27. Chart of high-fiber foods. *Mayo Clinic.* Retrieved November 7, 2018 from https://www.mayoclinic.org/healthy-lifestyle/nutrition-and-healthy-eating/in-depth/high-fiber-foods/art-20050948

28. Bjarnadottir, Adda. (2017, August 1) Everything you need to know about avocado. *Medical News Today.* Retrieved November 7, 2018 from https://www.medicalnewstoday.com/articles/318620.php

29. Chia Seeds. *Harvard T.H. Chan.* Retrieved November 7, 2018 from https://www.hsph.harvard.edu/nutritionsource/food-features/chia-seeds/

30. Winham, D.M., & Hutchins, A.M. (2011). Perceptions of flatulence from bean consumption among adults in 3 feeding studies. *Nutrition journal.* 2011 Nov 21;10:128. doi: 10.1186/1475-2891-10-128.

31. Food Dyes: A Rainbow of Risks. *Center for Science in the Public Interest.* 2010, June 1. Retrieved November 7, 2018 from https://cspinet.org/resource/food-dyes-rainbow-risks

32. Barański, M., Średnicka-Tober, D., Volakakis, N., Seal, C., Sanderson, R., Stewart, G., ... Leifert, C. (2014). Higher antioxidant and lower cadmium concentrations and lower incidence of pesticide residues in organically grown crops: A systematic literature review and meta-analyses. *British Journal of Nutrition*, 112(5), 794-811. doi:10.1017/S0007114514001366

33. Średnicka-Tober, D., Barański, M., Seal, C., Sanderson, R., Benbrook, C., Steinshamn, H., . . . Leifert, C. (2016). Higher PUFA and n-3 PUFA, conjugated linoleic acid, α-tocopherol and iron, but lower iodine and selenium concentrations in organic milk: A systematic literature review and meta- and redundancy analyses. *British Journal of Nutrition*, 115(6), 1043-1060. doi:10.1017/S0007114516000349

34. Velmurugan, G., Ramprasath, T., Swaminathan, K., Mithieux, G., Rajendhran, J., Dhivakar, M., Parthasarathy, A., Babu, D.D., Thumburaj, L.J., Freddy, A.J., Dinakaran, V., Puhari, S.S., Rekha, B., Christy, Y.J., Anusha, S.P., Divya, G., Suganya, K., Meganathan, B., Kalyanaraman, N., Vasudevan, V., Kamaraj, R., Karthik, M., Jeyakumar, B., Abhishek, A., Paul, E.K., Pushpanathan, M., Rajmohan, R.K., Velayutham, K., Lyon, A.R., & Ramasamy, S. (2016). Gut microbial degradation of organophosphate insecticides-induces glucose intolerance via gluconeogenesis. *Genome Biology.*

35. Reygner, J., Joly Condette, C., Bruneau, A., Delanaud, S., Rhazi, L., Depeint, F., Abdennebi-Najar, L., Bach, V., Mayeur, C., ... Khorsi-Cauet, H. (2016). Changes in Composition and Function of Human Intestinal Microbiota Exposed to Chlorpyrifos in Oil as Assessed by the SHIME® Model. *International journal of environmental research and public health*, 13(11), 1088. doi:10.3390/ijerph13111088

36. Myers, J. P., Antoniou, M. N., Blumberg, B., Carroll, L., Colborn, T., Everett, L. G., Hansen, M., Landrigan, P. J., Lanphear, B. P., Mesnage, R., Vandenberg, L. N., Vom Saal, F. S., Welshons, W. V., ... Benbrook, C. M. (2016). Concerns over use of glyphosate-based herbicides and risks associated with exposures: a consensus statement. *Environmental health : a global access science source*, 15, 19. doi:10.1186/s12940-016-0117-0

37. Brookie, K. L., Best, G. I., & Conner, T. S. (2018). Intake of Raw Fruits and Vegetables Is Associated With Better Mental Health Than Intake of Processed Fruits and Vegetables. *Frontiers in psychology*, 9, 487. doi:10.3389/fpsyg.2018.00487

38. Chan, Q., Stamler, J., Brown, I. J., Daviglus, M. L., Van Horn, L., Dyer, A. R., Oude Griep, L. M., Miura, K., Ueshima, H., Zhao, L., Nicholson, J. K., Holmes, E., Elliott, P., INTERMAP Research Group (2013). Relation of raw and cooked vegetable consumption to blood pressure: the INTERMAP Study. *Journal of human hypertension*, 28(6), 353-9. doi: [10.1038/jhh.2013.115]

39. Berg, G., Erlacher, A., Smalla, K., & Krause, R. (2014). Vegetable microbiomes: is there a connection among opportunistic infections, human health and our 'gut feeling'?. *Microbial biotechnology*, 7(6), 487-95. doi: [10.1111/1751-7915.12159]

40. Gibbons, Ann. The Evolution of Diet. *National Geographic Magazine.* Retrieved November 7, 2018 from https://www.nationalgeographic.com/foodfeatures/evolution-of-diet/

41. Lawton, Graham. 2016, November 2. Every human culture includes cooking – this is how it began. *New Scientist.* Retrieved November 7, 2018 from https://www.newscientist.com/article/mg23230980-600-what-was-the-first-cooked-meal/

42. Marco, M.L., Heeney, D.D., Binda, S., Cifelli, C.J., Cotter, P.D., Foligné, B., Gänzle, M.G., Kort, R., Pasin, G., Pihlanto, A., Smid, E.J., & Hutkins, R.W. (2017). Health benefits of fermented foods: microbiota and beyond. *Current opinion in biotechnology*, 44, 94-102.

43. Plotner, Becky. 2014, June 1. Sauerkraut Test Divulges Shocking Probiotic Count. *Nourishing Plot.* Retrieved November 7, 2018 from https://www.nourishingplot.com/2014/06/21/sauerkraut-test-divulges-shocking-probiotic-count/

44. Katrine Hass Rubin, Dorte Glintborg, Mads Nybo, Bo Abrahamsen, Marianne Andersen; Development and Risk Factors of Type 2 Diabetes in a Nationwide Population of Women With Polycystic Ovary Syndrome, *The Journal of Clinical Endocrinology & Metabolism*, Volume 102, Issue 10, 1 October 2017, Pages 3848–3857, https://doi.org/10.1210/jc.2017-01354

45. How Much Is Too Much? *Sugar Science*, a journal from University of California San Francisco. Retrieved November 7, 2018 from http://sugarscience.ucsf.edu/the-growing-concern-of-overconsumption.html

46. Umpleby, A.M., Shojaee-Moradie, F., Fielding, B.A., Li, X., Marino, A., Alsini, N., Isherwood, C.M., Jackson, N.C., Ahmad, A., Stolinski, M., Lovegrove, J.A., Johnsen, S., Mendis, A.S., Wright, J., Wilinska, M.E., Hovorka, R., Bell, J.D., Thomas, E.L., Frost, G.S., & Griffin, B.A. (2017). Impact of liver fat on the differential partitioning of hepatic triacylglycerol into VLDL subclasses on high and low sugar diets. *Clinical science*, 131 21, 2561-2573.

47. Knüppel, A., Shipley, M. J., Llewellyn, C. H., & Brunner, E. J. (2017). Sugar intake from sweet food and beverages, common mental disorder and depression: prospective findings from the Whitehall II study. *Scientific reports*, 7(1), 6287. doi:10.1038/s41598-017-05649-7

48. de la Monte, S. M., & Wands, J. R. (2008). Alzheimer's disease is type 3 diabetes-evidence reviewed. *Journal of diabetes science and technology*, 2(6), 1101-13. doi: [10.1177/193229680800200619]

49. Emilie Friberg, Alice Wallin and Alicja Wolk. Sucrose, High-Sugar Foods, and Risk of Endometrial Cancer—a Population-Based Cohort Study. *Cancer Epidemiology Biomarkers & Prevention*. September 1, 2011 (20) (9) 1831-1837; DOI: 10.1158/1055-9965.EPI-11-0402

50. Ken Peeters, Frederik Van Leemputte, Baptiste Fischer, Beatriz M. Bonini, Hector Quezada, Maksym Tsytlonok, Dorien Haesen, Ward Vanthienen, Nuno Bernardes, Carmen Bravo Gonzalez-Blas, Veerle Janssens, Peter Tompa, Wim Versées, Johan M. Thevelein. Fructose-1,6-bisphosphate couples glycolytic flux to activation of Ras. *Nature Communications*, 2017; 8 (1) DOI: 10.1038/s41467-017-01019-z

51. Jiang, Y., Pan, Y., Rhea, P. R., Tan, L., Gagea, M., Cohen, L., Fischer, S. M., ... Yang, P. (2016). A Sucrose-Enriched Diet Promotes Tumorigenesis in Mammary Gland in Part through the 12-Lipoxygenase Pathway. *Cancer research*, 76(1), 24-9.

52. Gao, Y., Bielohuby, M., Fleming, T., Grabner, G. F., Foppen, E., Bernhard, W., Guzmán-Ruiz, M., Layritz, C., Legutko, B., Zinser, E., García-Cáceres, C., Buijs, R. M., Woods, S. C., Kalsbeek, A., Seeley, R. J., Nawroth, P. P., Bidlingmaier, M., Tschöp, M. H., ... Yi, C. X. (2017). Dietary sugars, not lipids, drive hypothalamic inflammation. *Molecular metabolism*, 6(8), 897-908. doi:10.1016/j.molmet.2017.06.008

53. H. Knopp, Robert & Retzlaff, Barbara & Walden, Carolyn & Fish, Brian & Buck, Brenda & McCann, Barbara. (2000). One-Year Effects of Increasingly Fat-Restricted, Carbohydrate-Enriched Diets on Lipoprotein Levels in Free-Living Subjects. Proceedings of the Society for Experimental Biology and Medicine. *Society for Experimental Biology and Medicine* (New York, N.Y.). 225. 191-9. 10.1046/j.1525-1373.2000.22524.x.

54. Murphy, E. A., Velazquez, K. T., & Herbert, K. M. (2015). Influence of high-fat diet on gut microbiota: a driving force for chronic disease risk. *Current opinion in clinical nutrition and metabolic care*, 18(5), 515-20. doi: [10.1097/MCO.0000000000000209]

55. Teng, K. T., Chang, C. Y., Chang, L. F., & Nesaretnam, K. (2014). Modulation of obesity-induced inflammation by dietary fats: mechanisms and clinical evidence. *Nutrition journal*, 13, 12. doi:10.1186/1475-2891-13-12

56. Turnbaugh, P.J., Ley, R.E., Mahowald, M.A., Magrini, V., Mardis, E.R., & Gordon, J.I. (2006). An obesity-associated gut microbiome with increased capacity for energy harvest. *Nature*, 444, 1027-1031. DOI: 10.1038/nature05414

57. Zhang, C., Zhang, M., Pang, X., Zhao, Y., Wang, L., & Zhao, L. (2012). Structural resilience of the gut microbiota in adult mice under high-fat dietary perturbations. *The ISME Journal*, 6, 1848-1857. DOI: 10.1038/ismej.2012.27

58. Murphy, E. A., Velazquez, K. T., & Herbert, K. M. (2015). Influence of high-fat diet on gut microbiota: a driving force for chronic disease risk. *Current opinion in clinical nutrition and metabolic care*, 18(5), 515-20. doi: [10.1097/MCO.0000000000000209]

59. NIH National Cancer Institute. Top Food Sources of Saturated Fat Among U.S. Population, 2005-2006 NHANES. Retrieved November 7, 2018 from https://epi.grants.cancer.gov/diet/foodsources/sat_fat/sf.html

60. Nguyen, P. K., Lin, S., & Heidenreich, P. (2016). A systematic comparison of sugar content in low-fat vs regular versions of food. *Nutrition & diabetes*, 6(1), e193. doi:10.1038/nutd.2015.43

61. U.S. Food and Drug Administration. Final Determination Regarding Partially Hydrogenated Oils (Removing Trans Fat). Retrieved November 7, 2018 from https://www.fda.gov/food/ingredientspackaginglabeling/foodadditivesingredients/ucm449162.htm

62. Kleinewietfeld, M., Manzel, A., Titze, J., Kvakan, H., Yosef, N., Linker, R. A., Muller, D. N., ... Hafler, D. A. (2013). Sodium chloride drives autoimmune disease by the induction of pathogenic TH17 cells. *Nature*, 496(7446), 518-22. doi: [10.1038/nature11868]

63. M.J. O'Donnell, A. Mente, A. Smyth, S. Yusuf; Salt intake and cardiovascular disease: why are the data inconsistent?, *European Heart Journal*, Volume 34, Issue 14, 7 April 2013, Pages 1034–1040, https://doi.org/10.1093/eurheartj/ehs409

64. American Heart Association. (2017, Feb 12) Processed Foods: Where is all that salt coming from? Retrieved November 7, 2018 from http://www.heart.org/HEARTORG/Conditions/HighBloodPressure/PreventionTreatmentofHighBloodPressure/Where-is-all-that-salt-coming-from_UCM_426950_Article.jsp#.W-TTUHpKgWp

65. University of Rhode Island. (2010, March 25). Pure maple syrup contains medicinally beneficial compounds, pharmacy researcher finds. *ScienceDaily*. Retrieved November 8, 2018 from www.sciencedaily.com/releases/2010/03/100321182924.htm

66. D Schramm, Derek & Karim, Malina & R Schrader, Heather & Holt, Roberta & Cardetti, Marcia & Keen, Carl. (2003). Honey with High Levels of Antioxidants Can Provide Protection to Healthy Human Subjects. *Journal of agricultural and food chemistry.* 51. 1732-5. 10.1021/jf025928k.

67. Schneider, Andrew. (2011, November 7) Tests Show Most Store Honey Isn't Honey. *Food Safety News.* Retrieved November 7, 2018 from https://www.foodsafetynews.com/2011/11/tests-show-most-store-honey-isnt-honey/

68. 2015, July 28. Which oils are best to cook with? *BBC News.* Retrieved November 7, 2018 from https://www.bbc.com/news/magazine-33675975

69. Covas, María-Isabel & Konstantinidou, Valentini & Fitó, Montserrat. (2009). Olive Oil and Cardiovascular Health. *Journal of cardiovascular pharmacology.* 54. 477-82. 10.1097/FJC.0b013e3181c5e7fd.

70. Schwingshackl, L., Lampousi, A. M., Portillo, M. P., Romaguera, D., Hoffmann, G., & Boeing, H. (2017). Olive oil in the prevention and management of type 2 diabetes mellitus: a systematic review and meta-analysis of cohort studies and intervention trials. *Nutrition & diabetes,* 7(4), e262. doi:10.1038/nutd.2017.12

71. Kumarendran, B., O'Reilly, M. W., Manolopoulos, K. N., Toulis, K. A., Gokhale, K. M., Sitch, A. J., Wijeyaratne, C. N., Coomarasamy, A., Arlt, W., ... Nirantharakumar, K. (2018). Polycystic ovary syndrome, androgen excess, and the risk of nonalcoholic fatty liver disease in women: A longitudinal study based on a United Kingdom primary care database. *PLoS medicine,* 15(3), e1002542. doi:10.1371/journal.pmed.1002542

72. Petta S, Ciresi A, Bianco J, Geraci V, Boemi R, Galvano L, et al. Insulin resistance and hyperandrogenism drive steatosis and fibrosis risk in young females with PCOS. *PLoS One.* 2017;12(11): e0186136

73. Noreen Hossain, Maria Stepanova, Arian Afendy, Fatema Nader, Youssef Younossi, Nila Rafiq, Zachary Goodman & Zobair M. Younossi (2011) Non-alcoholic steatohepatitis (NASH) in patients with polycystic ovarian syndrome (PCOS), *Scandinavian Journal of Gastroenterology,* 46:4, 479-484, DOI: 10.3109/00365521.2010.539251

74. Sarkola, Taisto & Fukunaga, T & Mäkisalo, Heikki & Eriksson, Peter. (2000). Acute effect of alcohol on androgens in premenopausal women. *Alcohol and alcoholism* (Oxford, Oxfordshire). 35. 84-90. doi: 10.1093/alcalc/35.1.84.

75. The Overuse of Antibiotics in Food Animals Threatens Public Health. *Consumers Union,* the advocacy division of Consumer Reports. Retrieved November 7, 2018 from https://consumersunion.org/news/the-overuse-of-antibiotics-in-food-animals-threatens-public-health-2/

76. Suez, Jotham & Korem, Tal & Zeevi, David & Zilberman-Schapira, Gili & A Thaiss, Christoph & Maza, Ori & Israeli, David & Zmora, Niv & Gilad, Shlomit & Weinberger, Adina & Kuperman, Yael & Harmelin, Alon & Kolodkin-Gal, Ilana & Shapiro, Hagit & Halpern, Zamir & Segal, Eran & Elinav, Eran. (2014). Artificial Sweeteners Induce Glucose Intolerance by Altering the Gut Microbiota. *Nature.* 70. doi: 10.1038/nature13793.

77. Rajaeieh, G., Marasi, M., Shahshahan, Z., Hassanbeigi, F., & Safavi, S. M. (2014). The Relationship between Intake of Dairy Products and Polycystic Ovary Syndrome in Women Who Referred to Isfahan University of Medical Science Clinics in 2013. *International journal of preventive medicine,* 5(6), 687-94.

78. Adebamowo CA, Spiegelman D, Danby FW, et al. High school dietary dairy intake and teenage acne. *J Am Acad Dermatol.* 2005;52:207–214.

79. (2011). Acne: Diet and acnegenesis. *Indian dermatology online journal,* 2(1), 2-5.

80. W. Cramer, Daniel & Xu, Huijuan & Sahi, Timo. (1994). Adult Hypolactasia, Milk Consumption, and Age-specific Fertility. *American journal of epidemiology.* 139. 282-9. 10.1093/oxfordjournals.aje.a116995.

81. Moyana TN, Lalonde JM. Carrageenan-induced intestinal injury in the rat--a model for inflammatory bowel disease. *Ann Clin Lab Sci.* 1990 Nov-Dec;20(6):420-6.

82. Martino, J. V., Van Limbergen, J., & Cahill, L. E. (2017). The Role of Carrageenan and Carboxymethylcellulose in the Development of Intestinal Inflammation. *Frontiers in pediatrics,* 5, 96. doi:10.3389/fped.2017.00096

83. (2012). Zonulin, regulation of tight junctions, and autoimmune diseases. *Annals of the New York Academy of Sciences,* 1258(1), 25-33. doi: [10.1111/j.1749-6632.2012.06538.x]

84. Hyun-seok Kim, MD, MPH; Kalpesh G. Patel, MD; Evan Orosz, DO; et al. Time Trends in the Prevalence of Celiac Disease and Gluten-Free Diet in the US Population: Results From the National Health and Nutrition Examination Surveys 2009-2014. *JAMA Intern Med.* 2016;176(11):1716-1717. doi:10.1001/jamainternmed.2016.5254

85. Admou, B., Essaadouni, L., Krati, K., Zaher, K., Sbihi, M., Chabaa, L., Belaabidia, B., ... Alaoui-Yazidi, A. (2012). Atypical celiac disease: from recognizing to managing. *Gastroenterology research and practice,* 2012, 637187.

86. Losurdo, Giuseppe & Principi, Mariabeatrice & Iannone, Andrea & Amoruso, Annacinzia & Enzo, Ierardi & Di Leo, Alfredo & Barone, Michele. (2018). Extra-intestinal manifestations of non-celiac gluten sensitivity: An expanding paradigm. *World Journal of Gastroenterology.* 24. 1521-1530. 10.3748/wjg.v24.i14.1521.

87. Raffaella Barbaro, M & Cremon, Cesare & Caio, Giacomo & De Giorgio, Roberto & Volta, Umberto & Stanghellini, Vincenzo & Barbara, Giovanni. (2015). 247 Zonulin Serum Levels Are Increased in Non-Celiac Gluten Sensitivity and Irritable Bowel Syndrome With Diarrhea. *Gastroenterology*. 148. S-56. 10.1016/S0016-5085(15)30192-X.

88. Mobeen, H., Afzal, N., & Kashif, M. (2016). Polycystic Ovary Syndrome May Be an Autoimmune Disorder. *Scientifica*, 2016, 4071735. doi: [10.1155/2016/4071735]

89. Kechagia, M., Basoulis, D., Konstantopoulou, S., Dimitriadi, D., Gyftopoulou, K., Skarmoutsou, N., & Fakiri, E. M. (2013). Health benefits of probiotics: a review. *ISRN nutrition*, 2013, 481651. doi:10.5402/2013/481651

90. Hemarajata, P., & Versalovic, J. (2013). Effects of probiotics on gut microbiota: mechanisms of intestinal immunomodulation and neuromodulation. *Therapeutic advances in gastroenterology*, 6(1), 39-51. doi: [10.1177/1756283X12459294]

91. Glick-Bauer, M., & Yeh, M. C. (2014). The health advantage of a vegan diet: exploring the gut microbiota connection. *Nutrients*, 6(11), 4822-38. doi:10.3390/nu6114822

92. Wu, G. D., Chen, J., Hoffmann, C., Bittinger, K., Chen, Y. Y., Keilbaugh, S. A., Bewtra, M., Knights, D., Walters, W. A., Knight, R., Sinha, R., Gilroy, E., Gupta, K., Baldassano, R., Nessel, L., Li, H., Bushman, F. D., ... Lewis, J. D. (2011). Linking long-term dietary patterns with gut microbial enterotypes. *Science (New York, N.Y.)*, 334(6052), 105-8. doi: [10.1126/science.1208344]

93. Le, L. T., & Sabaté, J. (2014). Beyond meatless, the health effects of vegan diets: findings from the Adventist cohorts. *Nutrients*, 6(6), 2131-47. doi:10.3390/nu6062131

94. (2015). Evidence-Based Approach to Fiber Supplements and Clinically Meaningful Health Benefits, Part 1: What to Look for and How to Recommend an Effective Fiber Therapy. *Nutrition today*, 50(2), 82-89. doi: [10.1097/NT.0000000000000082]

95. (2015). Evidence-Based Approach to Fiber Supplements and Clinically Meaningful Health Benefits, Part 2: What to Look for and How to Recommend an Effective Fiber Therapy. *Nutrition today*, 50(2), 90-97. doi: [10.1097/NT.0000000000000089]

96. Lambeau, K. V., & McRorie, J. W. (2017). Fiber supplements and clinically proven health benefits: How to recognize and recommend an effective fiber therapy. *Journal of the American Association of Nurse Practitioners*, 29(4), 216-223. doi: [10.1002/2327-6924.12447]

97. Alcock, Joe & Maley, Carlo & Aktipis, C. (2014). Is eating behavior manipulated by the gastrointestinal microbiota? Evolutionary pressures and potential mechanisms. *BioEssays*. 36. 10.1002/bies.201400071.

98. Magrone, T., Russo, M. A., & Jirillo, E. (2017). Cocoa and Dark Chocolate Polyphenols: From Biology to Clinical Applications. *Frontiers in immunology*, 8, 677. doi:10.3389/fimmu.2017.00677

99. Sicherer, S.H., & Sampson, H.A. (2018). Food allergy: A review and update on epidemiology, pathogenesis, diagnosis, prevention, and management. *The Journal of allergy and clinical immunology*, 141 1, 41-58. doi: 10.1016/j.jaci.2017.11.003

100. Samadi, Nazanin & Klems, Martina & Untersmayr, Eva. (2018). The role of gastrointestinal permeability in food allergy. *Annals of Allergy, Asthma & Immunology*. 10.1016/j.anai.2018.05.010.

101. Ghose, Tia. (2015, March 15) High-Fiber Diet May Help Prevent Allergies. *Live Science*. Retrieved November 7, 2018 from https://www.livescience.com/50046-fiber-reduce-allergies.html

102. Andrew T. Stefka, Taylor Feehley, Prabhanshu Tripathi, Ju Qiu, Kathy McCoy, Sarkis K. Mazmanian, Melissa Y. Tjota, Goo-Young Seo, Severine Cao, Betty R. Theriault, Dionysios A. Antonopoulos, Liang Zhou, Eugene B. Chang, Yang-Xin Fu, Cathryn R. Nagler. Commensals protect against food allergy. *Proceedings of the National Academy of Sciences*. Sep 2014, 111 (36) 13145-13150; DOI:10.1073/pnas.1412008111

103. Kristian Hallundbæk Mikkelsen, Filip Krag Knop, Morten Frost, Jesper Hallas, Anton Pottegård; Use of Antibiotics and Risk of Type 2 Diabetes: A Population-Based Case-Control Study, *The Journal of Clinical Endocrinology & Metabolism*, Volume 100, Issue 10, 1 October 2015, Pages 3633-3640, https://doi.org/10.1210/jc.2015-2696

104. Francino, M. (2016). Antibiotics and the Human Gut Microbiome: Dysbioses and Accumulation of Resistances. *Frontiers in Microbiology*. 6. 10.3389/fmicb.2015.01543.

105. McFarland LV. Meta-analysis of probiotics for the prevention of antibiotic associated diarrhea and the treatment of Clostridium difficile disease. *Am J Gastroenterol*. 2006;101(4):812-822

106. Rodgers, B., Kirley, K., & Mounsey, A. (2013). PURLs: prescribing an antibiotic? Pair it with probiotics. *The Journal of family practice*, 62(3), 148-50.

107. Trifan, A., Stanciu, C., Girleanu, I., Stoica, O. C., Singeap, A. M., Maxim, R., Chiriac, S. A., Ciobica, A., ... Boiculese, L. (2017). Proton pump inhibitors therapy and risk of Clostridium difficile infection: Systematic review and meta-analysis. *World journal of gastroenterology*, 23(35), 6500-6515. doi: [10.3748/wjg.v23.i35.6500]

108. Minalyan A., Gabrielyan, L., Scott, D. et al. *Curr Gastroenterol Rep* (2017) 19: 42. https://doi.org/10.1007/s11894-017-0577-6

109. Chen, Y., Liu, B., Glass, K., Du, W., Banks, E., & Kirk, M. (2016). Use of Proton Pump Inhibitors and the Risk of Hospitalization for Infectious Gastroenteritis. *PloS one*, 11(12), e0168618. doi:10.1371/journal.pone.0168618

110. (2013). Proton pump inhibitors and risk of vitamin and mineral deficiency: evidence and clinical implications. *Therapeutic advances in drug safety*, 4(3), 125-33. doi: [10.1177/2042098613482484]

111. Sukhovershin, R. A., & Cooke, J. P. (2016). How May Proton Pump Inhibitors Impair Cardiovascular Health?. *American journal of cardiovascular drugs : drugs, devices, and other interventions*, 16(3), 153-61.

112. Cheung KS, Chan EW, Wong AYS, et al. Long-term proton pump inhibitors and risk of gastric cancer development after treatment for Helicobacter pylori: a population-based study. *Gut* 2018;67:28-35.

113. Hu, Q., Sun, T. T., Hong, J., Fang, J. Y., Xiong, H., & Meltzer, S. J. (2017). Proton Pump Inhibitors Do Not Reduce the Risk of Esophageal Adenocarcinoma in Patients with Barrett's Esophagus: A Systematic Review and Meta-Analysis. *PloS one*, 12(1), e0169691. doi:10.1371/journal.pone.0169691

114. Kandil, T. S., Mousa, A. A., El-Gendy, A. A., & Abbas, A. M. (2010). The potential therapeutic effect of melatonin in Gastro-Esophageal Reflux Disease. *BMC gastroenterology*, 10, 7. doi:10.1186/1471-230X-10-7

115. N Diebel, Lawrence & Liberati, David & Hall zimmerman, Lisa. (2011). H2 blockers decrease gut mucus production and lead to barrier dysfunction in vitro. *Surgery*. 150. 736-43. 10.1016/j.surg.2011.07.067.

Chapter 10

1. Dolan, L. C., Matulka, R. A., & Burdock, G. A. (2010). Naturally occurring food toxins. *Toxins*, 2(9), 2289-332. doi: [10.3390/toxins2092289]

2. Weiler, Nicholas. (May 24, 2018) Gut Bacteria Produce a Special Enzyme To Protect Us from Plant Toxins. *UCSF News Center*. Retrieved November 7, 2018 from https://www.ucsf.edu/news/2018/05/410461/gut-bacteria-produce-special-enzyme-protect-us-plant-toxins

3. Scialla, Mark. (2016, June 22) It could take centuries for EPA to test all the unregulated chemicals under a new landmark bill. PBS. Retrieved November 7, 2018 from https://www.pbs.org/newshour/science/it-could-take-centuries-for-epa-to-test-all-the-unregulated-chemicals-under-a-new-landmark-bill

4. Mendonca, K., Hauser, R., Calafat, A. M., Arbuckle, T. E., & Duty, S. M. (2012). Bisphenol A concentrations in maternal breast milk and infant urine. *International archives of occupational and environmental health*, 87(1), 13-20. doi: [10.1007/s00420-012-0834-9]

5. Caserta, D., Di Segni, N., Mallozzi, M., Giovanale, V., Mantovani, A., Marci, R., & Moscarini, M. (2014). Bisphenol A and the female reproductive tract: an overview of recent laboratory evidence and epidemiological studies. *Reproductive biology and endocrinology : RB&E*, 12, 37. doi:10.1186/1477-7827-12-37. doi: [10.1186/1477-7827-12-37]

6. Calafat, A.M., Kuklenyik, Z., Reidy, J.A., Caudill, S.P., Ekong, J., & Needham, L.L. (2005). Urinary Concentrations of Bisphenol A and 4-Nonylphenol in a Human Reference Population. *Environmental health perspectives*.

7. (2009). The politics of plastics: the making and unmaking of bisphenol a "safety". *American journal of public health*, 99 Suppl 3(Suppl 3), S559-66. doi: [10.2105/AJPH.2008.159228]

8. Corrales, J., Kristofco, L. A., Steele, W. B., Yates, B. S., Breed, C. S., Williams, E. S., & Brooks, B. W. (2015). Global Assessment of Bisphenol A in the Environment: Review and Analysis of Its Occurrence and Bioaccumulation. *Dose-response : a publication of International Hormesis Society*, 13(3), 1559325815598308. doi:10.1177/1559325815598308

9. Hewlett, M., Chow, E., Aschengrau, A., & Mahalingaiah, S. (2017). Prenatal Exposure to Endocrine Disruptors: A Developmental Etiology for Polycystic Ovary Syndrome. *Reproductive Sciences*, 24(1), 19-27. https://doi.org/10.1177/1933719116654992

10. Kwon, E. J., & Kim, Y. J. (2017). What is fetal programming?: a lifetime health is under the control of in utero health. *Obstetrics & gynecology science*, 60(6), 506-519.

11. Rutkowska, Aleksandra & Rachoń, Dominik. (2014). Bisphenol A (BPA) and its potential role in the pathogenesis of the polycystic ovary syndrome (PCOS). *Gynecological endocrinology : the official journal of the International Society of Gynecological Endocrinology*. 30. doi: 10.3109/09513590.2013.871517.

12. Klenke, U., & Hutchins, B. I. (2011). Using bisphenol-a to study the onset of polycystic ovarian syndrome. *Frontiers in endocrinology*, 2, 12. doi:10.3389/fendo.2011.00012

13. Rashidi, B.H., Amanlou, M., Lak, T.B., Ghazizadeh, M., Haghollahi, F., Bagheri, M., & Eslami, B. (2017). The Association Between Bisphenol A and Polycystic Ovarian Syndrome: A Case-Control Study. *Acta medica Iranica*, 55 12, 759-764 .

14. Kandaraki, Eleni & Chatzigeorgiou, Antonios & Livadas, Sarantis & Palioura, Eleni & Economou, Frangiscos & Koutsilieris, Michael & Palimeri, Sotiria & Panidis, Dimitrios & Diamanti-Kandarakis, Evanthia. (2010). Endocrine Disruptors and Polycystic Ovary Syndrome (PCOS): Elevated Serum Levels of Bisphenol A in Women with PCOS. *The Journal of clinical endocrinology and metabolism*. 96. E480-4. 10.1210/jc.2010-1658.

15. Do, M. T., Chang, V. C., Mendez, M. A., & de Groh, M. (2017). Urinary bisphenol A and obesity in adults: results from the Canadian Health Measures SurveyConcentration urinaire de bisphénol A et obésité chez les adultes : résultats de l'Enquête canadienne sur les mesures de la santé. *Health promotion and chronic disease prevention in Canada : research, policy and practice*, 37(12), 403-412. doi: [10.24095/hpcdp.37.12.02]

16. G Boucher, Jonathan & Boudreau, Adèle & Ahmed, Shaimaa & Atlas, Ella. (2015). In Vitro Effects of Bisphenol A ɑ-D-Glucuronide (BPA-G) on Adipogenesis in Human and Murine Preadipocytes. *Environmental health perspectives*. 123. doi: 10.1289/ehp.1409143.

17. (2017) ENDO 2017 Breaking News: Early-Life BPA Exposure Reprograms Gene Expression Linked to Fatty Liver Disease. *Endocrine News*. Retrieved November 7, 2018 from https://endocrinenews. endocrine.org/endo-2017-breaking-news-early-life-bpa-exposure-reprograms-gene-expression-linked-fatty-liver-disease/

18. Dallio M, Masarone M, Errico S, et al. Role of bisphenol A as environmental factor in the promotion of non-alcoholic fatty liver disease: in vitro and clinical study. *Aliment Pharmacol Ther*. 2018;47:826-837. https://doi.org/10.1111/apt.14499

19. Verstraete, S. G., Wojcicki, J. M., Perito, E. R., & Rosenthal, P. (2018). Bisphenol a increases risk for presumed non-alcoholic fatty liver disease in Hispanic adolescents in NHANES 2003-2010. *Environmental health : a global access science source*, 17(1), 12. doi:10.1186/s12940-018-0356-3

20. Lai, Keng Po & Chung, Yan-Tung & Li, Rong & Wan, Hin-Ting & Kong-Chu Wong, Chris. (2016). Bisphenol A alters gut microbiome: Comparative metagenomics analysis. *Environmental pollution* (Barking, Essex : 1987). 218. doi: 10.1016/j.envpol.2016.08.039.

21. Lavanya Reddivari, D. N. Rao Veeramachaneni, William A. Walters, Catherine Lozupone, Jennifer Palmer, M. K. Kurundu Hewage, Rohil Bhatnagar, Amnon Amir, Mary J. Kennett, Rob Knight, Jairam K. P. Vanamala. Perinatal Bisphenol A Exposure Induces Chronic Inflammation in Rabbit Offspring via Modulation of Gut Bacteria and Their Metabolites. *mSystems*, 2017; 2 (5): e00093-17 DOI: 10.1128/mSystems.00093-17

22. Salehi, Ashkan and Belsham, Denise. (2017, April 1) The Effect of the Endocrine Disrupting Chemical Bisphenol A on Pro-opiomelanocortin, Circadian Rhythm and Neuroinflammatory Marker Gene Expression in Hypothalamic Cell Models. *Physiology*.

23. Qiaoyun Yang, Yue Zhao, Xinghua Qiu, Chunmei Zhang, Rong Li, Jie Qiao; Association of serum levels of typical organic pollutants with polycystic ovary syndrome (PCOS): a case–control study, *Human Reproduction*, Volume 30, Issue 8, 1 August 2015, Pages 1964–1973, https://doi.org/10.1093/humrep/dev123

24. Vagi, Sara J. et al. "Exploring the potential association between brominated diphenyl ethers, polychlorinated biphenyls, organochlorine pesticides, perfluorinated compounds, phthalates, and bisphenol a in polycystic ovary syndrome: a case–control study." BMC *endocrine disorders* (2014).

25. Hewlett, M., Chow, E., Aschengrau, A., and Mahalingaiah, S. Prenatal exposure to endocrine disruptors: a developmental etiology for polycystic ovary syndrome. *Boston University Theses & Dissertations* [4932] Available from: https://open.bu.edu/handle/2144/16018

26. Michele Tordjman, K. Grinshpan, L., Novack, L., Segev, D., Stern, N., Goen, T., and Berman, T. (2015) Endocrine Disruptors Burden in Vegetarians/Vegans Is Characterized By a Lower Exposure to Phthalates. *Endocrine Society*. Available from: http://press.endocrine.org/doi/abs/10.1210/endo-meetings.2015.ED.1.FRI-291

27. Serrano, S. E., Braun, J., Trasande, L., Dills, R., & Sathyanarayana, S. (2014). Phthalates and diet: a review of the food monitoring and epidemiology data. *Environmental health : a global access science source*, 13(1), 43. doi:10.1186/1476-069X-13-43

28. Karami, Ali & Golieskardi, Abolfazl & Ho, Yu Bin & Larat, Vincent & Salamatinia, Babak. (2017). Microplastics in eviscerated flesh and excised organs of dried fish. *Scientific Reports*. 7. 10.1038/s41598-017-05828-6.

29. Julia R. Varshavsky, Rachel Morello-Frosch, Tracey J. Woodruff, Ami R. Zota. Dietary sources of cumulative phthalates exposure among the U.S. general population in NHANES 2005–2014, *Environment International*, Volume 115, 2018, Pages 417-429, https://doi.org/10.1016/j. envint.2018.02.029.

30. Monaco, Kristen. (2018, February 13) Nonstick Chemicals May Disrupt Metabolic Function in Women. *MedPage Today*. Retrieved November 7, 2018 from https://www.medpagetoday. com/publichealthpolicy/environmentalhealth/71128?xid=nl_mpt_DHE_2018-02-14&eun=g407528d0r&pos=0

31. Hartle, Jennifer & Navas-Acien, Ana & Lawrence, Robert. (2016). The consumption of canned food and beverages and urinary Bisphenol A concentrations in NHANES 2003-2008. *Environmental Research*. 150. 375-382. doi: 10.1016/j.envres.2016.06.008.

32. Bae, S., & Hong, Y.C. (2015). Exposure to bisphenol A from drinking canned beverages increases blood pressure: randomized crossover trial. *Hypertension*, 65 2, 313-9. DOI: 10.1161/HYPERTENSIONAHA.114.04261

33. Jennifer C. Hartle, Ana Navas-Acien, Robert S. Lawrence, The consumption of canned food and beverages and urinary Bisphenol A concentrations in NHANES 2003-2008, *Environmental Research*, Volume 150, 2016, Pages 375-382, https://doi.org/10.1016/j.envres.2016.06.008.

34. Sasada T, Hinoi T, Saito Y, Adachi T, Takakura Y, Kawaguchi Y, et al. (2015) Chlorinated Water Modulates the Development of Colorectal Tumors with Chromosomal Instability and Gut Microbiota in Apc-Deficient Mice. PLoS ONE 10(7): e0132435. https://doi.org/10.1371/journal.pone.0132435

35. Majd, Sanaz (2015, October 21) Should You Drink Tap or Bottled Water? *Scientific American.* Retrieved from: https://www.scientificamerican.com/article/should-you-drink-tap-or-bottled-water/

36. Blake, Mariah. (2014, April) The Scary New Evidence on BPA-Free Plastics. *Mother Jones.* Retrieved from: https://www.motherjones.com/environment/2014/03/tritan-certichem-eastman-bpa-free-plastic-safe/

37. Klepeis, N.E., Nelson, W.C., Ott, W.R., Robinson, J.P., Tsang, A., Switzer, P., Behar, J.V., Hern, S.C., & Engelmann, W.H. (2001). The National Human Activity Pattern Survey (NHAPS): a resource for assessing exposure to environmental pollutants. *Journal of Exposure Analysis and Environmental Epidemiology*, 11, 231-252.

38. (2008). The sick building syndrome. *Indian journal of occupational and environmental medicine*, 12(2), 61-4. doi: [10.4103/0019-5278.43262]

39. Apte, K., & Salvi, S. (2016). Household air pollution and its effects on health. F1000Research, 5, F1000 Faculty Rev-2593. doi:10.12688/f1000research.7552.1

40. Rudel, R. A., & Perovich, L. J. (2009). Endocrine disrupting chemicals in indoor and outdoor air. *Atmospheric environment (Oxford, England : 1994)*, 43(1), 170-181. doi: [10.1016/j.atmosenv.2008.09.025]

41. (2018). Overview of air pollution and endocrine disorders. *International journal of general medicine*, 11, 191-207. doi:10.2147/IJGM.S102230

42. Vijayan, V. K., Paramesh, H., Salvi, S. S., & Dalal, A. A. (2015). Enhancing indoor air quality -The air filter advantage. *Lung India : official organ of Indian Chest Society*, 32(5), 473-9. doi: [10.4103/0970-2113.164174]

43. Vijayan, V. K., Paramesh, H., Salvi, S. S., & Dalal, A. A. (2015). Enhancing indoor air quality -The air filter advantage. *Lung India : official organ of Indian Chest Society*, 32(5), 473-9. doi: [10.4103/0970-2113.164174]

44. Singla, Veena. (2016, September 13) Toxic Dust: The Dangerous Chemical Brew in Every Home. *National Resource Defense Council.* Available from: https://www.nrdc.org/experts/veena-singla/toxic-dust-dangerous-chemical-brew-every-home

45. Marcia G. Nishioka,*, Hazel M. Burkholder, and, Marielle C. Brinkman, and Robert G. Lewis. Distribution of 2,4-Dichlorophenoxyacetic Acid in Floor Dust throughout Homes Following Homeowner and Commercial Lawn Applications: Quantitative Effects of Children, Pets, and Shoes. *Environmental Science & Technology.* 1999 33 (9), 1359-1365. DOI: 10.1021/es980580o

46. Layton et al. Migration of Contaminated Soil and Airborne Particulates to Indoor Dust. *Environmental Science & Technology*, 2009; 090924111235017 DOI: 10.1021/es9003735

47. Bassil, K. L., Vakil, C., Sanborn, M., Cole, D. C., Kaur, J. S., & Kerr, K. J. (2007). Cancer health effects of pesticides: systematic review. *Canadian family physician Medecin de famille canadien*, 53(10), 1704-11.

48. Exposures add up – Survey results, *Environmental Working Group.* Retrieved November 7, 2018 from https://www.ewg.org/skindeep/2004/06/15/exposures-add-up-survey-results/#.W2NtW9hKjVo

49. La Merrill, M., Emond, C., Kim, M. J., Antignac, J. P., Le Bizec, B., Clément, K., Birnbaum, L. S., ... Barouki, R. (2012). Toxicological function of adipose tissue: focus on persistent organic pollutants. *Environmental health perspectives*, 121(2), 162-9. doi: [10.1289/ehp.1205485]

50. S Lim, J & Son, H-K & Park, S-K & R Jacobs, D & Lee, Duk-Hee. (2011). Inverse associations between long-term weight change and serum concentrations of persistent organic pollutants. *International journal of obesity* (2005). 35. 744-7. 10.1038/ijo.2010.188.

51. Lim, J.S., Son, H., Park, S., Jacobs, D.R., & Lee, D. (2011). Inverse associations between long-term weight change and serum concentrations of persistent organic pollutants. *International Journal of Obesity*, 35, 744-747.

Chapter 11

1. Abels, C. , Kaszuba, A. , Michalak, I. , Werdier, D. , Knie, U. and Kaszuba, A. (2011), A 10% glycolic acid containing oil-in-water emulsion improves mild acne: a randomized double-blind placebo-controlled trial. *Journal of Cosmetic Dermatology*, 10: 202-209. doi:10.1111/j.1473-2165.2011.00572.x

2. Wohlrab J, Kreft D: Niacinamide - Mechanisms of Action and Its Topical Use in Dermatology. *Skin Pharmacol Physiol* 2014;27:311-315. doi: 10.1159/000359974

3. Carson, C. F., Hammer, K. A., & Riley, T. V. (2006). Melaleuca alternifolia (Tea Tree) oil: a review of antimicrobial and other medicinal properties. *Clinical microbiology reviews*, 19(1), 50-62. doi: [10.1128/CMR.19.1.50-62.2006]

4.   Enshaieh S et al: "The efficacy of 5% topical tea tree oil gel in mild to moderate acne vulgaris: a randomized, double-blind placebo-controlled study." *Indian journal of dermatology, venereology and leprology*, vol. 73, no. 1, 2007 Jan-Feb, pp. 22-5.

5.   B Bassett, I & L Pannowitz, D & C. Barnetson, R.St. (1990). A comparative study of tea-tree oil versus benzoylperoxide in the treatment of acne. *The Medical journal of Australia*. 153. 455-8.

6.   M. Rahmati Roudsari, R. Karimi, S. Sohrabvandi & A. M. Mortazavian (2015) Health Effects of Probiotics on the Skin, *Critical Reviews in Food Science and Nutrition*, 55:9, 1219-1240, DOI: 10.1080/10408398.2012.680078

7.   Grant, P. (2010), Spearmint herbal tea has significant anti-androgen effects in polycystic ovarian syndrome. a randomized controlled trial. *Phytother. Res.*, 24: 186-188. doi:10.1002/ptr.2900

8.   Rostami Mogaddam, M., Safavi Ardabili, N., Maleki, N., & Soflaee, M. (2014). Correlation between the severity and type of acne lesions with serum zinc levels in patients with acne vulgaris. *BioMed research international*, 2014, 474108. doi: [10.1155/2014/474108]

9.   El-akawi, Z. , Abdel-Latif, N. and Abdul-Razzak, K. (2006), Does the plasma level of vitamins A and E affect acne condition?. *Clinical and Experimental Dermatology*, 31: 430-434. doi:10.1111/j.1365-2230.2006.02106.x

10.   Pei, S., Inamadar, A. C., Adya, K. A., & Tsoukas, M. M. (2015). Light-based therapies in acne treatment. *Indian dermatology online journal*, 6(3), 145-57. doi: [10.4103/2229-5178.156379]

11.   Michael H. Gold, Whitney Sensing & Julie A. Biron (2011) Clinical efficacy of home-use blue-light therapy for mild-to moderate acne, *Journal of Cosmetic and Laser Therapy*, 13:6, 308-314, DOI: 10.3109/14764172.2011.630081

12.   Aslihan Cakir, Gul & Gulru Erdogan, Fatma & Gurler, Aysel. (2013). Isotretinoin treatment in nodulocystic acne with and without polycystic ovary syndrome: Efficacy and determinants of relapse. *International Journal of Dermatology*. 52. doi: 10.1111/j.1365-4632.2012.05691.x.

13.   Torzecka, J. D., Dziankowska-Bartkowiak, B., Gerlicz-Kowalczuk, Z., & Wozniacka, A. (2017). The use of isotretinoin in low doses and unconventional treatment regimens in different types of acne: a literature review. *Postepy dermatologii i alergologii*, 34(1), 1-5. doi: [10.5114/ada.2017.65614]

14.   Charny, J. W., Choi, J. K., & James, W. D. (2017). Spironolactone for the treatment of acne in women, a retrospective study of 110 patients. *International journal of women's dermatology*, 3(2), 111-115. doi:10.1016/j.ijwd.2016.12.002

15.   Mazza, Angela & Fruci, Barbara & Guzzi, Pietro & D'Orrico, B & Malaguarnera, Roberta & Veltri, Pierangelo & Fava, A & Belfiore, Antonino. (2013). In PCOS patients the addition of low-dose spironolactone induces a more marked reduction of clinical and biochemical hyperandrogenism than metformin alone. *Nutrition, metabolism, and cardiovascular diseases : NMCD*. 24. 10.1016/j.numecd.2013.04.016.

16.   Avci, P., Gupta, G. K., Clark, J., Wikonkal, N., & Hamblin, M. R. (2013). Low-level laser (light) therapy (LLLT) for treatment of hair loss. *Lasers in surgery and medicine*, 46(2), 144-51. doi: [10.1002/lsm.22170]

17.   van Zuuren EJ, Fedorowicz Z, Carter B, Andriolo RB, Schoones J. Interventions for female pattern hair loss. *Cochrane Database of Systematic Reviews* 2012, Issue 5. Art. No.: CD007628. DOI: 10.1002/14651858.CD007628.pub3.

18.   Gogtay, J. A., & Panda, M. (2009). Minoxidil topical foam: a new kid on the block. *International journal of trichology*, 1(2), 142. doi: [10.4103/0974-7753.58560]

19.   Jamilian, M., Foroozanfard, F., Bahmani, F. et al. Effects of Zinc Supplementation on Endocrine Outcomes in Women with Polycystic Ovary Syndrome: a Randomized, Double-Blind, Placebo-Controlled Trial. *Biol Trace Elem Res* (2016) 170: 271. https://doi.org/10.1007/s12011-015-0480-7

20.   El Taieb MA, Ibrahim H, Nada EA, and Seif Al-Din M. Platelets rich plasma versus minoxidil 5% in treatment of alopecia areata: A trichoscopic evaluation. *Dermatologic Therapy*. 2017;30:e12437. doi: 10.1111/dth.12437.

21.   Garg, S., & Manchanda, S. (2017). Platelet-rich plasma-an 'Elixir' for treatment of alopecia: personal experience on 117 patients with review of literature. *Stem cell investigation*, 4, 64. doi:10.21037/sci.2017.06.07

22.   Levy, L. L., & Emer, J. J. (2013). Female pattern alopecia: current perspectives. *International journal of women's health*, 5, 541-56. doi:10.2147/IJWH.S49337

23.   Hoedemaker, C. , Van Egmond, S. and Sinclair, R. (2007), Treatment of female pattern hair loss with a combination of spironolactone and minoxidil. *Australasian Journal of Dermatology*, 48: 43-45. doi:10.1111/j.1440-0960.2007.00332.x

24.   In Young Choi, Laura Piccio, Patra Childress, Bryan Bollman, Arko Ghosh, Sebastian Brandhorst, Jorge Suarez, Andreas Michalsen, Anne H. Cross, Todd E. Morgan, Min Wei, Friedemann Paul, Markus Bock, Valter D. Longo. A Diet Mimicking Fasting Promotes Regeneration and Reduces Autoimmunity and Multiple Sclerosis Symptoms, *Cell Reports*, Volume 15, Issue 10, 2016, Pages 2136-2146 https://doi.org/10.1016/j.celrep.2016.05.009.

25.   Choi, I. Y., Lee, C., & Longo, V. D. (2017). Nutrition and fasting mimicking diets in the prevention and treatment of autoimmune diseases and immunosenescence. *Molecular and cellular endocrinology*, 455, 4-12. doi: [10.1016/j.mce.2017.01.042]

26. Mu, Q., Kirby, J., Reilly, C. M., & Luo, X. M. (2017). Leaky Gut As a Danger Signal for Autoimmune Diseases. *Frontiers in immunology*, 8, 598. doi:10.3389/fimmu.2017.00598

27. En-De Hu, Da-Zhi Chen, Jin-Lu Wu, Feng-Bin Lu, Lu Chen, Ming-Hua Zheng, Hui Li, Yu Huang, Ji Li, Xiao-Ya Jin, Yue-Wen Gong, Zhuo Lin, Xiao-Dong Wang, Lan-Man Xu, Yong-Ping Chen. High fiber dietary and sodium butyrate attenuate experimental autoimmune hepatitis through regulation of immune regulatory cells and intestinal barrier, *Cellular Immunology*, Volume 328, 2018, Pages 24-32, https://doi.org/10.1016/j.cellimm.2018.03.003.

28. (2014). A Potential Link between Environmental Triggers and Autoimmunity. *Autoimmune diseases*, 2014, 437231. doi: [10.1155/2014/437231]

29. Kleinewietfeld, Markus & Manzel, Arndt & Titze, Jens & Kvakan, Heda & Yosef, Nir & A Linker, Ralf & N Muller, Dominik & Hafler, David. (2013). Sodium Chloride Drives Autoimmune Disease by the Induction of Pathogenic Th17 Cells. *Nature*. 496. 10.1038/nature11868.

30. Shoda, H., Yanai, R., Yoshimura, T., Nagai, T., Kimura, K., Sobrin, L., Connor, K. M., Sakoda, Y., Tamada, K., Ikeda, T., ... Sonoda, K. H. (2015). Dietary Omega-3 Fatty Acids Suppress Experimental Autoimmune Uveitis in Association with Inhibition of Th1 and Th17 Cell Function. *PloS one*, 10(9), e0138241. doi:10.1371/journal.pone.0138241

31. Melissa A. Bates, Christina Brandenberger, Ingeborg I. Langohr, Kazuyoshi Kumagai, Adam L. Lock, Jack R. Harkema, Andrij Holian, James J. Pestka. Silica-Triggered Autoimmunity in Lupus-Prone Mice Blocked by Docosahexaenoic Acid Consumption. PLOS ONE, 2016; 11 (8): e0160622 DOI: 10.1371/journal.pone.0160622

32. Törmä, Hans et al. Skin Barrier Disruption by Sodium Lauryl Sulfate-Exposure Alters the Expressions of Involucrin, Transglutaminase 1, Profilaggrin, and Kallikreins during the Repair Phase in Human Skin In Vivo, *Journal of Investigative Dermatology*, Volume 128, Issue 5, 1212 - 1219. DOI:10.1038/sj.jid.5701170

33. Younger, J., Parkitny, L., & McLain, D. (2014). The use of low-dose naltrexone (LDN) as a novel anti-inflammatory treatment for chronic pain. *Clinical rheumatology*, 33(4), 451-9. doi: [10.1007/s10067-014-2517-2]

34. Zijian Li, Yue You, Noreen Griffin, Juan Feng, Fengping Shan, Low-dose naltrexone (LDN): A promising treatment in immune-related diseases and cancer therapy, *International Immunopharmacology*, Volume 61, 2018, Pages 178-184, https://doi.org/10.1016/j.intimp.2018.05.020.

35. Miriyala S., Panchatcharam M., Rengarajulu P. (2007) CARDIOPROTECTIVE EFFECTS OF CURCUMIN. In: Aggarwal B.B., Surh Y.J., Shishodia S. (eds) The Molecular Targets and Therapeutic Uses of Curcumin in Health and Disease. ADVANCES IN EXPERIMENTAL MEDICINE AND BIOLOGY, vol 595. Springer, Boston, MA. DOI: https://doi.org/10.1007/978-0-387-46401-5_16

36. Ware, Megan. (2017, 20 December) Why do we need magnesium? *Medical News Today*. Available from: https://www.medicalnewstoday.com/articles/286839.php

37. DiNicolantonio JJ, O'Keefe JH, Wilson W Subclinical magnesium deficiency: a principal driver of cardiovascular disease and a public health crisis. *Open Heart* 2018;5:e000668. doi: 10.1136/openhrt-2017-000668

38. Gareth Willis, Rosie Hocking, Maneesh Udiawar, Aled Rees, Philip James. Oxidative stress and nitric oxide in polycystic ovary syndrome, *Nitric Oxide*, Volume 27, Supplement, 2012, Page S28, https://doi.org/10.1016/j.niox.2012.04.101.

39. Kapil, V., Haydar, S. M., Pearl, V., Lundberg, J. O., Weitzberg, E., & Ahluwalia, A. (2013). Physiological role for nitrate-reducing oral bacteria in blood pressure control. *Free radical biology & medicine*, 55, 93-100. doi: [10.1016/j.freeradbiomed.2012.11.013]

40. Sukhovershin, R. A., & Cooke, J. P. (2016). How May Proton Pump Inhibitors Impair Cardiovascular Health?. *American journal of cardiovascular drugs : drugs, devices, and other interventions*, 16(3), 153-61. doi: [10.1007/s40256-016-0160-9]

41. Burkman R, Schlesselman JJ, Zieman M. Safety concerns and health benefits associated with oral contraception. *American Journal of Obstetrics and Gynecology* 2004; 190(4 Suppl):S5–22.

42. Bassuk SS, Manson JE. Oral contraceptives and menopausal hormone therapy: relative and attributable risks of cardiovascular disease, cancer, and other health outcomes. *Annals of Epidemiology* 2015; 25(3):193-200

43. Charlotte Wessel Skovlund, Lina Steinrud Mørch, Lars Vedel Kessing, Theis Lange, and Øjvind Lidegaard, Association of Hormonal Contraception With Suicide Attempts and Suicides. *American Journal of Psychiatry* 2018 175:4, 336-342

44. Bonnema, Rachel & Mcnamara, Megan & L Spencer, Abby. (2010). Contraception Choices in Women with Underlying Medical Conditions. *American family physician*. 82. 621-8.

45. Steven T. Bird, Abraham G. Hartzema, James M. Brophy, Mahyar Etminan, Joseph A.C. Delaney. Risk of venous thromboembolism in women with polycystic ovary syndrome: a population-based matched cohort analysis. *Canadian Medical Association Journal*, 2012; DOI: 10.1503/cmaj.120677

46. ParaGard (copper IUD), *Mayo Clinic*. Retrieved November 7, 2018 from https://www.mayoclinic.org/tests-procedures/paragard/about/pac-20391270

47. Achilles, S. L., Austin, M. N., Meyn, L. A., Mhlanga, F., Chirenje, Z. M., & Hillier, S. L. (2018). Impact of contraceptive initiation on vaginal microbiota. *American journal of obstetrics and gynecology*, 218(6), 622.e1-622.e10. doi: [10.1016/j.ajog.2018.02.017]

48. Allsworth, J. E., & Peipert, J. F. (2011). Severity of bacterial vaginosis and the risk of sexually transmitted infection. *American journal of obstetrics and gynecology*, 205(2), 113.e1-6.

49. Sarathi, V., Kolly, A., Chaithanya, H. B., & Dwarakanath, C. S. (2017). High rates of diabetes reversal in newly diagnosed Asian Indian young adults with type 2 diabetes mellitus with intensive lifestyle therapy. *Journal of natural science, biology, and medicine*, 8(1), 60-63. doi: [10.4103/0976-9668.198343]

50. Jiarong Lan, Yanyun Zhao, Feixia Dong, Ziyou Yan, Wenjie Zheng, Jinping Fan, Guoli Sun. Meta-analysis of the effect and safety of berberine in the treatment of type 2 diabetes mellitus, hyperlipemia and hypertension, *Journal of Ethnopharmacology*, Volume 161, 2015, Pages 69-81, https://doi.org/10.1016/j.jep.2014.09.049.

51. Yifei Zhang, Xiaoying Li, Dajin Zou, Wei Liu, Jialin Yang, Na Zhu, Li Huo, Miao Wang, Jie Hong, Peihong Wu, Guoguang Ren, Guang Ning; Treatment of Type 2 Diabetes and Dyslipidemia with the Natural Plant Alkaloid Berberine, *The Journal of Clinical Endocrinology & Metabolism*, Volume 93, Issue 7, 1 July 2008, Pages 2559-2565, https://doi.org/10.1210/jc.2007-2404

52. The Endocrine Society. (2018, March 18). High-energy breakfast promotes weight loss: Diet helps reduce total daily insulin dose for type 2 diabetes. *ScienceDaily*. Retrieved November 9, 2018 from www.sciencedaily.com/releases/2018/03/180318144831.htm

53. (2016). The concept of low glycemic index and glycemic load foods as panacea for type 2 diabetes mellitus; prospects, challenges and solutions. *African health sciences*, 16(2), 468-79. doi: [10.4314/ahs.v16i2.15]

54. Hang Sun, Xingchun Wang, Jiaqi Chen, et al., "Melatonin Treatment Improves Insulin Resistance and Pigmentation in Obese Patients with Acanthosis Nigricans," *International Journal of Endocrinology*, vol. 2018, Article ID 2304746, 7 pages, 2018. https://doi.org/10.1155/2018/2304746.

55. Pintaudi, B., Di Vieste, G., & Bonomo, M. (2016). The Effectiveness of Myo-Inositol and D-Chiro Inositol Treatment in Type 2 Diabetes. *International journal of endocrinology*, 2016, 9132052. doi: [10.1155/2016/9132052]

56. Kaumudi J. Joshipura, Francisco J. Muñoz-Torres, Evangelia Morou-Bermudez, Rakesh P. Patel. Over-the-counter mouthwash use and risk of pre-diabetes/diabetes, *Nitric Oxide*, Volume 71, 2017, Pages 14-20, https://doi.org/10.1016/j.niox.2017.09.004.

57. Arnason, T. G., Bowen, M. W., & Mansell, K. D. (2017). Effects of intermittent fasting on health markers in those with type 2 diabetes: A pilot study. *World journal of diabetes*, 8(4), 154-164. doi: [10.4239/wjd.v8.i4.154]

58. Noon, M. J., Khawaja, H. A., Ishtiaq, O., Khawaja, Q., Minhas, S., Niazi, A. K., Minhas, A., ... Malhi, U. R. (2016). Fasting with diabetes: a prospective observational study. *BMJ global health*, 1(2), e000009. doi:10.1136/bmjgh-2015-000009

59. (2011). Long-acting glucagon-like peptide 1 receptor agonists: a review of their efficacy and tolerability. *Diabetes care*, 34 Suppl 2(Suppl 2), S279-84. doi: [10.2337/dc11-s231]

60. Cappelli, C., Rotondi, M., Pirola, I., Agosti, B., Gandossi, E., Valentini, U., De Martino, E., Cimino, A., Chiovato, L., Agabiti-Rosei, E., ... Castellano, M. (2009). TSH-lowering effect of metformin in type 2 diabetic patients: differences between euthyroid, untreated hypothyroid, and euthyroid on L-T4 therapy patients. *Diabetes care*, 32(9), 1589-90. doi: [10.2337/dc09-0273]

61. R Aroda, Vanita & L Edelstein, Sharon & B Goldberg, Ronald & C Knowler, William & M Marcovina, Santica & J Orchard, Trevor & A Bray, George & S Schade, David & Temprosa, Marinella & H White, Neil & Crandall, Jill. (2016). Long-term Metformin Use and Vitamin B12 Deficiency in the Diabetes Prevention Program Outcomes Study. *The Journal of Clinical Endocrinology & Metabolism*. 101. jc.2015-3754. 10.1210/jc.2015-3754.

62. Kellesarian, S.V., Malignaggi, V.R., Kellesarian, T.V., Al-Kheraif, A.A., Alwageet, M.M., Malmstrom, H., Romanos, G.E., & Javed, F. (2017). Association between periodontal disease and polycystic ovary syndrome: a systematic review. *International Journal of Impotence Research*, 29, 89-95.

63. Shulman, Jay & Wells, Linda. (1997). Acute ethanol toxicity from ingesting mouthwash in children younger than 6-years of age. *Pediatric dentistry*. 19. 404-8.

64. Agarwal, Pooja et al. Comparative evaluation of efficacy of 0.2% Chlorhexidine, Listerine and Tulsi extract mouth rinses on salivary Streptococcus mutans count of high school children—RCT, *Contemporary Clinical Trials*, Volume 32, Issue 6, 802 - 808. DOI: 10.1016/j.cct.2011.06.007

65. Hosamane, M., Acharya, A. B., Vij, C., Trivedi, D., Setty, S. B., & Thakur, S. L. (2014). Evaluation of holy basil mouthwash as an adjunctive plaque control agent in a four day plaque regrowth model. *Journal of clinical and experimental dentistry*, 6(5), e491-6. doi:10.4317/jced.51479

66. Nayak, P. A., Nayak, U. A., & Khandelwal, V. (2014). The effect of xylitol on dental caries and oral flora. *Clinical, cosmetic and investigational dentistry*, 6, 89-94. doi:10.2147/CCIDE.S55761

67. Salminen, Seppo & Salminen, E & Koivistoinen, P & Bridges, J & Marks, Vincent. (1985). Gut microflora interactions with xylitol in the mouse, rat and man. *Food and chemical toxicology : an international journal published for the British Industrial Biological Research Association*. 23. 985-90. 10.1016/0278-6915(85)90248-0.

68. Chen, Chunqiu & Tao, Chunhua & Liu, Zhongchen & Lu, Meiling & Pan, Qiuhui & Zheng, Lijun & Li, Qing & Song, Zhenshun & Fichna, Jakub. (2015). A Randomized Clinical Trial of Berberine Hydrochloride in Patients with Diarrhea-Predominant Irritable Bowel Syndrome. *Phytotherapy Research*. 29. n/a-n/a. DOI: 10.1002/ptr.5475.

69. (2015). Evidence-Based Approach to Fiber Supplements and Clinically Meaningful Health Benefits, Part 2: What to Look for and How to Recommend an Effective Fiber Therapy. *Nutrition today*, 50(2), 90-97. doi: [10.1097/NT.0000000000000089]

70. Portincasa, P., Bonfrate, L., de Bari, O., Lembo, A., & Ballou, S. (2017). Irritable bowel syndrome and diet. *Gastroenterology report*, 5(1), 11-19. doi: [10.1093/gastro/gow047]

71. Siah, K. T., Wong, R. K., & Ho, K. Y. (2014). Melatonin for the treatment of irritable bowel syndrome. *World journal of gastroenterology*, 20(10), 2492-8. doi: [10.3748/wjg.v20.i10.2492]

72. Tarasiuk, A., Mosińska, P., & Fichna, J. (2018). Triphala: current applications and new perspectives on the treatment of functional gastrointestinal disorders. *Chinese medicine*, 13, 39. doi:10.1186/s13020-018-0197-6

73. Rogers, G. B., Keating, D. J., Young, R. L., Wong, M. L., Licinio, J., & Wesselingh, S. (2016). From gut dysbiosis to altered brain function and mental illness: mechanisms and pathways. *Molecular psychiatry*, 21(6), 738-48. doi: [10.1038/mp.2016.50]

74. Yueshan Hu, Erik A. Ehli, Julie Kittelsrud, Patrick J. Ronan, Karen Munger, Terry Downey, Krista Bohlen, Leah Callahan, Vicki Munson, Mike Jahnke, Lindsey L. Marshall, Kelly Nelson, Patricia Huizenga, Ryan Hansen, Timothy J. Soundy, Gareth E. Davies. Lipid-lowering effect of berberine in human subjects and rats, *Phytomedicine*, Volume 19, Issue 10, 2012, Pages 861-867, https://doi.org/10.1016/j.phymed.2012.05.009.

75. Li, Yan & Kuang, Hongying & Shen, Wenjuan & Ma, Hongli & Zhang, Yuehui & Stener-Victorin, Elisabet & Hung, Ernest & Ng, Yu & Liu, Jianping & Kuang, Haixue & Hou, Lihui & Wu, Xiao-Ke. (2013). Letrozole, berberine, or their combination for anovulatory infertility in women with polycystic ovary syndrome: Study design of a doubleblind randomised controlled trial. BMJ open. 3. e003934. DOI: 10.1136/bmjopen-2013-003934.

76. An, Y. , Sun, Z. , Zhang, Y. , Liu, B. , Guan, Y. and Lu, M. (2014), The use of berberine for women with polycystic ovary syndrome undergoing IVF treatment. *Clin Endocrinol*, 80: 425-431. doi:10.1111/cen.12294

77. Chan E: Displacement of Bilirubin from Albumin by Berberine. *Neonatology* 1993;63:201-208. doi: 10.1159/000243932

78. Hallman, Mikko & Bry, Kristina & Hoppu, Kalle & Lappi, Marjatta & Pohjavuori, Maija. (1992). Inositol Supplementation in Premature Infants with Respiratory Distress Syndrome. *The New England journal of medicine*. 326. 1233-9. 10.1056/NEJM199205073261901.

79. Regidor, P. A., & Schindler, A. E. (2016). Myoinositol as a Safe and Alternative Approach in the Treatment of Infertile PCOS Women: A German Observational Study. *International journal of endocrinology*, 2016, 9537632.

80. Kuşcu, N., Bizzarri, M., & Bevilacqua, A. (2016). Myo-Inositol Safety in Pregnancy: From Preimplantation Development to Newborn Animals. *International journal of endocrinology*, 2016, 2413857.

81. ANGIK, Riju et al. A comparative study of metabolic and hormonal effects of myoinositol vs. metformin in women with polycystic ovary syndrome: a randomised controlled trial. *International Journal of Reproduction, Contraception, Obstetrics and Gynecology*, [S.l.], v. 4, n. 1, p. 189-194, feb. 2017. Available at: <http://www.ijrcog.org/index.php/ijrcog/article/view/1838>. Date accessed: 09 nov. 2018.

82. R. D'Anna, V. Di Benedetto, P. Rizzo, E. Raffone, M. L. Interdonato, F. Corrado & A. Di Benedetto(2012) Myo-inositol may prevent gestational diabetes in PCOS women, *Gynecological Endocrinology*, 28:6, 440-442, DOI: 10.3109/09513590.2011.633665

83. Alessandro Pacchiarotti, Gianfranco Carlomagno, Gabriele Antonini & Arianna Pacchiarotti (2016)Effect of myo-inositol and melatonin versus myo-inositol, in a randomized controlled trial, for improving in vitro fertilization of patients with polycystic ovarian syndrome, *Gynecological Endocrinology*, 32:1, 69-73, DOI: 10.3109/09513590.2015.1101444

84. Fulghesu, Anna & Ciampelli, Mario & Muzj, Giuseppe & Belosi, Chiara & Selvaggi, Luigi & Franco Ayala, Gian & Lanzone, Antonio. (2002). N-acetyl-cysteine treatment improves insulin sensitivity in women with polycystic ovary syndrome. *Fertility and sterility*. 77. 1128-35. 10.1016/S0015-0282(02)03133-3.

85. Cheraghi, E., Soleimani Mehranjani, M., Shariatzadeh, M. A., Nasr Esfahani, M. H., & Ebrahimi, Z. (2014). Co-Administration of Metformin and N-Acetyl Cysteine Fails to Improve Clinical Manifestations in PCOS Individual Undergoing ICSI. *International journal of fertility & sterility*, 8(2), 119-28.

86. Yamamoto, M., Feigenbaum, S. L., Crites, Y., Escobar, G. J., Yang, J., Ferrara, A., & Lo, J. C. (2012). Risk of preterm delivery in non-diabetic women with polycystic ovarian syndrome. *Journal of perinatology : official journal of the California Perinatal Association*, 32(10), 770-6.

87. Ahmed Y. Shahin, Ibrahim M.A. Hassanin, Alaa M. Ismail, Jan S. Kruessel, Jens Hirchenhain. Effect of oral N-acetyl cysteine on recurrent preterm labor following treatment for bacterial vaginosis, *International Journal of Gynecology & Obstetrics*, Volume 104, Issue 1, 2009, Pages 44-48, https://doi.org/10.1016/j.ijgo.2008.08.026.

88. Jorge E. Chavarro, Lidia Mínguez-Alarcón, Yu-Han Chiu, Audrey J. Gaskins, Irene Souter, Paige L. Williams, Antonia M. Calafat, Russ Hauser. Soy Intake Modifies the Relation Between Urinary Bisphenol A Concentrations and Pregnancy Outcomes Among Women Undergoing Assisted Reproduction. *The Journal of Clinical Endocrinology & Metabolism*, 2016; jc.2015-3473 DOI: 10.1210/jc.2015-3473

89. Shaum, K. M., & Polotsky, A. J. (2013). Nutrition and reproduction: is there evidence to support a "Fertility Diet" to improve mitochondrial function?. *Maturitas*, 74(4), 309-12. doi: [10.1016/j.maturitas.2013.01.011]

90. Verma, A., & Shrimali, L. (2012). Maternal body mass index and pregnancy outcome. Journal of clinical and diagnostic research : JCDR, 6(9), 1531-3.

91. Redman, L. M., Elkind-Hirsch, K., & Ravussin, E. (2011). Aerobic exercise in women with polycystic ovary syndrome improves ovarian morphology independent of changes in body composition. *Fertility and sterility*, 95(8), 2696-9. doi: [10.1016/j.fertnstert.2011.01.137]

92. Kumar, P., Nawani, N., Malhotra, N., Malhotra, J., Patil, M., Jayakrishnan, K., Kar, S., Jirge, P. R., ... Mahajan, N. (2013). Assisted reproduction in polycystic ovarian disease: A multicentric trial in India. *Journal of human reproductive sciences*, 6(1), 49-53. doi: [10.4103/0974-1208.112382]

93. Legro, Richard & G Brzyski, Robert & Diamond, Michael & Coutifaris, Christos & Schlaff, William & Casson, Peter & M Christman, Gregory & Huang, Hao & Yan, Qingshang & Alvero, Ruben & Haisenleder, Daniel & T Barnhart, Kurt & Bates, Gordon & Usadi, Rebecca & Lucidi, Scott & Baker, Valerie & Trussell, J.C. & A Krawetz, Stephen & Snyder, Peter & Zhang, Heping. (2014). Letrozole Versus Clomiphene for Infertility in the Polycystic Ovary Syndrome. *The New England journal of medicine*. 371. 119-129. 10.1056/NEJMoa1313517.

94. Chakraborty, P., Goswami, S. K., Rajani, S., Sharma, S., Kabir, S. N., Chakravarty, B., & Jana, K. (2013). Recurrent pregnancy loss in polycystic ovary syndrome: role of hyperhomocysteinemia and insulin resistance. *PloS one*, 8(5), e64446. doi:10.1371/journal.pone.0064446

95. Hashim, H.A. (2017). Management of Women with Clomifene Citrate Resistant Polycystic Ovary Syndrome – An Evidence Based Approach.

96. Seyedoshohadaei, F., Zandvakily, F., & Shahgeibi, S. (2012). Comparison of the effectiveness of clomiphene citrate, tamoxifen and letrozole in ovulation induction in infertility due to isolated unovulation. *Iranian journal of reproductive medicine*, 10(6), 531-6.

97. Legro, Richard & Barnhart, Huiman & Schlaff, William & R Carr, Bruce & Diamond, Michael & A Carson, Sandra & P Steinkampf, Michael & Coutifaris, Christos & G McGovern, Peter & Cataldo, Nicholas & G Gosman, Gabriella & E Nestler, John & Giudice, Linda & Leppert, Phyllis & Myers, Evan. (2007). Clomiphene, Metformin, or Both for Infertility in the Polycystic Ovary Syndrome. *The New England journal of medicine*. 356. 551-66. 10.1056/NEJMoa063971.

98. JOHNSON, N. (2011), Metformin is a reasonable first-line treatment option for non-obese women with infertility related to anovulatory polycystic ovary syndrome – A meta-analysis of randomised trials. *Australian and New Zealand Journal of Obstetrics and Gynaecology*, 51: 125-129. doi:10.1111/j.1479-828X.2010.01274.x

99. (2014). Metformin use in women with polycystic ovary syndrome. *Annals of translational medicine*, 2(6), 56. doi: [10.3978/j.issn.2305-5839.2014.04.15]

100. Nicholas J. Niemuth, Rebecca D. Klaper. Emerging wastewater contaminant metformin causes intersex and reduced fecundity in fish. *Chemosphere*, 2015; 135: 38 DOI: 10.1016/j.chemosphere.2015.03.060

101. Liv Guro Engen Hanem, Solhild Stridsklev, Pétur B Júlíusson, Øyvind Salvesen, Mathieu Roelants, Sven M Carlsen, Rønnaug Ødegård, Eszter Vanky; Metformin Use in PCOS Pregnancies Increases the Risk of Offspring Overweight at 4 Years of Age: Follow-Up of Two RCTs, *The Journal of Clinical Endocrinology & Metabolism*, Volume 103, Issue 4, 1 April 2018, Pages 1612–1621, https://doi.org/10.1210/jc.2017-02419

102. Rasmussen, C. B., & Lindenberg, S. (2014). The effect of liraglutide on weight loss in women with polycystic ovary syndrome: an observational study. *Frontiers in endocrinology*, 5, 140. doi:10.3389/fendo.2014.00140

103. Mehta, A., Marso, S. P., & Neeland, I. J. (2016). Liraglutide for weight management: a critical review of the evidence. *Obesity science & practice*, 3(1), 3-14. doi: [10.1002/osp4.84]

104. Skovlund CW, Mørch LS, Kessing LV, Lidegaard Ø. Association of Hormonal Contraception With Depression. JAMA Psychiatry. 2016;73(11):1154–1162. doi:10.1001/jamapsychiatry.2016.2387

105. Chasan-Taber, Lisa & Willett, Walter & E. Manson, JoAnn & Spiegelman, Donna & J. Hunter, David & Curhan, Gary & Colditz, Graham & J. Stampfer, Meir. (1996). Prospective Study of Oral Contraceptives and Hypertension Among Women in the United States. *Circulation*. 94. 483-9. 10.1161/01.CIR.94.3.483.

106. Kaminski, Pawel & Szpotanska-Sikorska, Monika & Wielgos, Miroslaw. (2013). Cardiovascular risk and the use of oral contraceptives. *Neuro endocrinology letters*. 34. 587-9.

107. Daniel A. Dumesic, Rogerio A. Lobo. Cancer risk and PCOS, *Steroids*, Volume 78, Issue 8, 2013, Pages 782-785, https://doi.org/10.1016/j.steroids.2013.04.004.

108. C Bishop, Suzette & Basch, Samuel & Futterweit, Walter. (2009). Polycystic Ovary Syndrome, Depression, and Affective Disorders. *Endocrine practice : official journal of the American College of Endocrinology and the American Association of Clinical Endocrinologists*. 15. 475-82. DOI: 10.4158/EP09083.RAR.

109. Månsson, Mattias et al. Women with polycystic ovary syndrome are often depressed or anxious—A case control study. *Psychoneuroendocrinology* , Volume 33 , Issue 8 , 1132 - 1138

110. Blay, S. L., Aguiar, J. V., & Passos, I. C. (2016). Polycystic ovary syndrome and mental disorders: a systematic review and exploratory meta-analysis. *Neuropsychiatric disease and treatment*, 12, 2895-2903. doi:10.2147/NDT.S91700

111. Dokras A, Clifton S, Futterweit W, Wild R. Increased prevalence of anxiety symptoms in women with polycystic ovary syndrome: systematic review and meta-analysis. *Fertil Steril*. 2012 Jan;97(1):225-30. e2. doi: 10.1016/j.fertnstert.2011.10.022.

112. Paganini, C., Peterson, G.M., Stavropoulos, V., & Krug, I. (2018). The Overlap Between Binge Eating Behaviors and Polycystic Ovarian Syndrome: An Etiological Integrative Model. *Current pharmaceutical design*, 24 9, 999-1006.

113. Lee, Iris et al. Increased risk of disordered eating in polycystic ovary syndrome *Fertility and Sterility*, Volume 107, Issue 3, 796 - 802. DOI: 10.1016/j.fertnstert.2016.12.014

114. Baker, J. H., Girdler, S. S., & Bulik, C. M. (2012). The role of reproductive hormones in the development and maintenance of eating disorders. *Expert review of obstetrics & gynecology*, 7(6), 573-583. doi: [10.1586/eog.12.54]

115. Blay, S. L., Aguiar, J. V., & Passos, I. C. (2016). Polycystic ovary syndrome and mental disorders: a systematic review and exploratory meta-analysis. *Neuropsychiatric disease and treatment*, 12, 2895-2903. doi:10.2147/NDT.S91700

116. (2010). Pathophysiology of depression: do we have any solid evidence of interest to clinicians?. *World psychiatry : official journal of the World Psychiatric Association (WPA)*, 9(3), 155-61.

117. Chaudhari, N., Dawalbhakta, M., & Nampoothiri, L. (2018). GnRH dysregulation in polycystic ovarian syndrome (PCOS) is a manifestation of an altered neurotransmitter profile. *Reproductive biology and endocrinology : RB&E*, 16(1), 37. doi:10.1186/s12958-018-0354-x

118. Grieve, S. M., Korgaonkar, M. S., Koslow, S. H., Gordon, E., & Williams, L. M. (2013). Widespread reductions in gray matter volume in depression. *NeuroImage. Clinical*, 3, 332-9. doi:10.1016/j.nicl.2013.08.016

119. Basak Ozgen Saydam, Arzu Ceylan Has, Gurkan Bozdag, Kader Karli Oguz & Bulent Okan Yildiz(2017) Structural imaging of the brain reveals decreased total brain and total gray matter volumes in obese but not in lean women with polycystic ovary syndrome compared to body mass index-matched counterparts, *Gynecological Endocrinology*, 33:7, 519-523, DOI: 10.1080/09513590.2017.1295440

120. Hu, M., Richard, J. E., Maliqueo, M., Kokosar, M., Fornes, R., Benrick, A., Jansson, T., Ohlsson, C., Wu, X., Skibicka, K. P., ... Stener-Victorin, E. (2015). Maternal testosterone exposure increases anxiety-like behavior and impacts the limbic system in the offspring. *Proceedings of the National Academy of Sciences of the United States of America*, 112(46), 14348-53.

121. Chandrasekhar, K., Kapoor, J., & Anishetty, S. (2012). A prospective, randomized double-blind, placebo-controlled study of safety and efficacy of a high-concentration full-spectrum extract of ashwagandha root in reducing stress and anxiety in adults. *Indian journal of psychological medicine*, 34(3), 255-62. doi: [10.4103/0253-7176.106022]

122. Lam RW, Levitt AJ, Levitan RD, et al. Efficacy of Bright Light Treatment, Fluoxetine, and the Combination in Patients With Nonseasonal Major Depressive DisorderA Randomized Clinical Trial. *JAMA Psychiatry*. 2016;73(1):56–63. doi:10.1001/jamapsychiatry.2015.2235

123. Victor Blüml, Michael D. Regier, Gerald Hlavin, Ian R.H. Rockett, Franz König, Benjamin Vyssoki, Tom Bschor, Nestor D. Kapusta. Lithium in the public water supply and suicide mortality in Texas, *Journal of Psychiatric Research*, Volume 47, Issue 3, 2013, Pages 407-411, https://doi.org/10.1016/j.jpsychires.2012.12.002.

124. Sugawara, N.; Yasui-Furukori, N.; Ishii, N.; Iwata, N.; Terao, T. Lithium in Tap Water and Suicide Mortality in Japan. *Int. J. Environ. Res. Public Health* 2013, 10, 6044-6048.

125. Tammi R.A. Kral, Brianna S. Schuyler, Jeanette A. Mumford, Melissa A. Rosenkranz, Antoine Lutz, Richard J. Davidson. Impact of short- and long-term mindfulness meditation training on amygdala reactivity to emotional stimuli, *NeuroImage*, Volume 181, 2018, Pages 301-313, https://doi.org/10.1016/j.neuroimage.2018.07.013.

126. Mei-Kei Leung, Way K.W. Lau, Chetwyn C.H. Chan, Samuel S.Y. Wong, Annis L.C. Fung & Tatia M.C. Lee (2018) Meditation-induced neuroplastic changes in amygdala activity during negative affective processing, *Social Neuroscience*, 13:3, 277-288, DOI: 10.1080/17470919.2017.1311939

127. Qin, S., Young, C. B., Duan, X., Chen, T., Supekar, K., & Menon, V. (2013). Amygdala subregional structure and intrinsic functional connectivity predicts individual differences in anxiety during early childhood. *Biological psychiatry*, 75(11), 892-900. doi: [10.1016/j.biopsych.2013.10.006]

128.   Gotink, R.A., Vernooij, M.W., Ikram, M.A. et al. Meditation and yoga practice are associated with smaller right amygdala volume: the Rotterdam study, *Brain Imaging and Behavior* (2018). https://doi.org/10.1007/s11682-018-9826-z

129.   Hölzel, B. K., Carmody, J., Vangel, M., Congleton, C., Yerramsetti, S. M., Gard, T., & Lazar, S. W. (2010). Mindfulness practice leads to increases in regional brain gray matter density. *Psychiatry research*, 191(1), 36-43. doi: [10.1016/j.pscychresns.2010.08.006]

130.   Aboulafia Brakha, Tatiana et al. Cognitive-behavioural group therapy improves a psychophysiological marker of stress in caregivers of patients with Alzheimer's disease. In: *Aging & Mental Health*, 2014, vol. 18, n° 6, p. 801-8. https://archive-ouverte.unige.ch/unige:39270

131.   Baker, J. H., Girdler, S. S., & Bulik, C. M. (2012). The role of reproductive hormones in the development and maintenance of eating disorders. *Expert review of obstetrics & gynecology*, 7(6), 573-583. doi: [10.1586/eog.12.54]

132.   Naessén, S. et al. Effects of an antiandrogenic oral contraceptive on appetite and eating behavior in bulimic women. *Psychoneuroendocrinology*, Volume 32 , Issue 5 , 548 - 554

133.   Kamalanathan, S., Sahoo, J. P., & Sathyapalan, T. (2013). Pregnancy in polycystic ovary syndrome. *Indian journal of endocrinology and metabolism*, 17(1), 37-43. doi: [10.4103/2230-8210.107830]

134.   Stefano Palomba, Marlieke A. de Wilde, Angela Falbo, Maria P.H. Koster, Giovanni Battista La Sala, Bart C.J.M. Fauser; Pregnancy complications in women with polycystic ovary syndrome, *Human Reproduction Update*, Volume 21, Issue 5, 1 September 2015, Pages 575–592, https://doi.org/10.1093/humupd/dmv029

135.   Said, A. S., & Manji, K. P. (2016). Risk factors and outcomes of fetal macrosomia in a tertiary centre in Tanzania: a case-control study. *BMC pregnancy and childbirth*, 16(1), 243. doi:10.1186/s12884-016-1044-3. doi: [10.1186/s12884-016-1044-3]

136.   de Vries, Marjolein J et al., Higher risk of preeclampsia in the polycystic ovary syndrome. *European Journal of Obstetrics and Gynecology and Reproductive Biology*, Volume 76 , Issue 1, 91 - 95

137.   Roos, N., Kieler, H., Sahlin, L., Ekman-Ordeberg, G., Falconer, H., & Stephansson, O. (2011). Risk of adverse pregnancy outcomes in women with polycystic ovary syndrome: population based cohort study. *BMJ (Clinical research ed.)*, 343, d6309. doi:10.1136/bmj.d6309

138.   Kamalanathan, S., Sahoo, J. P., & Sathyapalan, T. (2013). Pregnancy in polycystic ovary syndrome. *Indian journal of endocrinology and metabolism*, 17(1), 37-43. doi: [10.4103/2230-8210.107830]

139.   Nas K, Tűű L. A comparative study between myo-inositol and metformin in the treatment of insulin-resistant women. *Eur Rev Med Pharmacol Sci*. 2017 Jun;21(2 Suppl):77-82.

140.   R. D'Anna, V. Di Benedetto, P. Rizzo, E. Raffone, M. L. Interdonato, F. Corrado & A. Di Benedetto(2012) Myo-inositol may prevent gestational diabetes in PCOS women, *Gynecological Endocrinology*,28:6, 440-442, DOI: 10.3109/09513590.2011.633665

141.   El Safoury, O., Rashid, L., & Ibrahim, M. (2010). A study of androgen and estrogen receptors alpha, beta in skin tags. *Indian journal of dermatology*, 55(1), 20-4. doi: [10.4103/0019-5154.60345]

142.   Zangeneh, F. Z., Jafarabadi, M., Naghizadeh, M. M., Abedinia, N., & Haghollahi, F. (2012). Psychological distress in women with polycystic ovary syndrome from imam khomeini hospital, tehran. *Journal of reproduction & infertility*, 13(2), 111-5.

143.   Patel, A., Sharma, P. S., Narayan, P., Binu, V. S., Dinesh, N., & Pai, P. J. (2016). Prevalence and predictors of infertility-specific stress in women diagnosed with primary infertility: A clinic-based study. *Journal of human reproductive sciences*, 9(1), 28-34. doi: [10.4103/0974-1208.178630]

144.   Tiago S. Pavão, Priscila Vianna, Micheli M. Pillat, Amanda B. Machado, Moisés E. Bauer. Acupuncture is effective to attenuate stress and stimulate lymphocyte proliferation in the elderly, *Neuroscience Letters*, Volume 484, Issue 1, 2010, Pages 47-50, https://doi.org/10.1016/j.neulet.2010.08.016.

145.   Case, L. K., Jackson, P., Kinkel, R., & Mills, P. J. (2018). Guided Imagery Improves Mood, Fatigue, and Quality of Life in Individuals With Multiple Sclerosis: An Exploratory Efficacy Trial of Healing Light Guided Imagery. *Journal of evidence-based integrative medicine*, 23, 2515690X17748744.

146.   Jallo, N., Ruiz, R. J., Elswick, R. K., & French, E. (2014). Guided imagery for stress and symptom management in pregnant african american women. *Evidence-based complementary and alternative medicine : eCAM*, 2014, 840923.

147.   Lee, M. H., Kim, D. H., & Yu, H. S. (2013). The effect of guided imagery on stress and fatigue in patients with thyroid cancer undergoing radioactive iodine therapy. *Evidence-based complementary and alternative medicine : eCAM*, 2013, 130324.

148.   Campeau, Marie-Pierre & Gaboriault, Réal & Drapeau, Martine & Nguyen, Thu Van & Roy, Indranath & Fortin, Bernard & Marois, Mariette & Nguyen-Tan, P. (2007). Impact of Massage Therapy on Anxiety Levels in Patients Undergoing Radiation Therapy: Randomized Controlled Trial. *Journal of the Society for Integrative Oncology*. 5. 133-8. 10.2310/7200.2007.018.

149.   Sherman, K. J., Ludman, E. J., Cook, A. J., Hawkes, R. J., Roy-Byrne, P. P., Bentley, S. , Brooks, M. Z. and Cherkin, D. C. (2010). Effectiveness of therapeutic massage for generalized anxiety disorder: a randomized controlled trial. *Depress. Anxiety*, 27: 441-450. doi:10.1002/da.20671

150.   Sherman, K. J., Ludman, E. J., Cook, A. J., Hawkes, R. J., Roy-Byrne, P. P., Bentley, S., Brooks, M. Z., ... Cherkin, D. C. (2010). Effectiveness of therapeutic massage for generalized anxiety disorder: a randomized controlled trial. *Depression and anxiety*, 27(5), 441-50.

151.   Slavin, Joanne L. Dietary fiber and body weight, *Nutrition*, Volume 21, Issue 3, 411 - 418.

152. Martin O Weickert, Andreas FH Pfeiffer; Impact of Dietary Fiber Consumption on Insulin Resistance and the Prevention of Type 2 Diabetes, *The Journal of Nutrition*, Volume 148, Issue 1, 1 January 2018, Pages 7–12, https://doi.org/10.1093/jn/nxx008

153. Courcoulas, A. P., Yanovski, S. Z., Bonds, D., Eggerman, T. L., Horlick, M., Staten, M. A., & Arterburn, D. E. (2014). Long-term outcomes of bariatric surgery: a National Institutes of Health symposium. *JAMA surgery*, 149(12), 1323-9. doi: [10.1001/jamasurg.2014.2440]

Chapter 12

1. Gardner, B., Lally, P., & Wardle, J. (2012). Making health habitual: the psychology of 'habit-formation' and general practice. *The British journal of general practice : the journal of the Royal College of General Practitioners*, 62(605), 664-6. doi: [10.3399/bjgp12X659466]

2. Gardner, B., Lally, P., & Wardle, J. (2012). Making health habitual: the psychology of 'habit-formation' and general practice. *The British journal of general practice : the journal of the Royal College of General Practitioners*, 62(605), 664-6. doi: [10.3399/bjgp12X659466]

3. Mrazek Michael D., Mooneyham Benjamin W., Mrazek Kaita L., Schooler Jonathan W. Pushing the Limits: Cognitive, Affective, and Neural Plasticity Revealed by an Intensive Multifaceted Intervention, *Frontiers in Human Neuroscience*. Volume 10 (2016) Page 117, DOI: 10.3389/fnhum.2016.00117

4. Corrine K. Welt, Enrico Carmina; Lifecycle of Polycystic Ovary Syndrome (PCOS): From In Utero to Menopause, *The Journal of Clinical Endocrinology & Metabolism*, Volume 98, Issue 12, 1 December 2013, Pages 4629–4638, https://doi.org/10.1210/jc.2013-2375

5. Corrine K. Welt, Enrico Carmina; Lifecycle of Polycystic Ovary Syndrome (PCOS): From In Utero to Menopause, *The Journal of Clinical Endocrinology & Metabolism*, Volume 98, Issue 12, 1 December 2013, Pages 4629–4638, https://doi.org/10.1210/jc.2013-2375

6. Li, J. et al. The pregnancy outcomes of pcos patients at advanced age under in vitro fertilization in China, *Fertility and Sterility*, Volume 108, Issue 3, e250.

7. Kalra, Suleena Kansal et al. Is the fertile window extended in women with polycystic ovary syndrome? Utilizing the Society for Assisted Reproductive Technology registry to assess the impact of reproductive aging on live-birth rate *Fertility and Sterility*, Volume 100, Issue 1, 208 - 213.

8. Stassek, J., Ohnolz, F., Hanusch, Y., Schmidmayr, M., Berg, D., Kiechle, M., & Seifert-Klauss, V. R. (2015). Do Pregnancy and Parenthood Affect the Course of PCO Syndrome? Initial Results from the LIPCOS Study (Lifestyle Intervention for Patients with Polycystic Ovary Syndrome [PCOS]). *Geburtshilfe und Frauenheilkunde*, 75(11), 1153-1160. doi: [10.1055/s-0035-1558186]

9. Ribero, Simone et al. Acne and Telomere Length: A New Spectrum between Senescence and Apoptosis Pathways, *Journal of Investigative Dermatology*, Volume 137, Issue 2, 513 - 515.

10. Corrine K. Welt, Enrico Carmina; Lifecycle of Polycystic Ovary Syndrome (PCOS): From In Utero to Menopause, *The Journal of Clinical Endocrinology & Metabolism*, Volume 98, Issue 12, 1 December 2013, Pages 4629–4638, https://doi.org/10.1210/jc.2013-2375

11. Akın, L. , Kendirci, M. , Narin, F. , Kurtoglu, S. , Saraymen, R. , Kondolot, M. , Koçak, S. and Elmalı, F. (2015), The endocrine disruptor bisphenol A may play a role in the aetiopathogenesis of polycystic ovary syndrome in adolescent girls. Acta Paediatr, 104: e171-e177. doi:10.1111/apa.12885

12. Birch, L., Savage, J. S., & Ventura, A. (2007). Influences on the Development of Children's Eating Behaviours: From Infancy to Adolescence. *Canadian journal of dietetic practice and research : a publication of Dietitians of Canada = Revue canadienne de la pratique et de la recherche en dietetique : une publication des Dietetistes du Canada*, 68(1), s1-s56.

13. Prescott, S. L., Larcombe, D. L., Logan, A. C., West, C., Burks, W., Caraballo, L., Levin, M., Etten, E. V., Horwitz, P., Kozyrskyj, A., ... Campbell, D. E. (2017). The skin microbiome: impact of modern environments on skin ecology, barrier integrity, and systemic immune programming. *The World Allergy Organization journal*, 10(1), 29. doi:10.1186/s40413-017-0160-5

14. Jhun, I., & Phipatanakul, W. (2016). Early exposure to dogs and farm animals reduces risk of childhood asthma. *Evidence-based medicine*, 21(2), 80. doi: [10.1136/ebmed-2015-110373]

15. Prescott, S. L., Larcombe, D. L., Logan, A. C., West, C., Burks, W., Caraballo, L., Levin, M., Etten, E. V., Horwitz, P., Kozyrskyj, A., ... Campbell, D. E. (2017). The skin microbiome: impact of modern environments on skin ecology, barrier integrity, and systemic immune programming. *The World Allergy Organization journal*, 10(1), 29. doi:10.1186/s40413-017-0160-5

16. Marshall, Lisa. (2018, March 5) How bright light keeps preschoolers wired at night, *CU Boulder Today*. Available from: https://www.colorado.edu/today/2018/03/05/how-bright-light-keeps-preschoolers-wired-night

17. Kathryn Turnbull, Graham J. Reid, J. Bruce Morton; Behavioral Sleep Problems and their Potential Impact on Developing Executive Function in Children, *Sleep*, Volume 36, Issue 7, 1 July 2013, Pages 1077–1084, https://doi.org/10.5665/sleep.2814

18. Martinelli, Katherine. ADHD and Sleep Disorders: Are Kids Getting Misdiagnosed? *Child Mind Institute*. Retrieved November 7, 2018 from https://childmind.org/article/adhd-sleep-disorders-misdiagnosed/

19. Gamble, Jessa. Puberty: Early starters, *Nature*. Volume 550, pages S10–S11 (05 October 2017)

20. Rajalakshmi Lakshman, Nita G. Forouhi, Stephen J. Sharp, Robert Luben, Sheila A. Bingham, Kay-Tee Khaw, Nicholas J. Wareham, Ken K. Ong; Early Age at Menarche Associated with Cardiovascular Disease and Mortality, *The Journal of Clinical Endocrinology & Metabolism*, Volume 94, Issue 12, 1 December 2009, Pages 4953–4960, https://doi.org/10.1210/jc.2009-1789

21. DAN APTER, REIJO VIHKO; Early Menarche, a Risk Factor for Breast Cancer, Indicates Early Onset of Ovulatory Cycles, *The Journal of Clinical Endocrinology & Metabolism*, Volume 57, Issue 1, 1 July 1983, Pages 82–86, https://doi.org/10.1210/jcem-57-1-82

22. Kleinman, R. E., Hall, S., Green, H., Korzec-Ramirez, D., Patton, K., Pagano, M. E., & Murphy, J. M. (2002). Diet, breakfast, and academic performance in children. *Annals of nutrition & metabolism*, 46 Suppl 1(0 1), 24-30. doi: [10.1159/000066399]

23. Hania Szajewska & Marek Ruszczyński (2010) Systematic Review Demonstrating that Breakfast Consumption Influences Body Weight Outcomes in Children and Adolescents in Europe, *Critical Reviews in Food Science and Nutrition*, 50:2, 113-119, DOI: 10.1080/10408390903467514

24. Burt Solorzano, C. M., & McCartney, C. R. (2010). Obesity and the pubertal transition in girls and boys. *Reproduction (Cambridge, England)*, 140(3), 399-410. doi: [10.1530/REP-10-0119]

25. Tsai, Min-Chien & Chen, Wenchieh & Cheng, Yu-Wen & Wang, Cheng-Yu & Chen, Guan-Yu & Hsu, Tzung-Jen. (2006). Higher body mass index is a significant risk factor for acne formation in schoolchildren. *European journal of dermatology* : EJD. 16. 251-3.

26. Sergio E. Recabarren, Rosita Smith, Rafael Rios, Manuel Maliqueo, Bárbara Echiburú, Ethel Codner, Fernando Cassorla, Pedro Rojas, Teresa Sir-Petermann; Metabolic Profile in Sons of Women with Polycystic Ovary Syndrome, *The Journal of Clinical Endocrinology & Metabolism*, Volume 93, Issue 5, 1 May 2008, Pages 1820–1826, https://doi.org/10.1210/jc.2007-2256

Appendices

1. Li, S., & Gupte, A. A. (2017). The Role of Estrogen in Cardiac Metabolism and Diastolic Function. *Methodist DeBakey cardiovascular journal*, 13(1), 4-8. doi: [10.14797/mdcj-13-1-4]

2. Jessup, J. A., Wang, H., MacNamara, L. M., Presley, T. D., Kim-Shapiro, D. B., Zhang, L., Chen, A. F., ... Groban, L. (2013). Estrogen therapy, independent of timing, improves cardiac structure and function in oophorectomized mRen2.Lewis rats. *Menopause (New York, N.Y.)*, 20(8), 860-8. doi: [10.1097/GME.0b013e318280589a]

3. Tata, Brooke & El Houda Mimouni, Nour & Barbotin, Anne-Laure & Malone, Samuel & Loyens, Anne & Pigny, Pascal & Dewailly, Didier & Catteau-Jonard, Sophie & Sundström-Poromaa, Inger & Piltonen, Terhi & Dal Bello, Federica & Medana, Claudio & Prevot, Vincent & Clasadonte, Jerome & Giacobini, Paolo. (2018). Elevated prenatal anti-Müllerian hormone reprograms the fetus and induces polycystic ovary syndrome in adulthood. *Nature Medicine*. 24. DOI: 10.1038/s41591-018-0035-5.

4. Rosemary Braun, William L. Kath, Marta Iwanaszko, Elzbieta Kula-Eversole, Sabra M. Abbott, Kathryn J. Reid, Phyllis C. Zee, Ravi Allada. Universal method for robust detection of circadian state from gene expression, *Proceedings of the National Academy of Sciences*. Sep 2018, 115 (39) E9247-E9256; DOI:10.1073/pnas.1800314115

5. Peeples, Lynne. Medicine's secret ingredient – it's in the timing. *Nature* 556, 290-292 (2018) doi: 10.1038/d41586-018-04600-8

6. Madhusoodanan, Jyoti. (2017, Apr 1) Circadian Rhythms Influence Treatment Effects. *The Scientist*. Available from: https://www.the-scientist.com/features/circadian-rhythms-influence-treatment-effects-31746

7. University of North Carolina School of Medicine. (2009, January 16). Chemotherapy Most Effective At Time Of Day When Particular Enzyme At Lowest Level. *ScienceDaily*. Retrieved November 10, 2018 from www.sciencedaily.com/releases/2009/01/090113090501.htm

8. Tremellen, Kelton & Pearce, Karma. (2012). Dysbiosis of Gut Microbiota (DOGMA) - A novel theory for the development of Polycystic Ovarian Syndrome. *Medical hypotheses*. 79. 104-12. 10.1016/j.mehy.2012.04.016.

9. Guo Y, Qi Y, Yang X, Zhao L, Wen S, Liu Y, et al. (2016) Association between Polycystic Ovary Syndrome and Gut Microbiota. PLoS ONE 11(4): e0153196. https://doi.org/10.1371/journal.pone.0153196

10. Cohen, P. A., Goday, A., & Swann, J. P. (2012). The return of rainbow diet pills. *American journal of public health*, 102(9), 1676-86. doi: [10.2105/AJPH.2012.300655]

11. Kaplan, Justin. (2018, June 13) Harvard Scientists Aim To Reverse Diabetes With 'Surgery In A Pill', *Common Health*. Available from: http://www.wbur.org/commonhealth/2018/06/13/study-pill-glucose-diabetes-bariatric-surgery

12. Lee, Yuhan & E. Deelman, Tara & Chen, Keyue & S. Y. Lin, Dawn & Tavakkoli, Ali & M. Karp, Jeffrey. (2018). Therapeutic luminal coating of the intestine. *Nature Materials*. 17. DOI: 10.1038/s41563-018-0106-5.

13. Delzo, Janissa. (2018, June 14) Pill May Help People With Type 2 Diabetes Lose Weight, Control Blood Sugar, Early Findings Suggest, *Everyday Health*. Available from: https://www.everydayhealth.com/type-2-diabetes/could-pill-replace-weight-loss-surgery-type-2-diabetics

14. (2018). The microbiome in precision medicine: the way forward. *Genome medicine*, 10(1), 12. doi:10.1186/s13073-018-0525-6

15. Formby, B., & Schmidt, F. (2011). Efficacy of biorhythmic transdermal combined hormone treatment in relieving climacteric symptoms: a pilot study. *International journal of general medicine*, 4, 159-63. doi:10.2147/IJGM.S16139

16. Tao, X., Zhang, X., Ge, S. Q., Zhang, E. H., & Zhang, B. (2015). Expression of SIRT1 in the ovaries of rats with polycystic ovary syndrome before and after therapeutic intervention with exenatide. *International journal of clinical and experimental pathology*, 8(7), 8276-83.

17. Rappou, Elisabeth & Jukarainen, Sakari & Rinnankoski-Tuikka, Rita & Kaye, Sanna & Heinonen, Sini & Hakkarainen, Antti & Lundbom, Jesper & Lundbom, Nina & Saunavaara, Virva & Rissanen, Aila & Virtanen, Kirsi & Pirinen, Eija & Pietiläinen, Kirsi. (2016). Weight loss is associated with increased NAD(+)/SIRT1 expression but reduced PARP activity in white adipose tissue. *The Journal of clinical endocrinology and metabolism*. doi: 10.1210/jc.2015-3054.

18. (2015). Sirtuin-dependent clock control: new advances in metabolism, aging and cancer. *Current opinion in clinical nutrition and metabolic care*, 18(6), 521-7. doi: [10.1097/MCO.0000000000000219]

19. Grabowska, W., Sikora, E., & Bielak-Zmijewska, A. (2017). Sirtuins, a promising target in slowing down the ageing process. *Biogerontology*, 18(4), 447-476. doi: [10.1007/s10522-017-9685-9]

20. Zhu, Y., Yan, Y., Gius, D. R., & Vassilopoulos, A. (2013). Metabolic regulation of Sirtuins upon fasting and the implication for cancer. *Current opinion in oncology*, 25(6), 630-6. doi: [10.1097/01.cco.0000432527.49984.a3]

21. Hung, C. , Chan, S. , Chu, P. and Tsai, K. (2015), Quercetin is a potent anti-atherosclerotic compound by activation of SIRT1 signaling under oxLDL stimulation. *Mol. Nutr. Food Res.*, 59: 1905-1917. doi:10.1002/mnfr.201500144

22. Grabowska, W., Sikora, E., & Bielak-Zmijewska, A. (2017). Sirtuins, a promising target in slowing down the ageing process. *Biogerontology*, 18(4), 447-476. doi: [10.1007/s10522-017-9685-9]

23. Martens, C. R., Denman, B. A., Mazzo, M. R., Armstrong, M. L., Reisdorph, N., McQueen, M. B., Chonchol, M., ... Seals, D. R. (2018). Chronic nicotinamide riboside supplementation is well-tolerated and elevates NAD+ in healthy middle-aged and older adults. *Nature communications*, 9(1), 1286. doi:10.1038/s41467-018-03421-7

Index

Z

Acknowledgments

*T*his book is the culmination of years of work with of an amazing team of people and an even bigger community of doctors, researchers, patients, PCOS advocates, friends, and family. Without all of your love, help, guidance, and support, this book would not exist.

I would like to acknowledge Julia Pastore, my editor and constant advisor. Your incredible attention to detail and thoughtful suggestions are the reason this book reads like a book. I am extremely grateful that my friend and fellow PCOS-advocate, Amy Medling, referred you to me.

I would like to thank Amy and the entire PCOS community. You are the chorus of voices who are demanding better care for PCOS women. I hope this book is a powerful addition to our movement. As with most books, this book took longer than I anticipated. Thank you for unabashedly cheering me on month after month after month.

Thanks to all who assist me with PCOS speaking and research opportunities - Joy Devins and the team at Pure Encapsulations, Jake Orville and the team at Cleveland HeartLab, Joseph Antoun and the team at L-Nutra, Professor Valter Longo at the USC Longevity Institute, speaking coach Dr. Mark Tager, Sasha Ottey and Megan Stewart and their wonderful non-profits PCOS Challenge and PCOS Awareness, Drs. Kate Placzek and David Zava at ZRT Labs, and the team at UBiome.

Thanks as well to Professor Kelton Tremellen for his innovative DOGMA hypothesis of PCOS and for his steadfast encouragement.

My office staff and the talented naturopathic doctors I work with at my practice, the Integrative Medical Group of Irvine, have always been the best cheerleaders one could want. And thanks to all of my patients for trusting me and allowing me to be a small part of each of your life stories. Without you, I would not be a doctor. I hope we can continue to pursue health together for many years to come.

My caring friends have been by my side every step of the way. In particular, I want to thank the Functional Medicine Babes, my little support group of functional medicine health care providers, for freely sharing your knowledge and opinions. We are always at our best when we are with our friends.

There is not enough gratitude in the world for my devoted husband, Bob, my kids, and my many other family members. Thank you for always being there, for putting up with all of my dinner table talk about gluten, uteruses, and supplements, and for constantly reminding me of the joy of non-work life.

And, of course, I must give a giant thanks and hug to Alexis, my co-writer and eldest daughter, who helped me turn my ideas into written words. Without you, I could not have written this wonderful book.

About the Authors

About Felice Gersh, M.D.

Felice Gersh, M.D. is a multi-award winning physician with dual board certifications in OB-GYN and Integrative Medicine. She is the founder and director of the Integrative Medical Group of Irvine, a practice that provides comprehensive health care for women by combining the best evidence-based therapies from conventional, naturopathic, and holistic medicine.

An active part of the PCOS community, Dr. Gersh is a member of the PCOS Challenge Medical/Scientific Advisory Board. She is the Director of Clinical Affairs for the Women's Hormone Network. And she is a member of the AE-PCOS Society.

She taught obstetrics and gynecology at Keck USC School of Medicine for 12 years as an Assistant Clinical Professor and received the Outstanding Volunteer Clinical Faculty Award.

She is also a prolific writer and lecturer and has been featured in several films and documentary series, including The Real Skinny on Fat with Montel Williams and Fasting.

Dr. Gersh lives with her husband, Bob, in Orange County, CA. Visit her online at www.felicelgershmd.com.

About Alexis Perella

Alexis Perella writes about medicine, education, and design. She loves to make complex topics simple. www.alexisperella.com.

CPSIA information can be obtained
at www.ICGtesting.com
Printed in the USA
LVHW011450180319
611006LV00005B/284